Children and Parents
Clinical Issues for Psychologists and Psychiatrists

Children and Parents

Clinical Issues for Psychologists and Psychiatrists

Edited by

RAJINDER M GUPTA PhD
Dudley Psychology and Counselling Services

and

DEEPA S PARRY-GUPTA MB, ChB
Avon and Wiltshire NHS Trust

W
WHURR PUBLISHERS
LONDON AND PHILADELPHIA

© 2003 Whurr Publishers Ltd
First published 2003
by Whurr Publishers Ltd
19b Compton Terrace
London N1 2UN England and
325 Chestnut Street, Philadelphia PA 19106 USA

British Library Cataloguing in Publication Data

A catalogue record for this book
is available from the British Library.

ISBN 1 86156 351 5

Typeset by Adrian McLaughlin, a@microguides.net
Printed and bound in the UK by Athenæum Press Ltd, Gateshead, Tyne & Wear.

Contents

Contributors

Dr Bernadette Marie Bullock, Department of Psychology, University of Oregon, USA.

Dr Zulfiqar Ahmed Bhutta, The Husein Lalji Dewraj Professor of Paediatrics and Child Health, The Aga Khan University, Karachi, Pakistan.

Dr Kirby Deater-Deckard, Department of Psychology, University of Oregon, USA.

Dr Claire Dorer, Formerly Lecturer in Psychology and Social Work, University of Birmingham, UK.

Ms Liz Goldthorpe, Solicitor, All Stretton, Shropshire, UK.

Dr Laurie A Greco, West Virginia University, Morgantown, USA.

Dr Rajinder M Gupta, Child Psychologist and Honorary Clinical Tutor, Dudley Priority Health NHS Trust, Dudley, UK.

Professor David Howe, School of Social Work, University of East Anglia, Norwich, UK.

Dr Catherine A Lavers-Preston, Salmons Centre for Applied Social and Psychological Research, Canterbury Christ Church University College, Canterbury, UK.

Dr Tracy L Morris, Department of Psychology, West Virginia University, Morgantown, USA.

Dr Thomas G O'Connor, Institute of Psychiatry, London, UK.

Dr Deepa S Parry-Gupta, Psychiatrist, Department of Psychotherapy, Blackberry Hospital, Bristol, UK.

Dr Stephen Scott, Senior Lecturer and Consultant Child and Adolescent Psychiatrist, Institute of Psychiatry, London, UK.

Professor Edmund J Sonuga-Barke, Department of Psychology, University of Southampton, UK.

Dr Anthony L Schwartz, Centre for Health Policy and Practice, Staffordshire University, Stafford, UK.

Dr Frederika Theus, Institute on Disability and Human Development, Department of Disability and Human Development, University of Illinois at Chicago, Chicago, USA.

Introduction

Most professional training courses are long and intellectually demanding. Invariably, they require both practical experience and academic study. Following training, one needs to keep abreast of the current developments in one's field in order to evolve and offer good-quality care, particularly in the present climate of clinical governance.

Clinical governance refers to the means by which all NHS organizations ensure that proper processes for monitoring standards and for ensuring high quality of clinical care are in place. The government's consultation paper 'A First Class Service' (Department of Health, 1998) provides the details of the rationale behind clinical governance. Some of the key components include:

- evidence-based clinical practice;
- change in clinical practice takes place in the light of audit and research;
- continuing education for all clinical staff;
- continuing professional development for all staff.

Of these, it is evidence-based clinical practice that has caused considerable controversy – and still continues to do so. We will address first, albeit very briefly, some of the issues surrounding this concept and what it means to us. However, for a detailed treatment of this topic the interested reader should consult some of the references mentioned below.

Historically, the term 'evidence-based practice' owes its origins, which date back to the 1980s, to McMaster Medical School in Canada (Rosenberg and Donald, 1995). However, according to Sackett et al. (1996) the philosophical origins of evidence-based medicine go back to the mid-nineteenth century and earlier. When the term originated is not of much consequence here. What is important to emphasize is that, these days, evidence-based practice has become *sine qua non*, especially in the NHS – and even in other professions as well (see Rushton and Dance, 2002, who provide a commentary on the government's agenda in introducing the notion of evidence-based practice into the social services). Evidence-based practice has its roots in hospital medicine (Rosenberg and Donald, 1995; Sackett et al., 1996) but the reasoning that underlies this book stems from the relevance and usefulness of such practice as it applies to some of the issues and problems that clinicians have to deal with in the child and adolescent mental health services.

The term 'evidence-based practice' is fairly self-explanatory. The working party of the British Psychological Society (BPS) has defined it as 'the integration of individual clinical expertise with the best available external evidence from systematic research in order to reach decisions about client care' (Wolpert, 2002, p. 5; see also, Rosenberg and Donald, 1995; Sackett et al., 1996, for their explanation of the term – an explanation that is very often quoted in the literature). As well as defining evidence-based practice, the BPS also points out limitations to using it in child and mental health services. They state, and we share their view, that evidence-based practice 'does not mean the wholesale application of findings from randomised controlled trials to all individuals with similar problems in a "one size fits all" policy' (Wolpert, 2002, p. 5; see a very balanced annotation on this topic written by Harrington et al., 2002).

We are, on the whole, in agreement with the BPS's definition, but we feel that we should also state our notion of evidence-based clinical practice. It is important that we outline our views about this because it is the *raison d'être* that underpins the genesis of this book. The way we interpret it is that the clinical practice of mental health professionals should be rooted in well-researched and carefully evaluated evidence and should not be based on discredited concepts, less effective treatments, or fads. One should remain open-minded and embrace new thinking and should not remain wedded to outmoded ideas (cf. Gupta and Coxhead, 1990). Above all, it is vital that the families and children who come to see us for our help do not end up as being worse off as a result of our intervention, as Harrington (2001) quite rightly puts it.

It is equally important to bear in mind that not everything that is new is necessarily better than what is currently being practised. It is common that

> an approach used by many [clinicians] for many years falls out of favour; an educator emphasizes the value of a different method, and if such method receives monetary support from a private foundation, government support, or media emphasis, then these different methods come into favour and so the cycle of acceptance and rejection continues. (Gredler, 1990, p. 2)

So long as a particular approach is not fashion driven, and has not gained currency for the reasons outlined by Gredler above, we subscribe to the view of evidence-based practice on the lines that we have described.

Notwithstanding the current emphasis on evidence-based practice in the NHS (and its full backing from the government), it does have its critics and this has led to considerable debate (see Parry, 2000, and several studies cited therein; see also Ramchandani et al., 2001; Straus and McAlister, 2000, who try to address several criticisms of evidence-based practice in medicine; Williams and Garner, 2002). Some of the criticisms of evidence-based practice include the view that it is too prescriptive, a cost-cutting exercise, too academic and remote from clinical practice, and inappropriate to disciplines such as psychiatry and psychology. In our experience, we have found that if a therapeutic intervention is too prescriptive and is difficult to implement, it is unlikely to be employed despite the availability of overwhelming evidence in its favour. Coxhead and Gupta (1989) carried out a survey of practising educational psychologists' views on the delivery of behaviour modification to determine to what extent it was implemented in the way it was intended. This demonstrated that most practising educational psychologists had little or no commitment to the traditional view of behaviour modification (that is the way the experimental evidence would suggest that behaviour modification should be used – for details see Gelfand and Hartmann, 1975). The survey also showed that few educational psychologists believed that traditional behaviour modification should be implemented without any adaptation. An interesting, and somewhat unexpected, finding was that a vast majority of the respondents held rather unfavourable attitudes towards the traditional form of behaviour modification, although more experienced educational psychologists were less antagonistic. This survey is somewhat dated, but our more recent experience of working in different clinics in the last 10 years would suggest that, were we to repeat this survey, we would be likely to obtain similar results again.

What relevance do these findings have in the current debate about evidence-based practice *in the child and mental health services?* The way we interpret these findings from our survey is simply that no matter how efficacious and empirically sound a therapeutic approach may be, if, in the clinical situation, it appears impractical to clinicians and unacceptable to the recipients (who may be families or teachers – often the population the professionals in the child and mental health services deal with) it is highly unlikely that it is going to be implemented and adhered to in the way it was developed or intended. In fact, Kazdin (2002, p. 54) notes that 'The ways in which psychotherapy is studied depart considerably from how treatment is implemented in clinic practice.' Kazdin goes on to explain why this is the case and, among other differences, draws attention to the differences in the clinical population and the populations employed in the research designs (see also Harrington et al., 2002; Hotopf et al., 1999; Wolpert, 2002).

From the foregoing discussion it should not be inferred that we are suggesting that the available evidence should not form the basis of one's clinical judgement, or one's decision making, and the information that one gives to people who come to seek advice. In fact, this should always be the case and therefore we welcome the current climate and debate about the evidence-based practice; to do anything otherwise, would be unprofessional and unethical. However, the point that is being made here is that in the situations where we, and many other professionals work, any new evidence or form of therapeutic intervention, if it appears impractical, and, if clinicians' experience shows that the recipients often put up barriers in accepting and implementing it, is probably not going to be used as intended, and would possibly be adapted. It is highly unlikely that it is going to be modified to such an extent that it stops being effective. For example, Gupta and Coxhead (1990) adapted behaviour modification to make it more user friendly compared with the way it had been tried in experimental and laboratory situations whilst retaining what they felt were the key aspects that helped in bringing about changes in behaviour. We feel the adapted version, although empirically less elegant, remains effective and acceptable (see also Connor-Smith and Weisz, 2003).

In addition to the difficulties in accepting and in implementing empirically sound practice, Firth-Cozens (1997) has identified some other factors that lead to professionals failing to adopt new ideas. These include time constraints, high levels of stress (see also Schwartz's chapter in this book) and general resistance to change. On the other hand Firth-Cozens also notes factors that are conducive to accepting change, for example rewards, education, feedback and so on.

Notwithstanding the difficulties related to accepting and rejecting change, in the current climate of evidence-based practice a number of sources have sprung up providing clinicians with access to information related to their respective fields. They include journals, the World Wide Web, departments in universities, books and so forth. Obviously, there are a number of ways of keeping abreast of the research evidence and current thinking pertaining to one's specialist field. One straightforward, efficient and parsimonious way of obtaining such information is to have summaries of the seminal and current literature written in an authoritative yet accessible style in one source and its implications examined for the practitioner. This book attempts to achieve that. With this aim in mind, a number of clinically relevant topics were selected. The main rationale that is the basis of the selection of the subject matter for this book stems from personal experience of working with children and their parents over a long period. Based on our joint clinical experience, it was felt that, firstly, the topics selected should be clinically relevant and should have some bearing on clinicians' day-to-day work. Secondly, clinicians may not have in-depth knowledge and may not be familiar with the current research or thinking about those topics, or some aspects of them. Thirdly, the topics should not be too esoteric but, equally, not too familiar either. Two examples illustrate our decision-making process in selecting the areas covered in this book. Take for instance, the effect of culture on symptom development. Referring to the work by Gibbs and Huang (1998), Dr Frederika Theus, in Chapter 1, notes that some ethnic groups reinforce 'acting in' neurotic symptoms whereas some other ethnic groups reinforce 'acting out' behaviours: 'thus children learn patterns of illness and dysfunctional behaviour[s] that are culturally reinforced and tolerated'. Furthermore, there would also appear to be some variation in the way the different cultural groups express their emotional difficulties. Japanese Americans are more likely to express their emotional problems through somatic symptoms and may attribute their personal problems to physical health rather than to psychological or emotional difficulties. Our own observations would suggest that this might be the case with the first-generation Asian women in the UK and older women in India and Pakistan. Lavers-Preston and Sonuga-Barke, in Chapter 7, look critically at the effect of grandparents, particularly grandmothers, on the grandchildren as a result of their involvement in their upbringing, and on their own daughters. Many professionals often deal with children and adolescents where grandmothers play quite a crucial role in their grandchildren's upbringing. However, many of them may not be quite aware of the relevant literature, which provides some research evidence about the impact the grandmothers have, or can have, in the adjustment or maladjustment of their grandchildren and the interactional difficulties that occur between mothers and grandmothers. Thus the chapters dealing with these issues endeavour to fill that gap and hopefully provide clinically relevant and helpful research evidence.

Using this reasoning, 11 topics have been identified that appear to be commensurate with the objectives of this book. Each chapter seeks to cover most of the important literature pertaining to its topic and, where possible, the implications of that literature for clinicians have also been suggested. It is, however, envisaged that an experienced clinician would use his or her own judgement and experience in deciding how best to use the information provided. Thus it is not the intention of the book to be prescriptive.

The book has been divided into three sections, purely for convenience. The first section deals with issues related to behaviour, the second section with family-related issues, and the last section deals with general issues that can arise during clinical practice and may have a direct or indirect bearing on one's practice, but that are nonetheless important.

This book is intended to be useful for professionals who deal particularly with children and families, including clinical child psychologists, child and adolescent psychiatrists, educational psychologists, paediatricians, school medical officers, and social workers. We feel the information provided would be both relevant and useful in their routine work.

Finally, we would like to express our sincere appreciation to all our contributors for their participation in the present book. It is a great pleasure to acknowledge the help and support the first editor has received from his line managers, Nicky Whitehead and Richard Toogood. It is true to say that without their backing and encouragement, it would not have been possible for the first editor to embark upon this project. Special thanks to our publishers for their wise counsel and guidance whenever we have needed it. Last but not least, our thanks to Rahul Gupta who often helped his father with computer-related problems, and also to Dr Surya Gupta and to Dr Alan Rushton who made very helpful comments about the evidence-based practice from their perspectives.

Rajinder M Gupta
Deepa S Parry-Gupta

References

Connor-Smith JK, Weisz JR (2003) Applying treatment outcome research in clinical practice: techniques for adapting interventions to the real world. Child and Adolescent Mental Health 8: 1.

Coxhead P, Gupta RM (1989) A survey of educational psychologists' views of the delivery of behaviour modification. Educational Studies 15: 1.

Department of Health (1998) A First Class Service: Quality in the New NHS. London: Department of Health.

Firth-Cozens JA (1997) Health promotion: changing behaviour towards evidence-based health care. Quality in Health Care 6: 205–11.

Gelfand DM, Hartmann DP (1975) Child Behaviour: Analysis and Therapy. New York: Pergamon Press.

Gibbs JT, Huang LK (1998) A conceptual framework for the psychological assessment and treatment of minority youth. In Gibbs JT, Huang LN (eds) Children of Color: Psychological Interventions with Culturally Diverse Youth. San Francisco, CA: Jossey Bass.

Gredler GR (1990) Approaches to the remediation of learning difficulties: a current assessment. In Gupta RM, Coxhead P (eds) Interventions with Children. London: Routledge.

Gupta RM, Coxhead P (1990) Interventions with Children. London: Routledge.

Harrington R (2001) Commentary: evidence based child and adolescent mental health services. Child Psychology and Psychiatry Review 6: 2.

Harrington RC, Cartwright-Hatton S, Stein A (2002) Annotation: randomised trials. Journal of Child Psychology and Psychiatry 43: 6.

Hotopf M, Churchill R, Lewis G (1999) Pragmatic randomised controlled trials in psychiatry. British Journal of Psychchiatry 175: 217–23.

Kazdin AE (2002) The state of child and adolescent psychotherapy research. Child and Adolescent Mental Health 7: 2.

Parry G (2000) Evidence based psychotherapy: an overview. In Rowland N, Goss S (eds) Evidence Based Counselling and Psychological Therapies. London: Routledge.

Ramchandani P, Joughin C, Zwi M (2001) Evidence based child and adolescent mental health services: oxymoron or brave new dawn. Child Psychology and Psychiatry Review 6: 2.

Rosenberg W, Donald A (1995) Evidence based medicine: an approach to clinical problem solving. British Medical Journal 310: 1122–5.

Rowland N, Goss S (eds) (2000) Evidence-Based Counselling and Psychological Therapies: Research and Applications. London: Routledge.

Rushton A, Dance C (2002) Quality protects: a commentary on the government's agenda and the evidence base. Child Psychology and Psychiatry Review 7: 2.

Sackett DL, Rosenberg WMC, Gray JAM, Haynes RB (1996) Evidence-based medicine: what it is and what it isn't. British Medical Journal 312: 71–3.

Straus SE, McAlister FA (2000) Evidence-based medicine: a commentary on common criticisms. Can Med Ass J 163: 839–41.

Williams DDR, Garner J (2002) The case against the evidence: a different perspective on evidence based medicine. British Journal of Psychiatry 180: 8–12.

Wolpert M (2002) Drawing on the Evidence: Advice for Mental Health Professionals Working with Children and Adolescents. Leicester: BPS.

SECTION 1

BEHAVIOUR-RELATED ISSUES

CHAPTER 1

Brain-behaviour relationships in childhood mood and behaviour disorders

FREDERIKA C THEUS

When children exhibit disturbing behaviour the first question often posed to mental health clinicians is 'why?' This question comes from a multitude of sources – puzzled parents, concerned teachers, and society as a whole. The occurrence of childhood behavioural and mood disturbances is a long-standing source of societal concern, and the attempts made to understand these disturbances are a long-standing source of confusion.

Overall, mental health professionals, unfortunately, have not provided clear, reasonable explanations of the causes of these disorders. Until recently, explanations tended to be posed in relatively simplistic terms with an emphasis on oversimplified, one-to-one causal relationships. Throughout the decades, proposed etiologies included heredity, parenting practices – particularly on the part of the mother, 'society', and a multitude of neurobiological factors of varying complexity. Further complicating the issues are the innumerable myths, misconceptions and points of contention that have permeated the literature on childhood psychopathology. The prevailing view in the 1950s and 1960s, for example, was that depression, as clearly manifested and diagnosed in adults, could not occur in children due to the immaturity of the childhood personality structure (Fuller, 1992; Harrington, 1993). Following this view was the notion that depression can indeed exist in children but that it is not expressed directly. Rather, depression in children would be 'masked' by other overt behaviours and symptoms. This concept was referred to as the theory of 'masked depression' and will be discussed in greater detail in the subsequent review of comorbidity issues.

Regarding behaviour and conduct disorders, perhaps the greatest confusion has grown out of a desire to find a clear, single cause. Hinshaw and Anderson (1996), for example, stated: 'In psychiatric nosologies the locus of deviant behaviour is, by definition, intraindividual. As a result, the clear

3

roles of poverty, traumatic stress, and violent communities in fostering antisocial behaviour may be greatly underappreciated.' They emphasized the importance of recognizing that 'deviant behaviour is multideter-mined, with no clear separation of cultural, environmental, or intraindividual causal factors.'

The fact that a variety of terms, such as antisocial behaviour, emotion-al disturbance, conduct disorder and behaviour disorder are often used in conjunction and/or interchangeably, contributes to confusion in devel-oping an understanding of the types of emotional and behaviour difficulties displayed by children, and the causes of such difficulties. This chapter will focus primarily on the relationship between neurobiological functioning and behaviour in children with depressive disorders, and/or behaviour disorders largely characterized by oppositional behaviours and more severe conduct problems.

Developmental course

Before neurobiological influences can be explored, the nature and devel-opment of these disorders must be understood. A brief review of the phenomenology of oppositional defiant and conduct disorders and depressive disorders follows.

Oppositional defiant and conduct disorders

Oppositional defiant and conduct disorders include a range of behaviours linked by a common difficulty with conformity to societal norms and/or to the expectations of an authority figure. These tendencies, in their mildest forms, may be expressed in behaviours such as temper tantrums and argu-mentativeness. Children experiencing more severe difficulties may exhibit behaviours such as initiating fights, physical cruelty to people and/or ani-mals, theft, muggings, and forced sexual activity with others.

It is typical for children at various stages of development to exhibit some oppositional behaviour but behaviours are considered to be indica-tive of a disorder based on their frequency and severity, as well as on the degree to which social, academic and occupational functioning is impaired. The range in the severity and types of specific behaviours exhib-ited can be quite varied, which is partially due to the hierarchical and developmental nature of the disorders. Some children with no history of behaviour problems do begin to exhibit oppositional behaviours and severe conduct problems as they enter adolescence. Those who exhibit severe conduct problems typically do not begin by displaying extreme behaviours such as assault or stealing. Rather, they often have a history of less severe oppositional behaviours as young children. Evidence suggests that those children with oppositional defiant disorder (ODD) who develop more severe behaviours do not cease exhibiting the milder behaviours, or change the types of behaviours they display (Lahey and Loeber, 1994; Frick, 1998). Conversely, many young children who exhibit relatively mild oppositional behaviours do not later development severe conduct problems. Hinshaw and Anderson (1996) reported a high level of sensitivity in predicting conduct disorder (CD) from an earlier diagnosis of ODD, with over 90% of those with CD previously meeting and continuing to meet criteria for ODD. Nevertheless, they emphasized that the majority of children with ODD do not appear to develop the more severe pattern of behaviours that are characteristic of CD.

Depressive disorders

The phenomenology of depressive disorders in children and adolescents is equally complex. It is now generally agreed that depression not only does indeed occur in children but is actually one of the most pervasive mental health disorders among individuals under age 18 (Reynolds, 1992). Yet, there continues to be considerable debate among researchers and clinicians as to how depression is actually manifested in children.

Many researchers suggest that the features of depression in children are quite similar to those observed in adults, with developmental issues only minimally affecting the expression of the disorder. This is, in fact, largely the perspective taken in the most recent revision of the Diagnostic and Statistical Manual of the American Psychiatric Association (DSM-IV). Developmental psychologists, on the other hand, argue that depression is manifested differently across developmental stages. A depressed 8-year-old, for example, is likely to express his or her affective state behaviourally. Therefore, overt behaviours such as lethargy, poor school performance, and irritability might be exhibited (Schwartz et al., 1998). An adolescent, in comparison, might also exhibit these behaviours; however, given the adolescent's higher level of cognitive development and increased independence, his or her symptoms are also likely to be broader and to have a cognitive expression. Therefore, symptoms might include concerns about the future and feelings of worthlessness, as well as significant self-destructive behaviour and serious conduct problems (Weiss et al., 1992; Reinherz et al., 1991).

Developmental issues in assessment

Regardless of which view is held regarding the role of development in the expression of symptoms, most researchers and clinicians agree that developmental issues play a significant role in the accurate assessment of both depressive and behaviour disorders. First, although behaviour disorders are defined by the observable behaviours exhibited, many of the symptoms of depressive disorders are not always obvious or easily observed by those interacting with the child. A child with a suspected conduct disorder may be brought for treatment by a parent due to frequent fighting at school and lying at home, for example. A child with a depressive disorder, however, may be struggling with feelings of worthlessness and sadness, which may go relatively unrecognized by his/her parents. Therefore, the child with depression might not be referred for assessment until the symptoms have become quite pronounced.

Once a child is available for evaluation and subsequent treatment, it is important to remember that children, and to a lesser extent adolescents, have difficulty being aware of and describing their inner states, and the duration of symptoms. Therefore, obtaining specific information on symptom status presents a unique challenge in comparison to working with adult clients, particularly in the case of children with depressive disorders. In addition, limited or complete lack of reading skills further limits the utility of written self-report questionnaires.

Effects of gender and culture on symptom development

Issues of gender and culture further complicate the understanding of the development of behaviour and mood disorders in children. There is evidence, for example, that gender plays a role in the developmental progression of behaviour disorders. Boys, for instance, tend to exhibit more aggressive behaviour and more neuropsychological deficits when onset begins in childhood in comparison with boys who first exhibit conduct problems in adolescence. The latter group, moreover, is much less likely to have a pattern of disordered behaviour continuing into adulthood (Lahey et al., 1993; Moffitt, 1993). Females, in contrast, are more likely than males to begin exhibiting conduct problems in adolescence, with no previous history of oppositional behaviour. Further, whether the onset of disordered behaviour is in childhood or in adolescence, girls tend to exhibit more severe behaviours, are more likely to exhibit neuropsychological deficits, and are more likely to have antisocial behaviour patterns continuing into adulthood (Moffitt, 1993; Frick, 1998).

Regarding depressive disorders, there is much documentation to suggest that adolescent girls appear to be at increased risk in comparison to boys (Reynolds, 1992; Angold and Rutter, 1992; Nolen-Hoeksema and Girgus, 1994). Possible explanations of this gender difference include differences in hormonal development, socialization differences, attachment issues, and differing responses to maltreatment or other life stresses (Reynolds, 1992; Peterson et al., 1993).

Research on cultural factors is even less conclusive, with many studies confounding issues of race/ethnicity and socioeconomic status (SES). Research has not definitively demonstrated a higher rate of behaviour disturbance in one ethnic/racial group in comparison to others. Nevertheless, several studies suggest that some groups of non-white children, in comparison to white children, are more likely to receive more serious diagnoses, such as conduct disorder and depressive disorders (Gibbs, 1998; Proctor et al., 1992). Regarding depressive disorders, some studies have found increased rates in populations of African American male children in comparison to white male children, whereas others indicated no differences between racial groups in regard to prevalence and phenomenology (Harrington, 1993). Bui and Takeuchi (1992), in their examination of utilization rates, found that Asian American adolescents and Mexican American adolescents tended to be underrepresented in mental health facilities, whereas African American adolescents tended to be overrepresented. Further, Asian American adolescents were most often given non-psychiatric diagnoses or deferred diagnoses, whereas African Americans and Mexican Americans were most often diagnosed with adjustment disorders, which by definition often involve disturbances of mood and/or conduct.

In addition to the differences in referral and diagnostic patterns, the way that symptoms are expressed may differ across various ethnic groups. Gibbs and Huang (1998) suggested that 'some ethnic groups reinforce "acting in" neurotic symptoms, others reward "acting out" characterological symptoms, and still others reward somatic symptoms; thus children learn patterns of illness and dysfunctional behaviour that are culturally reinforced and tolerated.' According to Nagata (1998), for example, Japanese Americans may be more likely to express their emotional difficulties through somatic symptoms, and may identify their major personal problems as being related to physical health rather than to emotional or psychological functioning.

In addition, many ethnic/cultural groups vary in the degree to which they perceive the physical, the emotional and the spiritual aspects of personal functioning to be connected. Gibbs and Huang (1998) suggested that, across cultural groups, the person initially sought for help may range from 'a priest or minister to a spiritualist or native healer to an herbalist or acupuncturist to a tribal council or family elder.' Further, religious beliefs may play a significant role in therapy utilization and the overall diagnostic process. Boyd-Franklin (1989) emphasized, however, that the training of most clinicians excludes and disregards religion and spirituality as a clinical issue. Further, she maintained that when the role of spirituality in a client's life is ignored, and differences in orientation and world view are disregarded, the clinical process can be brought to a halt.

Comorbidity

While disorders of mood and behaviour are classified as distinct entities, issues of symptom commonality and comorbidity have significant implications for both research and clinical practice. One of the first attempts to examine the relationship between mood and behaviour was the development of the theory of 'masked depression,' which maintains that depression in children typically is not expressed directly. Rather, the depression is masked by 'depressive equivalents,' such as aggression, overactivity or somatic complaints. According to this theory, depression must therefore be inferred from the masking behaviours (Harrington, 1993; Welner, 1978; Fuller, 1992; Carlson and Cantwell, 1980).

Carlson and Cantwell (1980), however, concluded that it is often issues such as aggression or conduct problems that bring children to clinical attention, and that such problems may draw attention away from depressive symptoms. They hypothesized that these are the children that some clinicians would consider to have 'masked depression'. The authors suggested, however, that 'the mask, if present, is very thin.' Harrington (1993) also noted that the concept of masked depression is difficult to prove. He suggested that a crucial problem with the theory is that criteria for reliably distinguishing between symptoms, such as aggression or overactivity that are due to depression, and those same symptoms that occur as part of another disorder are not currently established.

Currently, the concept of masked depression is often viewed as one of the common misconceptions about depressive disorders in children. Nevertheless, the theory of masked depression was perhaps the first recognition of a possible association between mood and conduct problems.

Whether one fully accepts or rejects the notion of conduct problems as a 'mask' for depression, few researchers or clinicians question that in examining severe pathology in children, it is impossible to deny the existence of comorbidity. Hinshaw and Anderson (1996) suggested that the frequency of co-occurrence of behaviour/conduct disorders and depression is what initially led to the creation of the confusing notion of masked depression. While the comorbidity of depressive disorders and anxiety disorders appears to be the most frequently studied, conduct disorders are also identified as a commonly occurring comorbid disorder in children with depressive disorders.

In the often-cited study by Puig-Antich (1982), for example, the author found that approximately one-third of the boys referred for clinical service who were diagnosed with major depression also met DSM-III criteria for conduct disorder. It is important to note the presence of significant gender differences, however, as this finding was not true for girls. Similarly, in a study of depressed adolescents taken from a community sample, Kashani et al. (1987) found that 33% were also diagnosed as having a conduct disorder, and 50% received a diagnosis of oppositional defiant disorder. These findings indicated that the majority of adolescents with a depressive disorder also exhibited at least mild levels of clinically significant problematic behaviour.

The exact nature of the relationship between these two diagnostic categories, however, remains unclear. Depression, for example, is often viewed as a secondary condition to conduct disorder, stemming from the negative experiences and isolation resulting from the behaviour problems (Capaldi, 1992; Panak and Garber, 1992). Puig-Antich (1982), however, reported that 87% of the children who met criteria for a depressive disorder and for a conduct disorder experienced the onset of the depressive disorder prior to the onset of the conduct disorder.

Hammen and Rudolph (1996) suggested that the frequency of comorbidity may be indicative of flaws in the diagnostic system. Specifically, they proposed that the diagnostic boundaries established for adults are not actually applicable to children. Therefore, it is important to consider that overlapping symptoms of depression and anger, for example, may reflect the true nature of how children express and experience depression. Indeed, as previously stated, the practice of applying adult diagnostic criteria to children without amendment is criticized by many for its failure to fully consider developmental research on how age influences the expression and the frequency of occurrence of depressive symptoms (Harrington, 1993; Cantwell, 1992).

Overall, these findings provide evidence for some type of clinical connection between these disorders and highlight the necessity to consider them in conjunction when exploring etiology. Nevertheless, they also serve to highlight the significant variability inherent in groups of children having a depressive and/or behaviour disorder. Further, issues of gender, culture and developmental stage add a great deal of complexity to the process of determining etiology.

Perhaps the most important realization that has facilitated recent advancements in research seeking to determine causality of childhood emotional and behaviour problems is that the nature, development and severity of the pathology exhibited by children included in this broad category is indeed quite heterogeneous. Therefore, any theory of causality and resulting intervention plan must reflect this heterogeneity. Some causal theories, in fact, may be appropriate for explaining the behaviour of certain groups of children, but not for others. Further, no causal theory pinpointing a single factor is likely to adequately explain how and why emotional and behavioural problems develop in some children, but not in others. Rather, a complex interaction among multiple factors is most likely responsible. While the focus of this chapter is on the relationship between neurobiological functioning and behaviour, the complex interaction among the many factors operating must always be considered.

Traumatic brain injury (TBI) and mood/behaviour disorders

Perhaps the clearest indications of the relationship between brain functioning and mood and behaviour disorders is found in the research on traumatic brain injury, which is now recognized as a leading cause of death and disability among children. Many studies focus on the neuropsychological effects of TBI (Ewing-Cobbs et al., 1997; Levin et al., 1995). The behavioural sequelae, however, can be equally devastating and are often evident even after impairments in intellectual and neuropsychological functioning have resolved (Yeates et al., 1997; Shaffer, 1995; Fletcher, et al., 1996).

Behavioural problems documented to occur frequently in children and adolescents with brain injury include difficulties related to attention and overactivity, as well as increased problems with anger control, aggression and tantrums (Deaton, 1987; Shaffer, 1995). Many studies, most notably the landmark Isle of Wight studies, have clearly demonstrated that an association exists between central nervous system (CNS) dysfunction and psychiatric disorders (Rutter, 1981). Most agree that direct causality is evident regarding the impact of brain injury on intellectual functioning, but causality has proven more difficult to establish regarding emotional/ behaviour disturbance. Indeed, even when injuries are severe, the nature and severity of the sequelea are quite varied, with emotional and behaviour disturbance not being observed in every case (Yeates et al., 1997; Levin et al., 1995). Most studies have focused on injury-related variables, such as injury severity and location of injury, in an attempt to determine the factors that contribute to outcome variability. It appears, however, that a combination of both medical or injury-related factors and social/environmental factors contribute to both intellectual and emotional/ behavioural outcomes.

Yeates et al. (1997), in a study of 109 six- to 12-year-old children with TBI resulting from blunt head trauma found that injury severity accounted for equal variance in both cognitive and behavioural outcomes, but that preinjury family environmental factors, such as SES, overall social stressors and resources, and general level of family functioning, were more directly related to behavioural outcomes. Further, they concluded that severity of injury is very important in determining rate of recovery during the first year after injury, but that long-term cognitive and behavioural outcome appears just as much or more related to environmental factors. Overall, they concluded that 'preinjury environment factors account for significant variability in neurobehavioural outcomes following TBI in children, over and above that explained by injury-related variables.' Shaffer (1995) also concluded that most recent studies provide evidence that the effect of brain injury is mediated by the psychosocial environmental factors present before the injury, as well as the presence or absence of preinjury mood or behavioural symptoms.

The development of neuroimaging techniques not available at the time of the Isle of Wight and other early studies has greatly aided the study of localization effects. Rutter (1981) reported that, in a sample of children with brain injury, an association between localization of injury and type of psychiatric symptoms could not be demonstrated in most cases, but that depression appeared most common in children with damage in the right frontal or left parieto-occipital regions. More recently, Mendelsohn et al. (1992) reported that difficulties in social behaviour and behavioural inhibition are often associated with damage occurring in the frontal lobe.

One methodological problem inherent in many TBI studies is that most involve subjects from a single clinic or treatment centre. As a result, findings may not necessarily generalize to the overall population of children with TBI. Yeates et al. (1997), for example, identified as a weakness in their study the underrepresentation of non-white families and families of low SES in the analysis of the data.

Perhaps the most important consideration when attempting to understand the impact of brain injury on the development of emotional/behaviour problems is that children who experience brain injury tend to share some characteristics of behaviour and family functioning. Shaffer (1995) raised concerns about his earlier study of psychiatric outcomes of head injury in children (Shaffer et al., 1975), noting that limited data were collected about preinjury behaviour. Many of the younger children in the study had sustained injuries from passing vehicles as they stood in the road. Similarly, some of the older children were injured while engaged in high-risk behaviours, such as playing on rooftops. These factors raised questions about their level of impulsivity or overactivity, for example, as well as the quality of environmental supervision that was being provided. A higher rate of preinjury aggression, overactivity and general behavioural concerns than is found in the general population of children is indeed indicated in the brain-injury population (Bijur and Haslum, 1995; Asarnow et al., 1995). Further, higher rates of psychiatric disorders, particularly depression, are identified in parents of children who sustained brain injury. The presence of psychiatric disorders in the parent may place the child at higher risk for also developing a psychiatric disorder that may contribute to increased aggression, impulsivity and therefore brain injury. In addition, parental psychiatric disorder may also hinder the parent's ability to provide appropriate supervision, thus placing the child at increased risk of sustaining injury (McGuire and Rothenberg, 1986; Bijur and Haslum, 1995).

Finally, the emotional impact and stress placed on the child and his or her family cannot be disregarded. Depression and anger may actually occur as a result of the child's frustration in dealing with environmental demands that are often not appropriately adjusted in coordination with the child's neuropsychological deficits. It is also common for parents, as well as the child, to feel guilty about their role in the occurrence of the injury, both of which can lead to emotional and behaviour difficulties for the child.

Overall, while there is much evidence to indicate that brain injury can lead to mood and behaviour problems in children, a direct effect cannot be assumed. The indirect effects of the injury, as well as preinjury functioning and environment must always be considered in attempting to understand the relationship between brain functioning and emotional/behavioural problems.

Brain tumour effects

The reported incidence of CNS tumours in children and adolescents in the US is estimated to be 22 per million per year, the majority of which occur without any apparent predisposing condition. Changes in mood and behaviour are often the first clinical sign of pediatric brain tumour. Some of the behavioural changes, particularly in young children, may be a result of periodic pain and discomfort resulting from increased intracranial pressure. Nevertheless, the clinical presentation in school-age children and adolescents is mainly related to the anatomical location of the tumour (Siffert et al., 1999).

Although the relationship is unclear, lesions in parts of the brainstem, for instance, sometimes initially present with behavioural signs such as increased irritability and significant personality changes. Mood changes may result from tumours affecting the endocrine system. Similar to the effects of frontal lobe brain injury, tumours in the frontal lobe may also result in behavioural/personality changes, and the presentation may be extremely difficult to distinguish from that observed in personality disorders, for example (Lezak, 1995; Siffert at al., 1999). Individuals with temporal lobe lesions may also exhibit extreme behavioural problems, including erratic disruptive behaviour and extreme mood swings. Periods of severe temper outbursts and disruptive behaviour may alternate with periods of controlled and appropriate behaviour. Outbursts may sometimes occur randomly, but may also occur in response to stressors; therefore, clinicians may falsely believe that the behaviours have a functional rather than an organic cause (Lezak, 1995).

In addition, mood difficulties and changes may also occur as the child attempts to cope with changes in cognitive and physical functioning caused by the tumour, as well as with the stress of hospitalization and painful medical procedures, changes in physical appearance, disruption of family roles and routines, isolation from peers, and so forth (Ostroff and Steinglass, 1996; Siffert et al., 1999). Some emotional and behavioural changes may actually result from the child's decreased opportunities to interact with peers, and to continue developing age-appropriate social skills and behaviours (Healey et al., 1991; Siffert et al., 1999). Further, similar to brain injury outcome data, various environmental factors such as low SES, young maternal age, and single-parent environments are also linked to increased risk of emotional and behavioural difficulties (Mulhern et al., 1993).

In addition to the direct effects of the tumour on mood and behaviour, and the social-emotional impact of dealing with a chronic illness, certain aspects of treatment may also contribute to emotional and behavioural difficulties, such as withdrawal from medications or side-effects of medications. Steroids, which are used for various symptoms related to the tumour, as well as medications used to control seizures, can result in mood disturbances, particularly irritability (Siffert et al., 1999).

Overall, similar to the brain injury outcome studies, there appears to be a direct association between pediatric tumours and behaviour. Many other factors, however, including environment, treatment effects, and stress and quality of life changes related to having a brain tumour appear to play a significant role.

Prenatal and perinatal factors

Research suggests that there are a number of prenatal and perinatal risk factors involved in the development of behaviour problems in children. Many hypotheses about prenatal factors are based on studies of infant mortality rates, with the reasoning being that factors causing mortality can also contribute to brain damage in those infants who survive. Experimental research on animals is also an important source of information.

Infections

Previously, the impact of maternal viral infections on the later development of unborn children focused on communicable diseases such as measles, mumps and particularly rubella, which increases the risk of several difficulties such as cleft palate and microcephaly (Erickson, 1998). Recently, however, much attention is being focused on the effects of HIV infection and AIDS.

The majority of children and adolescents with HIV-1 are infected vertically, through their mothers, with transmission occurring either prenatally or during delivery (Pontrelli et al., 1999; Erickson, 1998). While HIV-1 infection does not begin in the brain, the infection passes through the blood-brain barrier to the brain, eventually resulting in CNS disease. Central nervous system involvement is estimated to occur in between 78% and 93% of children with HIV (Teeter and Semrud-Clikeman, 1997). Emotional lability, increased activity level and conduct problems, along with decreased school performance are frequently among the first signs of HIV-related CNS disease in children (Pontrelli et al., 1999). While emotional lability is a sign of CNS involvement, it is important to recognize the resulting emotional impact of such a devastating illness on the individual and the entire family. In addition to the individual's reaction to his/her own illness, many children and adolescents with HIV-1 are also coping with the reality of their mother's illness. Therefore, it is not a surprising finding that depression is common. The effects on adolescents are less frequently studied; however, the CNS manifestations are thought to be similar to those observed in children. Scarmato et al. (1996) found a pattern of brain atrophy using MRI data that was distinct from patterns resulting from other etiologies, with brain atrophy primarily affecting the subcortical white matter of the basal ganglia regions.

Substance use

Substances used during pregnancy can also contribute to serious neurodevelopmental and behavioural concerns throughout childhood. The focus is primarily on the effects of substances taken by the mother, but recent studies have begun to indicate that substances taken by males can damage their reproductive systems, and result in birth defects in their unborn children (Erickson, 1998). In many outcome studies, the effects of SES and other social factors confound the results. Nevertheless, substances such as nicotine, alcohol and cocaine can result in CNS damage, and appear to contribute to emotional and behavioural difficulties in children.

Alcohol

The association between maternal alcohol use during pregnancy and specific patterns of physical malformation, as well as behavioural difficulties, is well documented. Prenatal and postnatal growth deficiency, abnormal cardiac development, craniofacial anomalies, such as widely spaced eyes and small nose, and limb defects are a part of a specific pattern of anomalies comprising foetal alcohol syndrome (FAS). When some of the features associated with prenatal alcohol consumption are present without the full expression of FAS, the term foetal alcohol effects (FAE) is applied.

Studies have demonstrated effects on the developing CNS. Early signs include brain-wave abnormalities, impaired sucking response and sleeping problems (Teeter and Semrud-Clikeman, 1997). Brain imaging studies also indicate a correlation between the facial features associated with FAS and underlying brain malformation (Walker et al., 1999). Decreased size in the anterior region of the cerebellar vermis (Sowell et al., 1996), and midline brain anomalies (Swayze et al., 1997) are among the anomalies identified using brain imaging techniques. Cognitive problems, including mental retardation, and behaviour problems, such as overactivity, irritability, poor impulse control and poor understanding of cause/effect relationships, including the consequences of behaviour, are common in the children of mothers who used alcohol.

In addition to the confounding effects of SES and other environmental factors, inaccurate bioassay techniques also impede the ability of researchers to determine the precise relationship between factors such as amount of alcohol consumed and timing of alcohol exposure, and the nature and degree of cognitive and behaviour problems occurring throughout childhood. The short half-life of alcohol in the tissues, for example, limits the utility of direct assay techniques. Therefore, most information regarding the specifics of alcohol consumption must be obtained retrospectively through self-report (Walker et al., 1999). Nevertheless, findings clearly indicate that at least moderate amounts of prenatal alcohol exposure negatively affect cognitive and behavioural development.

Cocaine

Bioassays of cocaine use in pregnant woman are more accurate than those of alcohol use. Nevertheless, there are a number of factors that hinder the ability to draw definite conclusions about the effects of *in utero* cocaine exposure on the CNS and the subsequent emotional and behavioural development of the unborn child. Urine assays completed at the time of delivery, for example, provide information only about cocaine used during the previous 72 hours. Therefore, as in studies of alcohol use, detailed information about timing and amount of cocaine used must be obtained through interviews. In addition, the majority of individuals using cocaine are also polysubstance users. Women who use cocaine are also at increased risk for exposure to a variety of other risk factors that can affect CNS development in the foetus, such as poor nutrition and HIV infection (Walker et al., 1999). It is therefore difficult to determine which effects are actually primary effects of the cocaine use.

Further, longitudinal studies on the effects of *in utero* cocaine exposure throughout childhood and beyond are rare, with most focusing on infancy. Continuing drug use is also likely to occur in mothers who used cocaine during pregnancy. Therefore, the effects of prenatal exposure are often difficult to differentiate from the negative environmental effects that accompany parental drug use. What is known about cocaine exposure, however, is that the effects on the CNS of the developing foetus appear to be quite significant and include microcephaly and cranial abnormalities, such as lesions in the basal ganglion, frontal lobes, and posterior fossa (Dixon and Bejar, 1989).

Regarding emotional and behavioural effects, Edmondson and Smith (1994) studied prenatally cocaine-exposed infants at 6 months of age. In comparison to a matched control group, the cocaine-exposed infants were reported by their mothers to be less cooperative and more difficult to manage, and by professionals as being less communicative and less responsive. Allen et al. (1991) suggested that cognitive and behavioural problems in some individuals may not be evident until later in childhood when effects of frontal lobe and basal ganglia damage become more apparent. Nevertheless, there are few well-controlled studies of older children, and in those that exist, the results are varied. Ostrea et al. (1992) compared 6-year-old children with light to moderate *in utero* exposure with matched controls and found no significant differences in classroom behaviours as rated by teachers. Delaney-Black et al. (1998), in contrast, also studied 6-year-old children with prenatal exposure and found that their teachers, who were blind to exposure status, rated the exposed group higher for problem behaviours.

Nicotine

Maternal cigarette smoking is recognized as posing a significant health risk to the developing foetus, including premature delivery and low birth weight. Direct brain effects are indicated by both animal and human studies. Decreased brain size, for example, was found in a study of nicotine exposure on rats (Roy and Sabherwal, 1994) and may be related to findings of considerably smaller head size in human children exposed to nicotine *in utero* (Walker et al., 1999). Functional alteration of receptors within the basal ganglia was identified as a possible effect of nicotine on foetal brain development (Weitzman et al., 1992). Similar environmental confounding factors present in studies of alcohol and cocaine effects also affect outcome studies of nicotine exposure. Use of other substances such as caffeine and alcohol is also often associated with smoking. Further, women who smoke during pregnancy are likely to continue smoking after giving birth. Therefore, it is difficult to determine if behaviour problems occurring in childhood are related to prenatal exposure or to exposure to second-hand smoke during infancy and early childhood.

Nevertheless, studies suggest a significant association between *in utero* nicotine exposure and behaviour disorders occurring throughout childhood (Whitaker et al., 1997; Weitzman et al., 1992). Weissman et al. (1999), for example, conducted a longitudinal study of children with prenatal exposure to nicotine, and compared them with children without prenatal exposure on measures of behaviour. They found an increased risk of prepubertal-onset conduct disorder in boys, and an increased risk of adolescent-onset drug dependence in girls. Further, the authors emphasized that these outcomes appeared unrelated to potential confounding variables such as parental psychiatric disorders, postnatal smoking, and whether or not the children/adolescents smoked.

In summary, prenatal and perinatal factors such as HIV infection and *in utero* substance exposure appear to have a significant effect on the developing CNS and on subsequent emotional and behavioural development. Significant social and environmental factors, however, such as maternal illness and/or continuing maternal substance use make it difficult to draw definite conclusions about direct effects of infections and substance exposure. In addition, inaccurate bioassay techniques, and the fact that prenatal exposure is often to polysubstances further hinders the understanding of the effects of individual substances. Further, the effects of paternal substance use are not well studied, and may also be a significant confounding variable in studies of the effects of maternal substance use.

Prenatal and perinatal brain insults

Nass and Koch (1991) studied the effects of congenital unilateral brain injury caused by intrauterine strokes, and compared the effects of left versus right hemisphere damage. Measures of temperament were administered to parents of toddlers and to parents of preschool/school-age children. The authors found a relationship between problems in mood/temperament and location of insult. Both toddlers and preschool/school-age children with right hemisphere damage demonstrated more negative temperament on most dimensions measured, including mood, than those with left hemisphere damage. Counter to findings in studies of adults with acquired brain injury, toddlers with right hemisphere lesions exhibited more negative mood and those with left lesions displayed more positive mood. This difference was not significant for the preschool/school-age group. The authors questioned whether these findings suggested incomplete hemispheric specialization or were related to measurement issues.

Nevertheless, the question of how these early temperament differences affect later mood and behavioural development remains. Outcome studies of depression resulting from left versus right hemisphere damage in adults are mixed. Some show greater risk for depression with left hemisphere injuries, whereas others show equal risk resulting from injury to either hemisphere. Nass and Koch (1991) suggested, however, that the differences in toddler temperament related to right hemisphere damage might have significant impact on later development. Therefore, mood/behaviour problems in later childhood may not necessarily be direct effects of brain damage. The preschool/school-age children with right hemisphere damage exhibited negative temperament characteristics similar to those evidenced by the toddlers with right hemisphere damage. The question arises, however, as to what degree the toddlers' early temperament difficulties affect their early interactions and social experiences, and therefore contribute to the later development of mood and behaviour problems.

Another significant risk factor for perinatal brain injury is low birth weight. Low birth weight can result from a number of factors such as premature birth or intrauterine growth retardation related to maternal age, maternal trauma, substance use, genetic factors, or toxemia. Low birth weight infants are particularly vulnerable to perinatal brain injuries, especially intracranial haemorrhage. Whitaker et al. (1997) examined the relationship between neonatal ultrasound abnormalities and emotional/behavioural disturbance in a sample of 6-year-old children who were low birth weight infants. Two classifications of US abnormalities were compared. The first was germinal matrix haemorrhage and/or intraventricular haemorrhage (GMH/IVH), which are suggestive of injury to glial precursors. The second was parenchymal lesion (PL), and/or ventricular enlargement (VE), which are associated with perinatal white-matter injury. The impact of environmental factors was also examined. The presence of psychiatric disorders at age six was assessed using parent interviews.

The GMH/IVH group did not differ significantly from a group of children evidencing no abnormalities (NA) regarding the development of any class of psychiatric disorders. The prevalence of several specific disorders and classes of disorders, including disruptive behaviour disorders, however, was greater for the PL/VE group, with ADHD being the most common. Overall, boys in all three groups were more likely than girls to have any disorder, including behaviour disorders, although gender did not modify the effects of brain injury on the development of psychiatric disorders. The authors suggested that, although the findings did not support a relationship between GMH/IVH and the presence of psychiatric disorders in childhood, it is possible that such insults did result in behavioural problems that were not captured by the psychiatric diagnostic categories of the DSM-III-R. In addition, it is also possible that they result in disorders that typically do not arise until a later age.

Further, while many investigators maintain that positive social environment appears to mediate some of the negative effects of brain injury, Whitaker et al. (1997) suggested that both PL/VE and environmental factors, such as low household income, increased the risk of psychiatric disorder independently. In addition, positive environmental factors did not appear to provide any type of buffering effects against the effects of PL/VE.

Similarly, Laucht et al. (2000) in a study of the relationship between perinatal risk factors, psychosocial risk factors and behavioural problems in German school-age children, found little evidence for interactional effects. Rather, both perinatal risk factors, such as very low birth weight, toxemia, or asphyxia, and psychosocial risk factors appeared to have independent adverse effects. As a measure of behavioural outcomes, a German version of the Child Behavior Checklist (CBCL) (Achenbach, 1991) was administered. The CBCL is a checklist that is completed by parents as a measure of behaviour across several domains, such as anxious/depressed, aggressive behaviour, attention problems, and social problems. Children in the biological risk group had significantly higher scores than children in the non-risk group on the social problems scale and on the attention problems scale. Children in the psychosocial risk group exhibited higher scores than the nonrisk group on the following domains:

- delinquent behaviour;
- aggressive behaviour;
- attention problems; and
- somatic complaints.

Overall, the authors concluded that 'children growing up with early biological or psychosocial hazards are at increased risk for behaviour problems at 8 years of age.' Nevertheless, just as Whitaker et al. (1997) suggested that GMH/IVH might possibly result in behavioural disturbances that are not captured by specific psychiatric diagnostic categories, Laucht et al. (2000) identified a 'heterogeneous and subtle pattern of disturbance'. He hypothesized that the behavioural impact of perinatal complications may not be adequately described by common diagnostic categories.

Overall, evidence suggests that at least certain types of prenatal and perinatal brain injury contribute to the development of mood and behaviour disturbance in children, with problems perhaps being evident as early as the toddler stage. The full impact of early brain insults throughout childhood, however, may not be apparent due to limitations in the applicability of current diagnostic categories and criteria. In addition, psychosocial factors appear to be an independent risk factor, with positive social factors not appearing to buffer the effects of prenatal and perinatal injury.

Metabolic disorders

Metabolic disorders of the brain occur secondarily to pathological changes occurring in other areas of the body (Lezak, 1995). Brain imaging and neurophysiological techniques, particularly MRI, are used in diagnosing metabolic disorders. Individually, specific metabolic disorders are rare, but as a group metabolic disorders are rather common. It is not yet possible to link specific mood and behavioural symptom constellations to each particular metabolic disorder, but patterns do emerge and are helpful diagnostic indicators.

The psychiatric symptoms associated with Wilson's disease, an autosomal recessive disorder characterized by excessive accumulation of copper in the brain and other tissues, appear to be better documented than most other disorders. Mood and behaviour disturbances typically do not become apparent until late childhood or adolescence, and may be the most predominant symptoms even in the absence of neurological signs (Jackson et al., 1994). Psychiatric symptoms may include changes in personality such as irritability, low anger threshold, and eventually depression, which may be severe enough to result in suicidal ideation and attempts (Trifiletti and Packard, 1999). Therefore, Jackson et al. (1994) emphasized the importance of obtaining a careful physical examination, a thorough medical history, and laboratory testing for clients who exhibit psychiatric symptoms and also have abnormal liver function test results, and/or neurological findings.

More research is needed regarding the effects of specific metabolic disorders on the development of mood and behaviour problems. Current findings suggest that metabolic disorders do not independently result in the development of mood or behavioural disorders. Nevertheless, changes in mood and behaviour are often among the first indications of a metabolic disturbance. Mental health professionals must be aware of this relationship, given that in many cases the changes in mood and behaviour may be so significant and problematic that a mental health clinician is the first professional to be consulted.

Neurochemical factors

While identifiable organic conditions may contribute to emotional/behavioural problems in children, many children and adolescents presenting for mental health services do not have identifiable biologic indicators, such as tumours or known brain insults. Studies have suggested a relationship between various aspects of brain functioning and emotional/behaviour problems in these children as well. Regarding depressive disorders, in a review of the literature, Rogeness et al. (1992) concluded that there is 'evidence for dysregulation of noradrenergic function in major depressive disorder in children, with evidence more consistent with increased noradrenergic function than with decreased noradrenergic function.' They also reported that either decreased or increased serotonergic function is suggested.

Serotonin is believed to be involved in emotion and behaviour primarily due to an inhibitory effect on the striatal and lymbic system, thereby affecting impulse control. The highest level of serotonin receptors is in the frontal lobes, and deficiencies appear to result in a variety of behaviour problems. While the effects of imbalances in serotonin are unclear, they appear to involve increased susceptibility to aggression, impulsivity and depression (Teeter and Semrud-Clikeman, 1997).

Hughes et al. (1996) measured whole-blood serotonin levels in children and adolescents between the ages of seven and 18 years who met criteria for mood and/or behaviour disorders according to the DSM-III-R, in comparison to a control group. They found low levels in those with mood disorders, even when the mood disorder occurred in combination with a behaviour disorder. Regarding children and adolescents diagnosed with behaviour disorders, Hughes et al. (1996) found higher levels of whole-blood serotonin. Comparatively, Rogeness et al. (1992) concluded that decreased noradrenergic and serotonergic functioning is associated with conduct disorder. Further, they clarified that high whole-blood serotonin may be related to decreased serotonergic functioning. It is also important to note that Hughes et al. (1996) found higher levels of serotonin in the African American participants in comparison to white participants, particularly for those in the group with behaviour disorders. Sample size was too small to draw definite conclusions but this finding highlights the importance of examining ethnic/racial factors.

Prosser et al. (1997) studied plasma gamma aminobutyric acid (GABA) levels in children between the ages of seven and 17 with mood and/or behaviour disorders in comparison with a control group without disorders. Findings indicated increased levels in those diagnosed with behaviour disorders (comorbid CD and ADHD). Those with CD only or ADHD only did not have significantly high levels in comparison to the control group, suggesting an 'interaction model of severity'. GABA levels were lower in those individuals receiving medication treatment, such as SSRIs. Lower GABA levels were also found in the subjects with mood disorders in comparison to the control group, but did not appear affected by medication treatment.

The finding of lower GABA levels in subjects being treated for behaviour disorders is in contrast to those of Kemph et al. (1993), who found increased GABA levels and decreased aggression in children between the ages of five and 15 years meeting DSM-III-R criteria for CD or ODD, and who were being treated with clonidine. Prosser et al. (1997) suggested that perhaps the clonidine had a non-GABA related effect, such as sedation, which contributed to decreased aggression. In addition, the effect of the comorbid diagnoses of ADHD and CD on their findings is unclear.

Overall, current data suggest that there is a relationship between neurochemical functioning and emotional/behavioural functioning in children; however, the exact nature of that relationship remains elusive. Continued research is needed to determine how both increased and decreased levels of specific neurotransmitters relate to the occurrence of psychiatric disturbance in general, as well as to specific disorders. In addition, the effects of medication on neurochemical imbalances and resulting psychiatric symptoms are also in need of further investigation.

Electroencephalogram (EEG) studies

Electroencephalogram studies on adults have demonstrated patterns associated with various psychiatric disorders. Hughes and John (1999) in a review of the literature reported an incidence of abnormal conventional EEG findings in 20% to 40% of those assessed with mood disorders, including patterns of small sharp spikes, 6/s spike wave complexes and positive spikes. They also reported that alpha and/or theta power were increased in depressed individuals in QEEG studies. Electroencephalogram findings in children can be quite variable and difficult to interpret. Many EEG studies in child and adolescent populations have focused on ADHD and autism. Some studies of mood and other behaviour disorders, however, have indicated positive EEG findings.

Drake et al. (1992) examined EEG findings in 23 adults and children, ages nine to 44, who demonstrated episodic rage or violent behaviour. Three subjects had histories of febrile convulsions and eight had experienced head injuries previously. The authors reported, however, that none of the subjects had identifiable neurological disorders and all had normal neurological examinations. They found that seven subjects, including three children, had abnormal EEGs. Deckel et al. (1996) administered EEGs to adult male subjects, ages 21-25, identified as having antisocial personality disorder (ASP). Childhood difficulties were assessed on the Wender Behavior Checklist (Wender, 1971), which is designed to assess childhood behaviour and symptoms, retrospectively. On this measure, elevations were indicated on the hyperactivity scale, the conduct scale and the composite scale.

Findings indicated that the diagnosis of ASP and elevated conduct and hyperactivity scores were associated with greater activation of right relative to left frontal EEG activity. The authors concluded that these findings suggested that 'either higher right-hemisphere activity, lower left-hemisphere activity or both were associated with greater behaviour disturbances during childhood/young adulthood'. Given that information on childhood functioning was obtained retrospectively, however, one must be cautious in assuming that these findings can actually be generalized to child/adolescent populations.

Matsuura et al. (1993) examined school-age children from Tokyo, Beijing and Korea and had contrasting results. They conducted EEG examinations on children identified as having 'deviant behaviour' based on the parent questionnaires, and compared findings with those of children identified as exhibiting 'normal behaviour.' They reported that for children from all three countries, the EEGs of children exhibiting emotional and behavioural difficulties did not differ in the frequency histogram patterns or other measures in comparison with the EEGs of children without emotional/behavioural problems.

Regarding findings in children with depressive disorders, specifically, Puig-Antich (1987) found that the EEG sleep records of prepubertal children experiencing a major depressive episode did not differ from those of 'normal' children. These findings were in contrast to the studies of EEG sleep patterns of adults with major depression. The author hypothesized that the differences in adult and child EEG patterns may be due to maturational factors, and that EEG sleep patterns may be an 'age-sensitive marker' of depression.

Research findings are not strong enough to draw definite conclusions about the role of EEG data in the diagnosis and treatment of mood and behavioural disorders in children. Results of current studies are mixed, and the EEG variability and abnormalities observed in some studies are not clearly pathognomic. Nevertheless, the abnormal findings in much of the existing literature suggest that this is an area worthy of more extensive investigation.

Clinical implications

Assessment

Clearly, the population of children and adolescents presenting with mood and behavioural concerns represents an extremely complex and hetero-geneous group. In the assessment phase, it is essential that a thorough history be obtained, including a mental health history and a general medical history of both the child and the family. The family history will help to determine mental health and medical risk factors, and prognosis, and will also assist in identifying additional services that might be beneficial to the family.

Moreover, a physical examination for the child exhibiting mood and/or behaviour problems should be recommended, if one was not obtained recently. Many of the children and adolescents presenting for treatment will not have a clear organic impairment or medical disorder needing treatment but the possibility remains and should always be ruled out. This issue is particularly important given that mood and behavioural changes, including increases in aggression, are often the first symptoms of a neurobiological problem, such as a tumour or metabolic disorder. Clinicians should be especially emphatic about recommending medical consultation if the onset of mood and behaviour problems was sudden and/or if symptom severity increased rapidly, particularly in the absence of environmental stressors or psychosocial risk factors. Conversely, when psychosocial risk factors are indicated, the clinician must use extreme caution not to overly attribute the child's emotional and behavioural difficulties to these environmental factors. The possibility that medical factors are contributing to mood or behavioural problems must always be considered, with environmental stressors viewed as independent factors also placing the child at risk.

The necessity for a neuropsychological evaluation should also be considered. Such an assessment may be particularly warranted if the child is having academic difficulties and/or has a history placing him or her at risk for neuropsychological problems, such as prenatal or perinatal complications. In some cases, the individual may have resulting subtle learning deficits, with the behaviour and mood difficulties occurring at least partially in response to feelings of failure and frustration, for example. The clinician may then be instrumental in collaborating with educators and caregivers to make sure that expectations at school and in all other environments are realistic, and that the appropriate educational services are in place. In addition, mood and/or behavioural disturbances may also be the result of previously unidentified brain pathology. A neuropsychological evaluation often provides important clues regarding brain impairment, even when EEGs or other neurological studies are inconclusive.

Developmental factors

The provision of early intervention is highly valuable. In some instances, early, minor behavioural and temperament disturbances in high-risk individuals are apparent during the toddler stage and early childhood. If not addressed, these difficulties may contribute to long-term parent/child interaction problems, which may further contribute to the development of emotional and behaviour problems. Further, if parents are not provided with assistance in learning effective ways of responding to problematic behaviour, such behaviour may become even more significant and ingrained by later childhood or adolescence.

Children who do receive behavioural treatment, psychotherapy services, and/or medication treatment at an early stage of development may exhibit improvement over time and no longer appear to require intervention. It is important that clinicians help caregivers to understand that different developmental stages present with different challenges, and that they should consider resuming treatment if difficulties arise. The need for resumed treatment should not necessarily be viewed as an increase in psychopathology severity or as a failure of previous intervention, but as part of the developmental process. A child at high risk for emotional or behaviour disturbance may function adequately, with only minor difficulties in the lower grades at school, for example, but may experience increased disturbance upon entering high school, where the academic and social demands are much greater. Further, as expectations increase, and as the brain fails to develop typically, the effects of brain damage may become apparent in some children and be evidenced by problematic behaviour. It is important to avoid providing parents with an overly pessimistic outlook on the child's future, and definitive predictions regarding a child's future development should not be made. It is important, however, that parents be aware that emotional and behaviour difficulties may later become more apparent in children with certain risk factors, such as perinatal insults, and that intervention should then be obtained.

Medication treatment

The presence of emotional and behaviour problems in children does not always necessitate the provision of medication treatment. Given the potential neurobiological correlates, however, it is important that medication treatment be considered, particularly if behaviours are extreme and place the individual and/or others at risk of harm. Further, when medication is being prescribed for a medical condition, such as a seizure disorder, for example, the psychiatrist may also be quite valuable in helping to recognize possible medication side effects and in determining if some aspects of mood and behaviour disturbance might actually be related primarily to medication effects.

In addition, the psychiatrist and other professionals involved may also be helpful in educating the caregiver regarding the role of medication in treatment. Understandably, parents and others involved with the child often have a strong desire to find fast and effective treatment, particularly if there are numerous environmental stressors. They may become invested in medication treatment to the exclusion of psychotherapy/counselling services and environmental changes. The likelihood of this stance often appears increased in cases where there is a significant medical history, such as prenatal and/or perinatal complications. In such instances, many caregivers reason that because there appears to be a medical cause, a purely medical intervention is the most logical and should be sufficient. The clinicians involved must help the caregivers to understand the potential benefits, as well as the limitations, of medication treatment and begin to help them recognize the complex factors contributing to the development and maintenance of the child's emotional and behavioural difficulties.

Individual and family therapy

Treatment must also include opportunities for individual and/or family therapy. Although more research is needed regarding therapy approaches and techniques, it is largely accepted that individual therapy provides a means to improve the child's coping and problem-solving, and to explore and to address internal and external factors contributing to their disturbance. Parents and teachers should also be given guidance in how to respond to and interact with the child, particularly in regard to aggressive and other inappropriate behaviours. The need for more extensive family intervention and assistance, however, is often overlooked. Most studies providing evidence of impaired brain functioning in children and adolescents with mood and behaviour problems also emphasize the impact on the social functioning of the family. The diagnosis of a child with a brain tumour or any other disorder affecting CNS functioning can be quite devastating for the entire family, and results in significant changes in family roles and quality of life.

Even when a child exhibits significant mood and behaviour problems in the absence of such medical factors, the financial and emotional stress placed on the family can be enormous. Parents may feel that they are somehow to blame for the child's problems, marital problems may be exacerbated and siblings may begin to feel neglected, as much attention is focused on the child exhibiting difficulties, for example. Therefore, the initiation of family therapy to assist in adjusting to new roles, and in understanding and coping with the effect of the child's difficulties on the family is an important consideration.

The notion of whether or not positive social and environmental factors can provide a buffering effect for children and adolescents with CNS impairment continues to be debated. The research strongly suggests, however, that certain environmental stresses are a significant independent risk factor for later development of emotional and behaviour difficulties (Yeates, et al., 1997; Shaffer, 1995; Whitaker et al., 1997; Laucht et al., 2000). In addition to direct individual and family therapy, it is important that treatment not only focuses on addressing the child's symptoms and the family's reaction to them but must also include helping the family to address other sources of environmental stress. Assisting a single parent with several children with issues such as finding affordable daycare services, for example, might be just as important as providing treatment to the child exhibiting the disturbance. The involvement of social work and/or case management services in the intervention process may be highly beneficial in this regard.

In conclusion, the need for a multidisciplinary and flexible approach cannot be emphasized strongly enough. When children and adolescents begin to exhibit significant emotional and behavioural problems they may first come to the attention of any number of professionals, such as psychologists, social workers, behaviour specialists, neuropsychologists, physicians, and/or psychiatrists for assessment and/or treatment. Any of these professionals might be able to provide a useful and effective service, but is likely to only address a portion of the issues involved. Further, the organization of many clinics and facilities makes it difficult to obtain the desired and necessary collaboration. Counselling centres often do not have the capabilities to conduct neuropsychological assessments, for example. Similarly, neuropsychology clinics typically do not include behavioural analysis as part of the assessment process. In addition, issues of religion and spirituality, and race/ethnicity are minimally explored in the literature. As clinicians, we must remain aware that such factors may affect symptom presentation, as well as service utilization and response to treatment. Children and adolescents presenting with mood and behaviour disturbances represent a challenging and diverse population. Clinicians must be willing to engage in ongoing and active collaboration and consultation with other professionals, and to take a flexible, multifaceted approach to assessment and treatment in order to maximize the chances of effective intervention.

References

Achenbach TM (1991) Manual for the Child Behavior Checklist/4-18 and 1991 Profile. Burlington VT: University of Vermont Department of Psychiatry.

Allen LF, Palomares RS, DeForest P, Sprinkle B, Reynolds CR (1991) The effects of intrauterine cocaine exposure: transient or teratogenic? Archives of Clinical Neuropsychology 6: 133–46.

Angold A, Rutter M (1992) Effects of age and pubertal status in a large clinical sample. Development and Psychopathology 4: 5–28.

Asarnow RF, Satz P, Light R, Zaucha K, Lewis R, McCleary C (1995) The UCLA study of mild closed head injury in children and adolescents. In Broman SH, Michel ME (eds) Traumatic Head Injury in Children. New York: Oxford University Press.

Bijur PE, Haslum M (1995) Cognitive, behavioural, and motoric sequelae of mild head injury in a national birth cohort. In Broman SH, Michel ME (eds) Traumatic Head Injury in Children. New York: Oxford University Press.

Boyd-Franklin N (1989) Black Families in Therapy: A Multisystems Approach. New York: Guilford Press.

Bui KT, Takeuchi DT (1992) Ethnic minority adolescents and the use of community mental health care services. American Journal of Community Psychology 20: 403–17.

Cantwell DP (1992) Clinical phenomenology and nosology. Child and Adolescent Psychiatric Clinics of North America 1: 1–11.

Capaldi DM (1992) Co-occurrence of conduct problems and depressive symptoms in early adolescent boys: II. A 2-year follow-up at grade 8. Development and Psychopathology 4: 125–44.

Carlson GA, Cantwell DP (1980) Unmasking masked depression in children and adolescents. American Journal of Psychiatry 137(4): 445–9.

Deaton AV (1987) Behavioural change strategies for children and adolescents with severe brain injury. Journal of Learning Disabilities 20(10): 581–9.

Deckel AW, Hesselbrock V, Bauer L (1996) Antisocial personality disorder, childhood delinquency, and frontal brain functioning: EEG and neuropsychological findings. Journal of Clinical Psychology 52(6): 639–50.

Delaney-Black V, Covington C, Templin T, Ager J, Martier S, Sokol R (1998) Prenatal cocaine exposure and child behaviour. Pediatrics 102(4): 945–50.

Dixon SD, Bejar R (1989) Echoencephalographic findings in neonates associated with maternal cocaine and methamphetamine use: incidence and clinical correlates. Journal of Pediatrics 115(5): 770–8.

Drake ME Jr, Hietter SA, Pakalnis A (1992) EEG and evoked potentials in episodic-dyscontrol syndrome. Neuropsychobiology 26: 125–8.

Edmondson R, Smith T (1994) Temperament and behaviour of infants prenatally exposed to drugs: clinical implications for the mother-infant dyad. Infant Mental Health Journal 15: 368–79.

Erickson MT (1998) Etiological factors. In Ollendick TH, Hersen M (eds) Handbook of Child Psychopathology. New York: Plenum Press.

Ewing-Cobbs L, Fletcher JM, Levin HS, Francis DJ, Davidson K, Miner ME (1997) Longitudinal neuropsychological outcome in infants and preschoolers with traumatic brain injury. Journal of the International Neuropsychological Society 3: 581–91.

Fletcher JM, Levin HS, Lacher D, Kusnerik L, Harward H, Mendelsohn D, Lilly MA (1996) Behavioural outcomes after pediatric closed head injury: relationships with age, severity, and lesion size. Journal of Child Neurology 11: 283–90.

Frick PJ (1998) Conduct disorders. In Ollendick TH, Hersen M (eds) Handbook of Child Psychopathology. New York: Plenum Press.

Fuller T (1992) Masked depression in maladaptive black adolescents. The School Counselor 40: 24–31.

Gibbs JT (1998) African American adolescents. In Gibbs JT, Huang LN (eds) Children of Color: Psychological Interventions with Culturally Diverse Youth. Updated edition. San Francisco CA: Jossey-Bass.

Gibbs JT, Huang LK (1998) A conceptual framework for the psychological assessment and treatment of minority youth. In Gibbs JT, Huang LN (eds) Children of Color: Psychological Interventions with Culturally Diverse Youth. Updated edition. San Francisco CA: Jossey-Bass.

Hammen C, Rudolph KD (1996) Childhood depression. In Mash EJ, Barkley RA (eds) Child Psychopathology. New York: Guilford Press.

Harrington R (1993) Similarities and dissimilarities between child and adult disorders: the case of depression. In Costello CG (ed.) Basic Issues in Psychopathology. New York: Guilford Press.

Healey EA, Barnes PD, Kupsky WJ, Scott RM, Sallan SE, Black PM, Tarbell NJ (1991) The prognostic significance of postoperative residual tumour in ependymoma. Neurosurgery 28(5): 666–72.

Hinshaw SP, Anderson CA (1996) Conduct and oppositional defiant disorders. In Mash EJ, Barkley RA (eds) Child Psychopathology. New York: Guilford Press.

Hughes CW, Petty F, Sheikh S, Kramer GL (1996) Whole-blood serotonin in children and adolescents with mood and behaviour disorders. Psychiatry Research 65(2): 79–95.

Hughes JR, John ER (1999) Conventional and quantitative electroencephalography in psychiatry. Journal of Neuropsychiatry and Clinical Neurosciences 11(2): 190–208.

Jackson GH, Meyer A, Lippmann S (1994) Wilson's disease. Psychiatric manifestations may be the clinical presentation. Postgraduate Medicine 95: 135–8.

Kashani JH, Carlson GA, Beck NC, Hoeper EW, Corcoran CM, McAllister JA, Fallahi C, Rosenberg TK, Reid JC (1987) Depression, depressive symptoms, and depressed mood among a community sample of adolescents. American Journal of Psychiatry 144: 931–4.

Kemph JP, DeVan L, Levin GM, Jarecke R, Miller RL (1993) Treatment of aggressive children with clonidine: results of an open pilot study. Journal of the American Academy of Child and Adolescent Psychiatry 32(3): 577–81.

Lahey BB, Hart EI, Pliszka A, Applegate B, McBurnett K (1993) Neurophysiological correlates of conduct disorder: a rationale and a review of research. Journal of Clinical Child Psychology 22: 141–53.

Lahey BB, Loeber R (1994) Framework for a developmental model of oppositional defiant disorder and conduct disorder. In Routh DK (ed.) Disruptive Behaviour Disorders in Childhood. New York: Plenum Press.

Laucht M, Esser G, Baving L, Gerhold M, Hoesch I, Ihle W, Steigleider P, Stock B, Stoehr RM, Weindrich D, Schmidt MH (2000) Behavioural sequelae of prenatal insults and early family adversity at eight years of age. Journal of the American Academy of Child and Adolescent Psychiatry 39(10): 1229–37.

Levin HS, Ewing-Cobbs L, Eisenberg HM (1995) Neurobehavioural outcome of pediatric closed head injury. In Broman SH, Michel ME (eds) Traumatic Head Injury in Children. New York: Oxford University Press.

Lezak MD (1995) Neuropsychological Assessment. 3 edn. New York: Oxford University Press.

Matsuura M, Okubo Y, Toru M, Kojima T, He Y, You Y, Shen Y, Lee CK (1993) A cross-national EEG study of children with emotional and behavioural problems: a WHO collaborative study in the western pacific region. Biological Psychiatry 34: 59–65.

McGuire TL, Rothenberg MB (1986) Behavioural and psychosocial sequelae of pediatric head injury. Journal of Head Trauma Rehabilitation 1(4): 1–6.

Mendelsohn D, Levin HS, Bruce D, Lilly M, Harward H, Culhane KA, Eisenberg HM (1992) Late MRI after head injury in children: relationship to clinical features and outcome. Childs Nervous System 8: 445–52.

Moffitt TE (1993) Adolescence-limited and life-course persistent antisocial behaviour: a developmental taxonomy. Psychological Review 100: 674–701.

Mulhern RK, Carpentieri S, Shema S, Stone P, Fairclough D (1993) Factors associated with social and behavioural problems among children recently diagnosed with brain tumour. Journal of Pediatric Psychology 18(3): 39–50.

Nagata DK (1998) The assessment and treatment of Japanese American children and adolescents. In Gibbs JT, Huang LN (eds) Children of Color: Psychological Interventions with Culturally Diverse Youth. Updated edition. San Francisco CA: Jossey-Bass.

Nass R, Koch D (1991) Innate specialization for emotion: temperament differences in children with early left versus right brain damage. In Amir N, Rapin I, Branski D (eds) Pediatric Neurology: Behaviour and Cognition of the Child with Brain Dysfunction. Basel: Karger.

Nolan-Hoeksema S, Girgus JS (1994) The emergence of gender differences in depression during adolescence. Psychological Bulletin 115: 424–43.

Ostrea EM Jr, Brady M, Gause S, Raymundo AL, Stevens M (1992) Drug screening of newborns by meconium analysis: a large-scale, prospective, epidemiologic study. Pediatrics 89(1): 107–13.

Ostroff J, Steinglass P (1996) Psychosocial adaptation following treatment: a family system. In Bader L, Cooper C, Kaplan De-Nour A (eds) Cancer and the Family. New York: John Wiley.

Panak WF, Garber J (1992) Role of aggression, rejection, and attributions in the prediction of depression in children. Development and Psychopathology 4: 145–66.

Peterson AC, Compas BE, Brooks-Gunn J, Stemmler M, Ey S, Grant KE (1993) Depression in adolescence. American Psychologist 48: 155–68.

Pontrelli L, Pavlakis S, Krilov LR (1999) Neurobehavioural manifestations and sequelae of HIV and other infections. Child and Adolescent Psychiatric Clinics of North America 8(4): 869–78.

Proctor EK, Vosler NR, Murty S (1992) Child demographics and DSM diagnosis: a multi-axis study. Child Psychiatry and Human Development 22: 165–83.

Prosser J, Hughes CW, Sheika S, Kowatch RA, Kramer GL, Rosenbarger N, Trent J, Petty F (1997) Plasma GABA in children and adolescents with mood, behaviour, and comorbid mood and behaviour disorders: a preliminary study. Journal of Child and Adolescent Psychopharmacology 7(3): 181–99.

Puig-Antich J (1982) Major depression and conduct disorder in prepuberty. Journal of the American Academy of Child Psychiatry 21(2): 118–28.

Puig-Antich J (1987) Sleep and neuroendocrine correlates of affective illness in childhood and adolescence. Journal of Adolescent Health Care 8: 505–29.

Reinherz HZ, Frost K, Pakiz B (1991) Changing faces: correlates of depressive symptoms in late adolescence. Family and Community Health 14: 52–63.

Reynolds WM (1992) Internalizing Disorders in Children and Adolescents. New York: John J. Riley & Sons.

Rogeness GA, Javors MA, Pliszka SR (1992) Neurochemistry and child and adolescent psychiatry. Journal of the American Academy of Psychiatry 31(5): 765–81.

Roy TS, Sabherwal U (1994) Effects of prenatal nicotine exposure on the morphogenesis of somatosensory cortex. Neurotoxicology and Teratology 16(4): 411–21.

Rutter M (1981) Psychological sequelae of brain damage in children. American Journal of Psychiatry 138(12): 1533–44.

Scarmato V, Frank Y, Rozenstein A, Lu DF, Hyman R, Bakshi S, Pahwa S, Pavlakis S (1996) Central brain atrophy in childhood AIDS encephalopathy. AIDS 10(11): 1227–31.

Schwartz JAJ, Gladstone TRG, Kaslow NJ (1998) Depressive disorders. In Ollendick TH, Hersen M (eds) Handbook of Child Psychopathology. New York: Plenum Press.

Shaffer D (1995) Behaviour sequelae of serious head injury in children and adolescents: the British studies. In Broman SH, Michel ME (eds) Traumatic Head Injury in Children. New York: Oxford University Press.

Shaffer D, Chadwick O, Rutter M (1975) Psychiatric outcome of localized head injury in children. Amsterdam: Excerpa Medica.

Siffert J, Greenleaf M, Mannis R, Allen J (1999) Pediatric brain tumors. Child and Adolescent Psychiatric Clinics of North America 8(4): 879–903.

Sowell ER, Jernigan TL, Mattson SN, Riley EP, Sobel DF, Jones KL (1996) Abnormal development of the cerebellar vermis in children prenatally exposed to alcohol: size reduction in lobules I-V. Alcoholism: Clinical and Experimental Research 20(1): 31–4.

Swayze VW, Johnson VP, Hanson JW, Piven J, Sato Y, Giedd JN, Mosnik D, Andreasen NC (1997) Magnetic resonance imaging of brain anomalies in fetal alcohol syndrome. Pediatrics 99(2): 232–40.

Teeter PA, Semrud-Clikeman M (1997) Child Neuropsychology: Assessment and Interventions for Neurodevelopmental Disorders. Needham Heights MA: Allyn & Bacon.

Trifiletti RR, Packard AM (1999) Metabolic disorders presenting with behavioural symptoms in the school-age child. Neurologic Disorders 8(4): 791–806.

Walker A, Rosenberg M, Balaban-Gil K (1999) Neurodevelopmental and neurobe-
    havioural sequelae of selected substances of abuse and psychiatric medications
    in utero. Child and Adolescent Psychiatric Clinics of North America 8(4):
    845–67.
Weiss B, Weisz JR, Politano M, Carey M, Nelson WM, Finch AJ (1992) Relations
    among self-reported depressive symptoms in clinic-referred children versus
    adolescent. Journal of Abnormal Psychology 101: 361–87.
Weissman MM, Warner V, Wickramaratne PJ, Kandel DB (1999) Maternal smoking
    during pregnancy and psychopathology in offspring followed to adulthood.
    Journal of the American Academy of Child and Adolescent Psychiatry 38(7):
    892–9.
Weitzman M, Gortmaker S, Sobl A (1992) Maternal smoking and behaviour prob-
    lems of children. Pediatrics 90: 342–9.
Welner A (1978) Childhood depression: an overview. Journal of Nervous and
    Mental Disease 166(8): 588–93.
Wender PH (1971) Minimal Brain Dysfunction in Children. New York: Wiley.
Whitaker AH, Van Rossem R, Feldman JF, Schonfeld IS, Pinto-Martin JA, Torre C,
    Shaffer D, Paneth N (1997) Psychiatric outcomes in low-birth-weight children
    at age 6 years: relation to neonatal cranial ultrasound abnormalities. Archives
    of General Psychiatry 54: 847–56.
Yeates KO, Taylor HG, Drotar D, Wade SL, Klein S, Stancin T, Schatschneider C
    (1997) Preinjury family environment as a determinant of recovery from trau-
    matic brain injuries in school-age children. Journal of the International
    Neuropsychological Society 3: 617–30.

CHAPTER 2
Social phobia in children: clinical considerations

TRACY L MORRIS, LAURIE A GRECO

Michael is a 9-year-old boy who dreads informal interactions with his peers. He experiences dizziness and a pounding heart prior to lunch time at school and fears he might say or do something embarrassing in front of the other children. To avoid appearing socially inept Michael pretends to be sick during his lunch period. Rather than eating and socializing with his peers, Michael spends the hour lying down in the nurse's office.

Amy is a 16-year-old who admits to having been shy her entire life. As an infant and toddler, she clung to her mother and was slow to warm up in the presence of unfamiliar children and adults. During preschool, Amy frequently played alone while quietly watching her more sociable peers. This pattern of shyness and inhibition intensified throughout elementary and middle school, reaching debilitating levels when Amy entered high school. Amy currently is refusing to attend school because she cannot bear the thought of giving an oral presentation in her English class. Amy is terrified of making a mistake and humiliating herself in front of her classmates.

What is social phobia?

The cases above paint a picture of a relatively common and often long-lasting disorder affecting between 2% and 13% of the US population (lifetime prevalence estimates vary greatly due to methodological differences across studies). Social phobia, also known as social anxiety disorder (SAD) is defined in the fourth edition of the Diagnostic and Statistical Manual of Mental Disorders (DSM-IV) as a 'marked and persistent fear of one or more social or performance situations in which the person is exposed to unfamiliar people or to possible scrutiny by others' (American Psychiatric Association (APA), 1994, p. 416). Social anxiety and 'fear of negative evaluation' have been regarded as hallmark features of social phobia. Individuals with this diagnosis fear they will say or do something embarrassing in the presence of others and as a result they avoid anxiety-inducing situations or endure them with extreme distress.

Children diagnosed with social phobia must demonstrate the capacity for age-appropriate social relationships (for example, with family members) and experience anxiety-related symptoms in the presence of other children (symptoms must extend beyond interactions with adults). The peak age of onset for social phobia is in adolescence, perhaps due to the heightened importance of peers during this time period.

Researchers and clinicians have identified behavioural, cognitive and somatic symptoms characterizing childhood social phobia. Escape and avoidance behaviours, such as those demonstrated by Amy and Michael, are particularly salient. Responses such as 'freezing', clinging and tantrums also may be observed, particularly when children are unable to avoid the feared situation. Maladaptive cognitions, such as self-deprecating beliefs or intense fear of negative evaluation, are common. Children and adolescents with social phobia, for example, may perceive themselves as socially inept and interpret even the most benign social events (such as birthday parties) as threatening. Finally, children and adolescents with social phobia often experience intense physiological responses, including heart palpitations, trembling, sweating and blushing. In Michael's case, anticipation of unstructured social encounters during lunchtime elicited bodily sensations such as a 'pounding heart' and dizziness.

Is social anxiety 'normal'?

Some level of social anxiety may be both universal and adaptive (for example, Menzies and Harris, 2001). Many of us, for example, can recall instances of heightened anxiety in social situations (such as first dates) and performance situations (such as public speaking) without ever meeting criteria for social phobia. Similarly, childhood shyness is a relatively common phenomenon that some children simply outgrow. How, then, do clinicians distinguish between normal and adaptive versus clinically relevant social anxiety?

Generally speaking, individuals must demonstrate impaired functioning and/or experience significant levels of distress to receive a diagnosis of social phobia. In the opening scenarios, Michael seeks refuge in the nurse's office to avoid unstructured peer interactions and Amy avoids giving a speech by refusing to attend school. Both cases reflect instances of functional impairment with the potential for severe consequences, including peer relationship difficulties and decreased academic functioning. Thus, both Michael and Amy appear to be potential candidates for receiving a diagnosis of social phobia.

Developmental course

The mean age of onset for social phobia typically has been reported as from early- to mid-adolescence (Turner and Beidel, 1989). However, most adults with social phobia will report having been extremely 'shy' most all of their lives. Retrospective investigations (Stemberger et al., 1995) indicate that the developmental pattern of social phobia often reflects an early onset and progressive generalization of social fear. It is quite common for adults to report long intervals (over 20 years on average) between the reported onset of social anxiety and initial attempts to seek treatment. Such findings suggest a high degree of stability for social phobia in the absence of intervention.

Comorbidity

Social phobia is a highly comorbid disorder. The most common comorbid conditions include other anxiety disorders (particularly generalized anxiety disorder) and depression. Children who meet criteria for multiple anxiety disorders often show earlier onset, longer chronicity, and higher intensity of their anxiety symptoms than those meeting criteria for a single anxiety disorder. When multiple forms of anxiety are present, the clinician should suggest a longer course of treatment in which exposure is implemented across multiple contexts. The presence of depression also complicates the picture. When depressive symptoms are severe it is generally necessary to treat those as a primary target before implementing treatment for social anxiety. Pharmacological treatments often are useful adjuncts in such cases.

Social phobia as a risk factor

A number of negative and long-lasting conditions have been linked with childhood social phobia. There is evidence to suggest that early social anxiety may increase an individual's risk for certain conditions. For example, Stein et al. (1990) found that depression began after the onset of social phobia in the majority of cases. Children experiencing clinical levels of social anxiety also tend to have fewer close friendships and are less accepted by their peer group compared with their sociable classmates.

Restriction of social activities in an effort to avoid or reduce feelings of social anxiety impedes the development of interpersonal relationships (Schneier et al., 1992) and may adversely impact academic and occupational functioning (Turner et al., 1986). As social withdrawal increases and functioning becomes more impaired, depression becomes more likely.

Social anxiety may also increase risk for substance abuse. Page and Andrews (1996) reported a 27% rate of alcohol problems for adults with social phobia, representing risk ratios three (males) to five (females) times those of the ECA population estimates. Individuals who experience high levels of social anxiety may use alcohol in an attempt to lower inhibition and general physiological arousal. Social phobia has been found to precede alcohol abuse in the majority of comorbid cases (Kushner et al., 1990).

Further research is necessary to elucidate patterns of risk associated with social anxiety. However, at this point it seems clear that high levels of social anxiety do little to promote wellbeing and may seriously reduce an individual's quality of life. In light of such adverse consequences, the early identification and subsequent treatment of children and adolescents at risk for social phobia appears a worthy pursuit.

How does social phobia develop?

As with nearly every childhood disorder, social phobia presumably results from the complex interaction between environmental and biological influences. Due to the nature of this chapter, we provide only a cursory summary of general findings within both domains, placing relative emphasis on the potential role of family factors. For more thorough coverage of social phobia etiology, we refer the reader to Morris (2001) and Hudson and Rapee (2000).

Genetic and biological factors

There is considerable evidence supporting the role of genetic and temperamental factors in the origin of social phobia. Family studies, for example, suggest that social phobia is relatively more common among first-degree relatives, with monozygotic twins evincing the highest concordance rates. In short, it appears that a genetic predisposition towards anxiousness may put individuals at risk for anxiety disorders, including social phobia. Thus, when biologically vulnerable individuals encounter stressful environmental conditions, they are more prone to develop an anxiety disorder.

Behavioural inhibition is a biologically based temperament style characterized by fear of novel stimuli, such as unfamiliar people, objects and events. Behaviourally inhibited children may be withdrawn and overly cautious in their interactions, putting them at increased risk of pervasive social difficulties. As illustrated in Amy's case, it is possible for behaviourally inhibited toddlers to become shy children. In the absence of intervention, these children may go on to develop debilitating levels of social and evaluative fears characteristic of social phobia. Indeed, temperament research points to a link between behavioural inhibition and social-evaluative concerns in both children and adults (Turner and Beidel, 1989).

Environmental influences

Behavioural theories have emphasized the potential role of conditioning, modelling and information transfer in the development of social phobia. The *conditioning* of fears can occur through direct or indirect (vicarious) exposure to a traumatic situation or event. *Modelling* involves 'learning by example,' such as when children imitate avoidance behaviour demonstrated by a socially anxious parent. Finally, *information transfer* refers to the verbal or nonverbal transmission of information regarding social situations. Parents, for example, may directly or indirectly communicate information regarding the 'dangerousness' of social situations (for example 'if you make a mistake when reading aloud, you will get a bad grade and children will laugh at you').

In general, direct and vicarious conditioning appear to trigger more circumscribed or situation-specific fears, such as anxiety experienced exclusively during oral presentations. Conversely, individuals experiencing more generalized and pervasive social anxiety often have a long history of shyness, with its chronicity and severity influenced by environmental factors. Due to the tremendous amount of learning that occurs in the home, we turn next to parental influences related to the development of social phobia.

Parental influence

It is crucial to assess the family environment when considering environmental factors that may be involved in the development or maintenance of social phobia. Three central avenues have been identified as playing an important role in the formation of social fears:

- children's restricted exposure to social situations;
- parental modelling of social and evaluative concerns; and
- parent child-rearing style (see Masia and Morris, 1998 for review).

Restricted exposure

Early on, children rely on parents for initiating and maintaining their social contacts. Parents who fail to set up 'play dates' and who do not make social arrangements restrict their child's exposure to important peer experiences. By doing so, parents may place their child at risk for later social difficulties, including social anxiety. Such parental restriction may be unintentional; however, some findings indicate that parents of socially anxious adults discouraged family sociability and sought to isolate them as they were growing up.

Modelling

In ambiguous and novel situations, children may use their parents' verbal and nonverbal behaviour as cues or guides for appropriate responding. Parents of socially anxious children tend to be overly concerned with the opinions of others and may experience their own social evaluative fears. Moreover, such parents may interpret social situations as threatening and demonstrate avoidance and reticent behaviour in the presence of their children. By modelling such behaviour, parents may be inadvertently encouraging their children's social fears. Children, for example, may imitate their parents' avoidance and distress-related behaviour when confronted with similar social situations. Conversely, parents who model positive behaviour during social discourse may encourage their children to behave accordingly.

Parenting style

Certain types of parenting styles may contribute to the formation and intensification of social phobia and related difficulties. Some anxiety research has focused on the potential role of parental rejection and over-protection/control. Although definitions may vary, *rejection* refers to low affection and warmth, often co-occurring with parental negativity and/or indifference. Parental *overprotection* refers to over-controlling and intrusive behaviour, in which parents may exhibit excessive vigilance and prohibit age-appropriate levels of autonomy. A growing body of literature suggests that overprotective and rejecting parenting may put children at risk for current or future internalizing symptoms, including social anxiety and depression (see, for example, Dadds and Barrett, 1996; Greco and Morris, 2001). Our studies focusing on parent-child interactions, for example, suggest that both mothers and fathers of socially anxious children demonstrate controlling behaviour (such as physical takeovers) and rejecting behaviour (such as criticisms) during joint tasks (Greco and Morris, 2001; Spaulding and Morris, 1997).

In summary, the complex interaction between biological and environmental factors may lead to the formation and maintenance of childhood social phobia. Due to the chapter aims, we focused primarily on environmental and parental influences. We would like to stress, however, that no single factor (such as parenting style) *causes* social phobia. It is more likely to be the case that multiple factors interact with one another, with certain factors ameliorating or exacerbating the effects of others. Much research is needed to help us gain a more thorough understanding of the various pathways to social phobia.

Assessment of social phobia

As with any disorder, a careful assessment includes the use of multiple methods (for example, self-report and behavioural observations). When working with children and families, it is important to solicit information from multiple sources, such as parents, teachers and peers. We also recommend careful evaluation of children's cognitive, behavioural and somatic responses in a variety of social contexts, such as home and school. Using a multi-method, multi-modal approach will allow for a thorough description of the presenting problem, which can be used to guide case conceptualization and treatment planning. Schniering et al. (2000) provide a thorough review of diagnostic issues and assessment methods for childhood anxiety disorders. Below we emphasize measures developed (in whole or in part) to assess social anxiety and social phobia.

Structured interview

The Anxiety Disorders Interview Schedule for DSM-IV Child Version (ADIS-C) (Silverman and Albano, 1996) is a semi-structured interview developed to assist with the differential diagnoses of DSM-IV anxiety disorders. Even though the ADIS-C focuses primarily on childhood anxiety disorders, interview questions are included to screen for affective and externalizing disorders as well. The child and parent(s) are interviewed separately and the resulting information combined to determine diagnostic status.

The ADIS-C includes items assessing children's cognitive, behavioural and physiological responses across a range of potentially anxiety-provoking situations (for example, interacting with peers, being separate from a parent). To assess clinical significance, intensity ratings are obtained to indicate the extent to which particular fears interfere with daily functioning. The social phobia section on the ADIS-C asks the child and parent(s) to provide fear, avoidance and interference ratings across 13 social and performance situations. We would advise taking the time to administer the full interview prior to initiating treatment as it can be quite useful in differential diagnosis and in obtaining relevant targets for treatment planning.

Self-report measures

Self-report questionnaires are a common means of obtaining information on anxiety symptoms among children over 8 years of age. The two most widely used (and psychometrically sound) measures of social anxiety in children are the SPAI-C and the SASC-R.

Social Phobia and Anxiety Inventory for Children (SPAI-C)

The SPAI-C (Beidel, Turner and Morris, 1995, 1998) is an empirically derived self-report measure developed to assess the frequency and range of social fears experienced by children and adolescents (8–14 years) in multiple social settings, such as home and school. The SPAI-C consists of 26 items evaluating cognitions (for example, 'what if I make a mistake and look stupid'), behaviour (for example, avoiding social situations), and somatic responses (for example, 'feel sweaty', 'heartbeat fast') across a range of potentially fear-inducing situations (such as school plays or parties). The measure has demonstrated excellent internal consistency and high test-retest reliability across two-week and 10-month intervals.

Beidel, Turner, Hamlin and Morris (2000) provide data on the external and discriminative validity of the SPAI-C among 254 children aged eight to 14 years. Behavioural validation was examined through read-aloud and role-play tasks. Independent observers' ratings of the children's anxiety and effectiveness in the behavioural tasks and the children's ratings of their own distress were significantly associated with SPAI-C scores. More importantly, the measure successfully discriminated not only between children with social phobia and normal controls, but also between children with social phobia and children with other anxiety disorders. This is quite notable given that other anxiety assessment instruments generally have failed to differentiate among children of varying diagnostic groups.

Social Anxiety Scale for Children-Revised (SASC-R)

The SASC-R (La Greca and Stone, 1993) is a 22-item measure of social anxiety that focuses on both subjective experiences and behavioural consequences (such as avoidance or withdrawal) associated with social anxiety. The SASC-R is comprised of three factors: Fear of Negative Evaluation (FNE), and two subscales reflecting Social Avoidance and

Distress (SAD) with new or unfamiliar peers (SAD-New) and more generalized social avoidance and distress (SAD-G). Scores on the SASC-R and
SASC-A (adolescent version) have been associated with peer relationship
difficulties, such as peer rejection and neglect, and low self-esteem (for
example, La Greca and Stone, 1993). The measure has been shown to
have good reliability and validity.

Morris and Masia (1998) examined the association of the SPAI-C and
the SASC-R among 277 grade-school children. A moderate association was
found indicating that the two measures do not assess identical constructs.
One consideration is that the SPAI-C was developed specifically to assess
the construct of social phobia as defined in the DSM-IV whereas the SASC-R
was designed to assess the general construct of social anxiety.

Parent report

In most settings clinicians rely heavily on information provided by parents
(and often to a lesser extent on information provided directly by the
child) when conducting an assessment and formulating a treatment plan.
However, parents should not be considered the gold standard for all
information about their children. Information should be obtained from
pertinent individuals present in situations in which the problem behaviours occur (for example, teachers provide valuable data on the child's
academic performance and interactions with peers). It is common to find
inconsistencies in information provided by the parents, children and
teachers – the bases for such discrepancies should be explored as they
may provide important contextual information for treatment planning.

Behavioural observation

Behavioural observation is an important component of the assessment of
anxiety. Ideally, the child will be observed in the natural setting in which
the anxiety manifests. For example, in the case of social phobia, it may be
particularly useful to observe the child during school recess periods.
However, with consideration and preparation, clinicians may set up situations in and around their offices that provide the proper setting events
in which the relevant behaviours may be displayed (for example, reading
aloud, delivering a speech).

Treatment of social phobia

Behavioural approaches to the treatment of childhood anxiety have gar-
nered strong empirical support. A thorough review of behavioural

treatment strategies is beyond the scope of this chapter (see March, 1995 and Vasey and Dadds, 2001 for more complete coverage). Below, we present an overview of the most common strategies used to decrease anxiety and improve social functioning of anxious children. Comprehensive treatment of childhood anxiety generally involves the use of several of these treatment strategies within an organized framework.

Relaxation

Procedures to promote relaxation may involve training progressive tensing and relaxing of each of the major muscle groups, use of pleasant imagery, or a combination of both. When working with very young children the clinician must be mindful of cognitive limitations. It is generally most effective to present the relaxation skills in the form of a game – such as having the child pretend he is a turtle, stretching out his neck and limbs, and then pulling them back into the shell. Although relaxation training in itself is not considered sufficient for the treatment of social phobia, when practised regularly relaxation may be useful in lowering the child's overall level of arousal.

Exposure

Exposure-based approaches involve exposing the child to the feared situation(s) in a sufficient manner to allow for habituation and extinction of anxious responding. Such approaches include systematic desensitization, graduated exposure and flooding. The empirical literature suggests that exposure is a necessary component of the successful treatment of all anxiety disorders including social phobia.

Systematic desensitization

This approach involves training in relaxation and the development of a fear hierarchy. Once the children are able to learn to put themselves in a relaxed state, items from the fear hierarchy are presented (from least to most anxiety producing). These pairings may be presented through imagery or live in the clinic or natural setting. With repeated pairings, the child is able to remain in the presence of successively more salient fear stimuli for progressively longer periods of time.

Graduated exposure

This approach is similar to systematic desensitization, however relaxation procedures are not implemented during the presentation of the feared stimuli. Most clinicians prefer to use a graduated exposure approach when working with children (rather than sustained flooding), working slowly through a hierarchy, gradually exposing children to more challenging situations for increasing periods of time. No evidence is available to suggest that the inclusion of relaxation training (as in systematic desensitization) is a necessary component or even adds incrementally to the success of exposure in the treatment of social phobia. However, when working with an extremely fearful child the clinician may find that the process of relaxation training helps establish rapport and, as such, may foster more cooperation among children during subsequent exposure work.

Contingency management

Contingency management strategies are used one way or another in the treatment of most childhood disorders. This approach involves stipulation of consequences for performing target behaviours. Contracts are formulated that explicitly state what the child is to do in order to receive certain levels of reinforcement (and often a response cost for failure to meet a given goal). This generally requires training parents and/or teachers to administer consequences, although some adolescents may be able to self-contract. Contingency management is a useful adjunct to exposure-based strategies in that it facilitates completion of homework assignments specified in the treatment plan.

Social skills training

Many anxious children exhibit social skills deficits. This of course is particularly the case with social phobia. These children often avoid social situations in which they may miss out on opportunities to learn age-appropriate skills. Most social skills training (SST) programmes involve coaching, modelling and social problem-solving components. Typical skills taught include joining in activities with peers, establishing and maintaining conversations, developing friendships, and communicating assertiveness.

Multicomponent treatment programmes

Social effectiveness therapy for children

Beidel, Turner and Morris (2000) provide the first published study of a controlled trial of behavioural treatment for social phobia in preadolescent children. Fifty children (ages eight to 12) were randomized to social effectiveness therapy for children (SET-C) or an active treatment for improving test taking and study skills. Each programme lasted 12 weeks and the programmes were equivalent in terms of therapist-participant

contact. Components of the SET-C programme included parent education, social skills training, peer generalization and graduated *in vivo*
exposure. One group social skills training session and one individual
graduated *in vivo* exposure session were held each week. Instruction,
modelling, behaviour rehearsal, feedback and social reinforcement were
used to teach and reinforce appropriate social behaviour. Topic areas
included nonverbal social skills, initiating and maintaining conversations, joining groups of children, friendship establishment and
maintenance, positive assertion and negative assertion. A unique and
essential component of SET-C is the use of formalized peer interaction
experiences to assist in the generalization of social skills to situations
outside the clinic. 'Normal' child volunteers were recruited from the
community to serve as peer facilitators in the peer generalization experiences (developmentally appropriate group recreational activities – for
example, roller skating).

Following treatment, children receiving SET-C demonstrated statistically and clinically significant improvements across various domains (for
example, decreased levels of social and general anxiety, increased social
skill and performance ratings, and more adaptive functioning in daily
situations). These improvements were maintained 6 months post-
treatment. Notably, 67% of children who participated in the SET-C
programme no longer met diagnostic criteria for social phobia after
treatment compared to only 5% of those receiving the active control
treatment.

Cognitive-behavioural group treatment for adolescents

Albano and Barlow (1996) developed a cognitive-behavioural group
treatment for adolescents diagnosed with social phobia. Cognitive-
behavioural group treatment for adolescents (CBGT-A) is a modified
version of CBGT for adults (see Heimberg et al., 1990). More specifically, the adolescent version of CBGT is a 16-week programme that includes
psychoeducation, exposure-based activities (for example structured
snack time, role-plays), and a variety of skill-building techniques (for
example, SST, social problem-solving, cognitive restructuring).

To date, two pilot studies have examined the short-term efficacy of
CBGT-A (Albano et al., 1995; Hayward et al., 2000). Albano et al. reported 3- and 12-month follow-up data for five adolescents; four were
completely diagnosis free at both follow-up evaluations, and the fifth
improved to the point of only expressing subclinical levels of social anxiety. In a subsequent investigation, Hayward and colleagues randomly
assigned 35 female adolescents (M = 15. 8 years) diagnosed with social
phobia to a treatment (n = 12) or control (n = 23) group. Similar to

findings reported by Albano et al., significantly fewer teens participating in CBGT-A met diagnostic criteria for social phobia post-treatment. Notably, however, there were no diagnostic differences between the treated and untreated groups at 1-year follow-up, highlighting the need to investigate further the long-term efficacy of CBGT-A.

Inclusion of parents

Consideration of the family context is essential for effective assessment and treatment of social anxiety. Parents who experience high levels of anxiety are more likely to model strategies of avoidance in an effort to reduce discomfort and inadvertently may contribute to the development of anxiety in children by providing information that may promote heightened states of arousal and hypervigilance.

Dadds and his colleagues have conducted a series of studies demonstrating that parents of anxious children are more likely to model threat interpretations to ambiguous cues and to provide and reinforce avoidant solutions in response to hypothetical social scenarios than parents of aggressive or nonclinical control children (Barrett et al., 1996; Dadds et al., 1996). Given the role of parents in potentially maintaining anxious behaviour, efforts toward incorporating parents in treatment are becoming more common.

Spence, Donovan and Brechman-Toussaint (2000) investigated the effectiveness of an integrated cognitive-behavioural treatment (CBT) package with and without parental involvement for children and adolescents diagnosed with social phobia. Fifty children (aged seven to 14 years) were randomly assigned to CBT, CBT plus parent training, or a waiting-list control condition. The CBT package included SST, relaxation training, positive self-instruction, cognitive challenge and graded exposure. The programme included 12 weekly small group sessions and two booster sessions (3 months and 6 months post-treatment). The parent involvement component was designed to help parents learn to model and reinforce the social skills taught in the CBT package; to ignore avoidance and socially anxious behaviour; to encourage child participation in social activities; and to reinforce homework completion. Parents observed the children's group sessions behind a one-way mirror and participated in a 30-minute weekly training session while their children were practising skills in another room. At a 12-month follow-up 81% of children in the CBT plus parental involvement group no longer met criteria for social phobia (in contrast to 53% of children in the CBT only group). Results of these studies provide preliminary data supporting the incorporation of parents in the treatment of childhood anxiety disorders.

Conclusions

Social phobia tends to be an early onset, chronic and comorbid disorder. Early identification and treatment may help to spare children from a lifetime of distress. The last decade has witnessed advances in our understanding of etiological factors as well as the development of psychometrically sound self-report measures and empirically supported treatments. We strongly encourage clinicians to include parents in the treatment of children presenting with social phobia. Exposure-based approaches appear to be crucial for successful remediation of social fears. Clinicians should give strong consideration to observing children in natural settings (for example, at school) and designing opportunities for exposure in the natural environment. The more elements of the natural environment that may be incorporated the greater likelihood of facilitating skill acquisitions, maintenance and generalization.

References

Albano AM, Barlow DH (1996) Breaking the vicious cycle: cognitive behavioral group treatment for socially anxious youth. In Hibbs ED, Jensen PS (eds) Psychosocial Treatments for Child and Adolescent Disorders: Empirically based Strategies for Clinical Practice. Washington-DC: American Psychological Association, pp. 43–62.

Albano AM, Marten PA, Holt CS, Heimberg RG, Barlow DH (1995) Cognitive-behavioral group treatment for social phobia in adolescents: a preliminary study. Journal of Nervous and Mental Disease 183: 649–56.

American Psychological Association (1994) Diagnostic and Statistical Manual of Mental Disorders. 4 edn. Washington DC: APA.

Barrett PM, Rapee RM, Dadds MR, Ryan SM (1996) Family enhancement of cognitive style in anxious and aggressive children: threat bias and the FEAR effect. Journal of Abnormal Child Psychology 24: 187–203.

Beidel DC, Turner SM, Morris TL (1995) A new inventory to assess child social phobia: The Social Phobia and Anxiety Inventory for Children. Psychological Assessment 7: 73–9.

Beidel DC, Turner SM, Morris TL (1998) Social Phobia and Anxiety Inventory for Children. North Tonawanda, NY: Multi-Health Systems Ltd.

Beidel DC, Turner SM, Morris TL (2000) Behavioral treatment of childhood social phobia. Journal of Consulting and Clinical Psychology 68: 1072–80.

Beidel DC, Turner SM, Hamlin K, Morris TL (2000) The Social Phobia and Anxiety Inventory for Children (SPAI-C): external and discriminant validity. Behavior Therapy 31: 75–87.

Dadds MM, Barrett PM (1996) Family processes in child and adolescent anxiety and depression. Behaviour Change 13: 231–9.

Dadds MM, Barrett PM, Rapee RM (1996) Family process and child anxiety and aggression: an observational analysis. Journal of Abnormal Child Psychology 24: 715–34.

Greco LA, Morris TL (2001) Father-child interactions and child social anxiety: laboratory findings and clinical implications. Manuscript submitted for publication.

Hayward C, Varady S, Albano AM, Thienemann M, Henderson L, Schatzberg AE (2000) Cognitive-behavioral group therapy for social phobia in female adolescents: results of a pilot study. Journal of American Academy of Child and Adolescent Psychiatry 39: 721–6.

Heimberg RG, Dodge CS, Hope DA, Kennedy CR, Zollo LJ (1990) Cognitive behavioral group treatment for social phobia: comparison with a credible placebo control. Cognitive Therapy Resource 14: 1–23.

Hudson JL, Rapee RM (2000) The origins of social phobia. Behavior Modification 24(1):102–29.

Kushner MG, Sher KJ, Beitman BD (1990) The relation between alcohol problems and the anxiety disorders. American Journal of Psychiatry 147: 685–95.

La Greca AM, Stone WL (1993) Social anxiety scale for children-revised: factor structure and concurrent validity. Journal of Clinical Child Psychology 22: 17–27.

March J (ed.) (1995) Anxiety Disorders in Children and Adolescents. New York: Guilford Press.

Masia CL, Morris TL (1998) Parental factors associated with social anxiety: methodological limitations and suggestions for integrated behavioral research. Clinical Psychology Science and Practice 5: 211–28.

Menzies RG, Harris LM (2001) Nonassociative factors in the development of phobias. In Vasey MW, Dadds MR (eds) The Developmental Psychopathology of Anxiety. Oxford: Oxford University Press, pp. 183–204.

Morris TL (2001) Social phobia. In Vasey MW, Dadds MR (eds) The Developmental Psychopathology of Anxiety. Oxford: Oxford University Press, pp. 435–58.

Morris TL, Masia CL (1998) Concurrent validity of the Social Phobia and Anxiety Inventory for Children and the Social Anxiety Scale for Children-Revised. Journal of Clinical Child Psychology 27: 452–8.

Page AC, Andrews G (1996) Do specific anxiety disorders show specific drug problems? Australian and New Zealand Journal of Psychiatry 30: 410–14.

Schneier FR, Johnson J, Hornig CD, Liebowitz MR, Weissman MM (1992) Social phobia: comorbidity and morbidity in an epidemiologic sample. Archives of General Psychiatry 49: 282–8.

Schniering CA, Hudson JL, Rapee RM (2000) Issues in the diagnosis and assessment of anxiety disorders in children and adolescents. Clinical Psychology Review 20: 453–78.

Silverman WK, Albano AM (1996) Anxiety Disorders Interview Schedule for DSM-IV Child Version. San Antonio: Psychological Corporation.

Spaulding S, Morris TL (1997) Direct observation of mother-child interaction: an etiological pathway for social anxiety. In Masia CL, Morris TL (eds) Assessment of Anxiety Disorders in Youth: Innovative Techniques for Comprehensive Assessments of Anxiety Symptomatology. Symposium presented at the annual meeting of the Anxiety Disorders Association of America, New Orleans.

Spence SH, Donovan C, Toussaint-Brechman M (2000) The treatment of childhood social phobia: the effectiveness of a social skills training-based, cognitive-
behavioural intervention, with and without parental involvement. Journal of
Child Psychology and Psychiatry and Allied Disciplines 41: 713–26.

Stein MB, Tancer ME, Gelernter CS, Vittone BJ, Uhde TW (1990) Major depression
in patients with social phobia. American Journal of Psychiatry 147: 637–9.

Stemberger RT, Turner SM, Beidel DC, Calhoun KS (1995) Social phobia: an
analysis of possible developmental factors. Journal of Abnormal Psychology
104: 526–31.

Turner SM, Beidel DC (1989) Social phobia: clinical syndrome, diagnosis, and
comorbidity. Clinical Psychology Review 9: 3–18.

Turner SM, Beidel DC, Dancu CV, Keys DJ (1986) Psychopathology of social phobia and comparison to avoidant personality disorder. Journal of Abnormal
Psychology 95: 389–94.

Vasey MW, Dadds MR (eds) (2001) The Developmental Psychopathology of
Anxiety. Oxford: Oxford University Press.

CHAPTER 3

Effective treatment for conduct disorder

STEPHEN SCOTT

Overview

The term 'conduct disorder' refers to persistent antisocial behaviour in a child or adolescent according to the World Health Organization system of classification (ICD 10). In the US the term is restricted to more severe behaviours seen in adolescents (DSM IV criteria). Here 'conduct disorder' will be used to cover all persistent antisocial behaviours across children and adolescents because the evidence to suggest that the phenomena differ fundamentally according to age group is weak (Scott, 2000). Many clinicians experience a certain sinking feeling when they see children with conduct disorder, believing that there is little that they can do that will be effective. In fact behaviourally based parenting programmes that teach behavioural principles of child management by following a specific curriculum over several weeks are the most widely researched psychological intervention in child and adolescent mental health. This intervention is the single most effective treatment for conduct problems in children, and is solidly based on extensively researched models of parent-child interaction. From early beginnings that focused on techniques for managing child misbehaviour at home, it has spread to include the promotion of child problem-solving skills, improvement of peer relationships, and the enhancement of literacy and school relationships. The content of programmes now goes beyond behaviour to address beliefs, emotions and the wider social context, and to address issues that can impair parents' effectiveness such as poor self-confidence, depression, an unsupportive partner and social isolation. Yet despite being highly effective and well received by parents, parenting programmes are still not routinely available as a treatment in any country in the world.

For younger children there is now a great deal of evidence to show that parenting programmes with a behavioural component are very effective, and so this chapter will concentrate primarily on parenting programmes and their developments. These however include programmes for teachers in schools and programmes to help children acquire social skills and literacy. For teenagers there is far less convincing evidence of robust interventions, as many a worker in a Youth Offending Team is only too aware. However, three approaches have been shown to reduce offending somewhat, namely functional family therapy, multi-systemic therapy and treatment foster care, each of which will be discussed.

Summary of research since 1992

Distinction of behaviourally based parenting programmes from other approaches

Because there are now so many ways of working with parents, it is worthwhile defining them before considering the evidence. Some characteristics of behaviourally based parenting programmes are:

Content

- Structured sequence of topics, introduced in set order over eight to 12 weeks;
- subjects include play, praise, incentives, setting limits and discipline;
- emphasis on promoting sociable, self-reliant child behaviour and calm parenting;
- constant reference to parents' own experience and predicament;
- theoretical basis informed by extensive empirical research and made explicit;
- detailed manual available to enable replicability.

Delivery

- Collaborative approach acknowledging parents' feelings and beliefs;
- difficulties normalized, humour and fun encouraged;
- parents supported to practise new approaches during session and through homework;
- parent and child seen together in individual family work; just parents in some group programmes;
- crèche, good quality refreshments and transport provided if necessary;
- therapists supervised regularly to ensure adherence and to develop skills.

These programmes differ from other psychological interventions in important ways. A *psychoeducational* approach is used by many clinicians, whereby parents are informed about the nature of their child's difficulties and advised on management but are not expected to practise specific skills. *Individual behavioural work* is used by many clinicians for a wide range of presenting conditions (for example, see Herbert, 1987). It has the advantage of flexibility so that content, pace and duration can be tailored to the specific needs of a family. However, it may not match the range and depth of coverage of techniques found in a systematic programme. *Counselling* of a Rogerian type (Rogers, 1961) is widely used in non-medical settings, with an emphasis on non-judgemental positive regard and respect for the parent. Listening well to parents helps engagement and is popular but unless there are other elements such as helping them to find new solutions to their difficulties, as for example in the Parent Adviser Model (Davis and Spurr, 1998) the gain for child mental health may be little. *Family therapy* shares with parent training an interactional view of the maintenance of child behaviour problems. Exploration of families' beliefs and interrelationships may lead them to greater understanding of their predicament. Skills are not, as a rule imparted, the theoretical model is not usually made explicit to the family and has less research backing and there are fewer evaluations (Chamberlain and Rosicky, 1995). *Humanistic parenting programmes* often focus on the improvement of parent-child relationships, particularly how to talk and communicate with a child (see review by Smith, 1996). A strength of these programmes is that they are often delivered by voluntary sector organizations in community settings which can make them more accessible and acceptable than clinic services (Cunningham et al., 1995). A disadvantage is that sometimes staff are less well trained and the programmes have seldom been rigorously evaluated using child outcomes.

Research basis on the causes of conduct disorder relevant for planning rational treatment

Longitudinal course, nature and nurture

Studies of the natural history of serious antisocial behaviour used to suggest that it peaks in late teenage or young adulthood, when most offending occurs. However, as Tremblay (2000) has pointed out, the age when physical aggression is maximal is around 22 months (and not 22 years!). From this perspective, it may be pertinent to ask not what causes antisocial behaviour to develop, but rather, why did the usual peak at around 2 years of age not reduce? What are the usual mechanisms that cause antisocial behaviour to diminish after this age? They may turn out to be the same mix of parent and child factors already identified, but studies are needed to see whether antisocial schoolchildren were more disruptive than others before the age of two, or only after.

Better characterization of antisocial behaviour has revealed at least two reliable subtypes. In one, antisocial behaviour is manifest early, typically by 3 years of age, carries on throughout life ('early onset lifetime persistent' pattern) (Moffitt, 1993), and is associated with hyperactivity, impulsiveness, irritability and emotional problems, and lower IQ. In the other, antisocial behaviour begins in adolescence often as part of peer group rebelliousness, and reduces in adulthood ('adolescence-limited' type). The early-onset pattern appears to have a substantially higher heritability than the adolescence-limited type, where environmental influences, especially shared ones, are more prominent. More complex typologies of antisocial behaviour usually include a type with multiple comorbid psychopathology and neuropsychological deficits, where the heritability can be as high as 96% (Silberg et al., 1996). Some might conclude that changing the parental environment will have little effect where genetic influence is high.

This is erroneous for several reasons. Firstly, the cause of a problem and solutions to ameliorate it may operate through quite different mechanisms – thus phenylketonuria is a genetically caused condition but responds to environmental manipulation, namely a phenylalanine low diet. Secondly, genetic studies measure the variation in environment occurring naturally in the study population, which may not be very great for most members, whereas intervention often allows the level to be experimentally changed to a greater extent. Thus early-onset type antisocial behaviour might not vary much across the range of environments found in most families, but if very different environments are applied (as say in treatment foster-care or an in-patient unit) it may change substantially. Thirdly, there is now good evidence of an interaction between child predisposition to antisocial behaviour and rearing environment. Infants with more negative temperaments (assessed independently from their parents) are more susceptible to poor parenting as shown by the development of more externalizing problems by the age of three than would be predicted from just adding the effects of temperament and parenting (Belsky et al., 1998). Likewise adoption studies suggest that children with higher genetic risk (as indexed by parental criminality, antisocial personality or substance misuse) are far more likely to develop criminal behaviour in families with difficulties (for example, criminal, psychiatric or legal problems) than predicted by just adding the genetic and rearing risks (Cadoret et al., 1995; Bohman, 1996). The implication for parent training is that rather than being *less* effective for children with severe types of antisocial behaviour with high genetic liability, it may be *more* effective for them.

Taylor et al. (1996) conducted a community study of 7-year-old children with hyperactivity who were followed up aged 17. Subsequent analyses have shown that the 7-year-old hyperactive children whose parents were highly critical had developed far higher levels of conduct problems by 17 than those whose parents were not unduly critical. This suggests that children with disruptive behaviour that has a substantial inherited component can nonetheless be parented in a way that makes a considerable difference to their psychosocial outcome.

Evidence that parenting practices affect child behaviour

A note of caution before examining the association between child-rearing styles and child behaviour! Some pundits assert confidently the 'right' and 'wrong' ways to bring up children. However, judging by the changes in the last 100 years, what we assert today may be dramatically overturned in future. For example in Victorian Britain it was stated that children should be 'seen and not heard' and a popular motto was 'spare the rod and spoil the child', whereas today emphasis is on listening to children and there is pressure to make any physical punishment illegal. Parenting beliefs and practices vary over time and across cultures and research findings need to be interpreted bearing this in mind. For example, the work of Deater-Deckard and colleagues (1996) suggests that while for white Americans not smacking children is associated with the lowest rates of conduct problems, in African Americans not smacking is associated with an *increase* in antisocial behaviour.

Nonetheless, a strong association has repeatedly been found between particular styles of parenting and child antisocial behaviour. Harsh, inconsistent discipline, high criticism, rejection and neglect are implicated for children at all ages with lack of supervision becoming especially important as the young person spends more time out of the home (Patterson et al., 1992). Longitudinal studies indicate that these factors are predictive of later antisocial behaviour even after allowing for the initial level of aggression (Patterson et al., 1992), suggesting a possible causal role, although other explanations are possible. The role of positive parenting practices has more recently been shown to make an independent contribution, with warmth, involvement in children's activities, praise and encouragement being associated with lower levels of antisocial behaviour (Pettit et al., 1997). Once a moderate level of positive parenting practice is present, however, it appears to be the presence of negative parenting that seems most influential.

Factors that impede effective parenting

Not all parents start with the same level of skills for parenting, and not all are able to change the same amount. A number of risk factors are relevant, and the question arises whether outcome is better if they are addressed through adding specific components to parenting programmes.

Generalized learning disability

There is no intrinsic reason why people with IQs under 70 should parent poorly, although as IQ gets lower, especially below 60, general impairment of social functioning becomes more and more evident (Scott, 1994). Empirical evidence is patchy, but children deemed by local authorities to be at risk from parental abuse or neglect are more likely to have parents of lower IQ (Dowdney and Skuse, 1993). Parental IQ has not been studied as a predictor of outcome in parent training, though as with any new learning task, it is likely to have a moderating effect.

Parental mental disorder

Any mental disorder of moderate or severe degree may interfere with parenting ability. However harm does not appear to be done through the parent having a mental disorder unless it leads to poorer care for the child (Quinton and Rutter, 1988). Conversely, getting the disorder better will not necessarily lead to a great improvement in parenting skills, unless they were at a good enough level previously. Maternal depression leads to less sensitive responding and less cognitive stimulation for the child (Murray and Cooper, 1997), but unless the maternal deprivation is severe then this is not a contra-indication to parent training. Indeed, some studies have shown significant improvement in depression levels compared with controls after parent training (Sanders and McFarland, 2000). One mechanism may be the increased sense of self-efficacy and reduced helplessness about child management the parents report after programmes (Sanders, Markie-Dadds, Tully and Bor, 2000).

Interparental discord

Cross-sectional studies have found that interparental discord adds to the prediction of child antisocial behaviour, over and above parenting practices (Webster-Stratton and Hammond, 1999). Whilst genetic transmission of aggressiveness may well be a component, the child is also likely to learn antisocial habits of conflict resolution and see fewer examples of prosocial skills and negotiation. Therefore gains from a parenting programme may be limited if the child is still exposed to interparental conflict. Some programmes have a specific component to address interparental relationships, as reviewed below.

Poor living conditions

In the UK there is a gradient of increasing prevalence of child disorders with lower social class as defined by occupation of chief breadwinner in the household (Meltzer et al., 2000). This gradient is especially marked for conduct problems. The extent to which this has a direct effect on children, or is a marker for other mechanisms is not fully resolved. In some studies, once quality of parenting is allowed for, poor living conditions are not associated with further levels of disorder (reviewed in Rutter et al., 1998). However, such an analysis does not allow for the possibility that poor conditions *lead to* poorer parenting. It is not difficult to imagine that living in adverse housing conditions with few facilities and no money to buy practical support such as child minding could disrupt calm and constructive parenting, especially for, say, a lone parent with a mental heath problem. Studies indicate that child psychopathology increases with psychosocial adversity (Rutter, 1995), and Patterson et al. (1992) showed a strong association between deprivation and poor parenting. Improving living conditions is usually beyond parenting programmes, although some offer practical support to help parents engage with housing and benefits agencies.

Social isolation

Social isolation is associated with poorer parenting and with a worse response to parent training (Dumas and Wahler, 1983). Amongst what Wahler termed 'insular mothers', most adult contacts were with official agencies and their own mothers who were critical and negative. On days when this occurred, the mothers' harsh and inconsistent parenting of the children rose severalfold. Moreover whilst they did as well as non-insular mothers in the immediate outcome of parent training, at follow-up nearly all the gains had been lost. Attempts have been made to add social support systems to parent training programmes (Dadds and McHugh, 1992), and to address their despondent cognitions and narratives about themselves (Wahler et al., 1993), as discussed below.

Parents who experienced poor parenting as children themselves

Many neglectful or abusing parents experienced little good care themselves, so have little experience to draw upon with their own children. However, this does not mean that they inevitably are unable to become good enough parents. Quinton and Rutter (1988) studied girls who had been brought up in children's homes who subsequently became mothers. Their own experience of parenting had been poor in two ways, first the reason they were in the homes was their parents' inability to care for them adequately; second, at the time children's homes were run on very

institutional lines without a great deal of close personal contact between
staff and children, and a high turnover of staff that made the development
of long-term trusting relationships with them unlikely. Despite this and
probable associated genetic risk factors, half the women with this background were parenting satisfactorily as judged by interview and direct
observation measures. Current attachment research using the Adult
Attachment Interview is linking parents' own attachment status to the
quality of their upbringing (Main 1996). There do not appear to be studies using parents' own upbringing (as opposed to parents' attachment
status) as a predictor of intervention outcome.

Particular beliefs about a child

So far, parenting has been discussed as a general ability. However, the
quality of relationship between the same parent and different children in
the family varies. Adoption studies show that children who were scapegoated in comparison to their siblings in their family of origin do
especially badly in terms of outcomes (Rushton et al., 2000). Whilst some
of this may be due to inherent characteristics of the child, which led them
to become criticized or scapegoated, nonetheless it is likely that the negative environment further added to their difficulties, particularly in light
of the evidence of the interaction between child vulnerability and harsh
parenting described above. In clinical practice it is common to uncover
resentments around what the child represents – for example, an antisocial
boy who is seen by his mother to resemble his father whom she hates
since he beat her. The implication for intervention is that in addition to
imparting skills, beliefs about the child need to be explored and attempts
made to help the parent view the child more positively.

Child cognitive processes

The behaviourist approach is mainly concerned with the external events
impinging on an individual, and takes less account of how they may be
thinking or feeling. Indeed a central tenet is the lack of a need for intro-
spection or understanding of what is in the 'black box' inside an organism
(Skinner, 1953). This has made it especially useful for dealing with animals and babies but ignores the fundamentally human phenomena of
language and thought. In contrast, since the 1970s, particular cognitive
styles have been shown to be characteristic of children and young people
with disorders such as depression and conduct problems. In interpersonal encounters, the latter are more likely to perceive the intentions of
others as hostile, generate fewer solutions to conflicts, and to believe an
aggressive solution will be more effective (Dodge and Schwartz, 1997).

Individual cognitive and problem-solving programmes have been developed (Lochman and Wells, 1996), and can be used with parent training programmes, as discussed below.

Less work has been done mapping the cognitive processes of parents with disruptive children. Unsurprisingly, parents of antisocial children have more negative beliefs about them and attribute more negative intentions to them; rates of depression amongst mothers are high (Sanders and McFarland, 2000). Some parent training programmes incorporate techniques from cognitive therapy. Thus parents may be encouraged to monitor their own 'self-talk' or 'inner voice' and to check on hopeless and defeatist cognitions, and be helped to find ways of replacing these with more positive statements that facilitate coping (Webster-Stratton and Hancock, 1998).

However, parents of children with behaviour problems may not just think differently, they may perceive events differently too. Experiments showing videotapes found that these parents not only failed to see many episodes of positive child behaviour, but surprisingly also saw fewer episodes of *negative* child behaviour. This suggests that rather than just being biased towards seeing child behaviour in a bad light, these parents are also less attuned to perceiving *any* child behaviour accurately, and hold global, non-specific negative feelings towards their children (Wahler and Dumas, 1989). The implication for parent training may be that parents need to be helped to perceive their children's behaviour more accurately and become more attuned to nuances of their children's mental state, rather than just being offered management skills. Parent training programmes that use videotaped sequences of parent-child interaction incorporate this.

The influence of the child's peers and academic attainments

Longitudinal studies have shown that independent of the initial level of antisocial behaviour and parenting quality, deviant peer associations (Fergusson et al., 1999; Poulin et al., 1999) and lower IQ and academic underachievement further influence antisocial behaviour (Patterson et al., 1992; Hinshaw, 1992; Fergusson and Lynskey, 1997; Rutter et al., 1998). While some programmes aimed at antisocial outcomes have added on components to address these issues, for example, by promotion of prosocial peer affiliation (Conduct Problems Prevention Research Group, 1992; Dishion and Andrews, 1995) and special tuition (Conduct Problems Prevention Research Group, 1992; Barkley et al., 2000), parents can also have some influence on these processes, which could be incorporated into parenting programmes. This would envisage a model of parenting that goes beyond a good interactional style and prudent management

within the home to playing a role in helping the child cope with the outside world. This may include programme elements to enable the parent
to negotiate with school (Webster-Stratton and Hancock, 1998), to coach
better peer relationships through 'play dates' (Frankel et al., 1997) or to
raise child literacy through training parents to use specific reading techniques with their child (Scott and Sylva, 2002). At a broader level, parents
can help select the environment to which the child is exposed, by encouraging certain friendships to flourish and discouraging others, by choosing
an appropriate school for the child's needs, and by helping learning
through providing a facilitative home environment. These aspects of parenting are seldom parts of parent training programmes, although they
feature in some 'self-help' books on parenting.

Research evidence on treatment programmes

Methodological considerations

Several general issues are relevant before discussing particular trials
(Kazdin, 2001). Firstly, different measurement methods and informants
will give different effect sizes (Scott, 2001). As a rule, teacher-rated questionnaire ratings of child antisocial behaviour are more predictive of later
antisocial behaviour than those that are parent rated, and methods that
use objective, standardized criteria, such as semi-structured interviews or
direct observation, are more predictive than questionnaires (Bank et al.,
1993).

Secondly, statistical significance does not equate to clinical significance.
The latter can be assessed from the original dimensional measure of psychopathology statistically in terms of the *effect size* (the mean change in
the treated group minus the change in the control group, divided by the
pooled pretreatment standard deviation; according to Cohen's (1988)
guidelines that are widely accepted, an effect size of 0.2 standard deviations is small, one of 0.5 standard deviations moderate, and one of 0.8
standard deviations is large); or by the proportion of the groups that
improve by more than 30% (Webster-Stratton et al., 1989), or by more
complex formulae that compare the change in the treated sample with
general population means (Jacobson and Truax, 1991). Clinically significant change can also be assessed in terms of the proportion of the sample
that no longer meets criteria for a diagnosis, or by using a measure that
assesses the impact of the problem on social functioning or quality of life
(Gowers et al., 2000). Clinical significance has only relatively recently
become reported in studies, but for most described below it was possible
to calculate an effect size.

Thirdly, there is usually substantial attrition in trials with families of conduct problem children. Two reporting strategies artificially inflate effectiveness, namely only reporting those who attend the majority of treatment sessions, and dropping those who are lost to assessment after entering the trial. The former is becoming less common, but the latter is still widespread. It should be mandatory at least to publish both the results for all those on whom data was collected, and a second analysis including those on whom post-treatment data are missing but adjustments made, for example assuming no change since the last data point. Otherwise it is impossible to estimate how much change one can expect if a treatment modality is introduced to a service.

Fourthly, the sample used is crucial. Volunteers who respond to advertising campaigns are more likely to be motivated, to have space to think about and implement programmes, and be better off financially. Those referred to specialist parenting clinics may also have been deemed suitable by the referrer, or be self-referred. Some university-based trials exclude children with significant comorbidity, thus dropping those who are likely to do worst. This is in contrast to those referred to generic mental health clinics, who may be more multiply disadvantaged and have more severe and comorbid symptoms (Woodward et al., 1997). Even these clinics may miss the most disadvantaged. This is particularly important now that services are starting to target whole populations.

Lastly, many of the cited trials have taken place in university clinics run by highly motivated originators of programmes who supervise carefully chosen therapists intensively in demonstration projects. In the meta-analysis of child psychotherapy trials by Weisz et al. (1995) those trials conducted in university clinics had a large mean effect-size of 0.7 standard deviations, whereas all the clinic-based studies reviewed since 1950 did not have any significant effects. It might be concluded 'the good news is that child psychotherapies work, but the bad news is that they don't work in real life'. Therefore to be considered robust, findings need to be replicated in ordinary clinical settings by therapists who are part of the routine service and independent of the originator of the programme (Kendall, 1998) as occurred for example in the replication of the Webster-Stratton programme by Scott, Spender, Doolan, Jacobs and Aspland (2001).

Outcome studies

Individual parent training programmes

For the programmes given individually, several well-designed studies showed substantial changes in observed parent practices and in reported and observed child oppositional behaviour, in comparison to untreated controls (Patterson et al., 1982; Forehand et al., 1980; Eyberg and Robinson, 1982; Webster-Stratton, 1984; Sanders, Markie-Dadds, Tully and Bor, 2000). Improvements have typically been of the order of 0.5 to 0.6 standard deviations on direct observation measures, and 0.6 to 0.9 standard deviations on parent report measures. The gains have been substantially maintained at follow-up a year later (Patterson, 1974; Kazdin et al., 1992; Webster-Stratton et al., 1989) and, over the longer term, Forehand and Long (1988) reported follow-ups of 4 to 10 years.

Group parent training programmes

For group programmes, again there are several good studies. The meta-analysis by Serketich and Dumas (1996) calculated a mean effect size of 0.86 standard deviations for child behaviour change; that by Hoag and Burlingame (1997) 0.69 standard deviations. The systematic review by Barlow (1999) found 255 studies of group parent training, but only 16 were of a high standard methodologically. In these, the mean effect size of child behaviour change compared to waiting-list controls rated by *parents* ranged from 0.4 standard deviations to 1.0 standard deviation. *Direct observation* showed an effect size of 0.4 to 0.6 standard deviations, somewhat smaller than parent report results. Surprisingly, none of these studies used semi-structured interviews or structured ones. Follow-up at 1 to 3 years has shown that significant gains remain, with rather little loss in most programmes. Drop-out rates were typically in the range of 10% to 20%, lower than the 30% plus or so found in usual clinical practice. Weisz et al. (1995) have pointed out the lack of effectiveness studies in 'real life' clinics, but the UK multicentre trial by Scott, Spender, Doolan, Jacobs and Aspland (2001) found an effect size of 1.06 standard deviations for clinically referred cases using regular clinic staff to administer the intervention.

Self-administered programmes

Sending parents a book and then offering regular telephone advice led to reasonable gains on parent questionnaires and direct observation in two small studies by Sutton (1992, 1995). In a larger study Webster-Stratton (1984) invited parents to come into the clinic regularly and follow the self-administered version of her videotape series with clinicians on hand to offer help if requested. Gains of around 1.0 standard deviation compared to waiting-list controls were found on parent report, which was as great a gain as in the clinician led comparison group. However, on direct observation there was no change, whereas the clinician led group format fared 0.4 standard deviations better than controls.

Multi-level programmes

Sanders and colleagues in Brisbane, Australia (Sanders, 1999) have developed a comprehensive set of ways of delivering their positive parenting programme (Triple P). Level 1 comprises a universal strategy of providing an entire population with information through television advertisements and entertaining TV programmes specifically made to reinforce good parenting practice, with the opportunity to call for a tip sheet. Level 2 comprises brief (one or two 20-minute consultations) with a primary healthcare worker who has three days training, reinforced for the parent with four videotapes on parenting and tipsheets. Level 3 is similar but offers more consultations in primary care. Level 4 offers a fuller 10-week traditional parenting programme, which can be delivered as self-administered, individualized at clinic, or group. The self-administered programme comprises a book of instruction and a workbook of exercises, which can be supplemented by telephone calls. Level 5, enhanced, is a further 10-week programme added on to the individually administered clinic programme that comprises addressing in an individualized way parental factors that get in the way of effective parenting, and addresses marital communication, mood management and stress coping skills. It is given to those who have not progressed sufficiently with lower levels of intervention, and includes home visits.

Evaluation of the different ways of delivering the standard level 4 programme has been carried out in a trial with 305 3-year-olds (Sanders, Markie-Dadds, Tully and Bor, 2000). Participants were volunteers screened to meet criteria that included having an elevated score on the Eyberg Child Behaviour Inventory and at least one index of family adversity; parents were predominantly lower class, but mostly not highly disadvantaged. They were allocated to receive the standard basic clinician administered 10-week programme, self-administered, or an abbreviated version of the enhanced programme. The results showed that on direct observation, only the enhanced condition reduced antisocial behaviour (effect size (es) 0.5 sd) compared to waiting-list controls. However, on the Eyberg questionnaire all treatment conditions produced an improvement, with a trend towards a larger effect in the enhanced (enhanced 1.0 standard deviation, basic 0.7 standard deviations, self-administered 0.5 standard deviations). However, the self-administered programme showed improvements on only two of five child behaviour measures. One-year follow-up showed further improvements in all three treatment groups, but there were no controls at this stage. A possible problem when interpreting this study was the differential attrition rates in getting post-intervention data collection between treatment and control groups. The attrition rates were enhanced 40%, basic 29%, self-administered 31%, but controls 8%. Careful analysis was carried out that showed attrition to be more likely in children with more severe behaviour problems, and mothers who were more depressed and had worse relationships with their partners. These are some of the risk factors associated with less change. The difference in attrition rates of 32% between the reportedly most effective intervention (enhanced) and the controls could be disguising a much smaller treatment effect, if the missing 32% changed less than those followed up.

Sanders, Montgomery and Brechman-Toussaint (2000) evaluated an innovative 13 episode television series (*Families*) that included elements of the Triple P programme interwoven into an 'infotainment'. The series had been broadcast to millions in New Zealand. In this study however, volunteers with children aged two to eight in Australia were allocated to watch the programmes on video at home, or were allocated to a waiting list. Parents were reasonably advantaged. Evaluation was by questionnaire only, and showed an effect size of 0.4 to 0.5 standard deviations in anti-social behaviour, increased sense of parenting competence, and no loss at 6-month follow-up. Attrition was not reported.

In conclusion, there is reasonable evidence that self-administered programmes may help some families. Further research is needed to see whether more disadvantaged families could benefit. This mode of delivery has the potential to be a cost-effective way of disseminating parent training widely.

Humanistic programmes

There have been a number of methodologically acceptable studies of humanistic programmes, although they have tended to use volunteer samples with better motivated parents and less severe child problems than in clinical samples. Sheeber and Johnson (1994) studied 3 to 5-year-olds with 'difficult temperaments' and compared a parenting group based on understanding of child characteristics with waiting-list controls and found no difference in child CBCL scores on externalizing behaviour, although an effect size of 0.6 on internalizing problems. Freeman (1975) compared an Adlerian group with a 'traditional' mothers' discussion group and a no-treatment control and found that both treatment groups displayed significant reductions in total CBCL scores but were not significantly different. These studies used volunteer samples with moderate levels of child difficulty; none used interviews or direct observation to evaluate outcome.

Direct comparison of behaviourally based with humanistic programmes

In head-to-head comparisons of humanistic versus behavioural programmes, findings are mixed. Pinsker and Geoffrey (1981) compared a behavioural group with Parent Effectiveness Training (PET), a humanistic approach. They found that on parent report the behavioural group showed a significant reduction in child problem behaviour whereas PET and controls did not, but on direct observation, both treatment groups did better than controls. Bernal et al. (1980) compared a client-centred group with behavioural management and waiting-list controls and found on parent report the behavioural group did better than the other two, but on direct observation no group changed. Frasier and Matthes (1975) compared behavioural with Adlerian parenting groups and had a no treatment control; on parent report, none of the groups changed significantly. Again, all these studies used volunteer samples. In contrast, Nicol et al. (1988) studied 38 families referred by local social services for active physical abuse and allocated them to individual play therapy for the child plus support from social worker for the mother (a traditional child guidance approach), or home-based work that offered elements of parent training plus parent support through 'casework'.

Drop-out was high in both groups, at 45%, but the intervention with parent training led to a greater reduction in parental coerciveness and aversive behaviour towards their children, measured using direct observation. Overall, the evidence for humanistic programmes is weak.

Generalization to home, siblings and school

Several studies used direct observation to show generalization of parent training from clinic to home (for example, Peed et al., 1977; Forehand and McMahon, 1981) confirming parental reports of improved behaviour. Moreover, studies suggest that parents use the newly learned parenting behaviours with other children in the family, as well as the index child (Humphries et al., 1978; Eyberg and Robinson, 1982).

Studies looking for transfer of improved behaviour to the school setting have been inconsistent. For example, Horn et al. (1987), Cox and Matthews (1977), Webster-Stratton et al. (1988) and McNeil et al. (1991) all found reduced antisocial behaviour in the school setting following parent training, whereas Forehand et al. (1979), Kazdin et al. (1992), Webster-Stratton et al. (1989), and Webster-Stratton and Hammond (1997), Webster-Stratton and Hancock (1998) and Taylor et al. (1998) found no change. This is important because if only questionnaires are used, teacher reports predict later antisocial behaviour better than parent ones (Bank et al., 1993). Therefore in the development of programmes to prevent antisocial behaviour, school-based elements are now often included (Conduct Problems Prevention Research Group, 1999; Barkley et al., 2000).

Adding behavioural components to increase parental adherence

Studies suggest that adding explicit teaching of social learning principles to a programme (McMahon et al., 1981), or adding explicit monitoring of the achievement of parenting goals followed by self-reward (Wells et al., 1980) improves the change in parental behaviour and child compliance on direct observation.

Programmes that address factors interfering with effective parenting

General approaches

Wahler and colleagues (1993) developed an adjunctive treatment called 'synthesis training' for isolated mothers. Parents are guided to identify and label their reactions to stressful events, understand their own reactions and feelings and the way they explain events to themselves, and change the way they treat their children accordingly. Studies suggest that this is an effective treatment and prevents drop-off in gains seen in insular mothers offered standard programmes. Blechman (1998) included communication skills and stepwise problem-solving to help identify and resolve problems arising from broad extrafamilial factors that interfere with parenting; Pfiffner et al. (1990) found a similar intervention enhanced the maintenance of gains with moderately aggressive children.

Multisystemic therapy (MST) was developed by Henggeler and colleagues (1998). It is a home-based clinical intervention that is intensive (only three or four clients per therapist), relatively short (3 months) and highly supervised. Therapy is given according to the 'system' that is assessed as showing weaknesses, for example, parent-child, marital, peer relationship, or social. The precise form of intervention may vary, but the approach incorporates many elements of structural family therapy. Brunk et al. (1987) compared MST with group parent training for abusive and neglectful families. Both interventions were associated with improvements in parental psychiatric symptoms, overall stress and identified problems. Those receiving MST showed more improvement on observed parent-child interactions, whereas those receiving parent training showed more reduction in social problems, which the authors attributed to the group format. The parent training offered was described by the authors as 'mechanistic' and had no role-play element, sticking strictly to parental management. Therefore it would seem useful to take the best elements of both approaches, and offer MST with a major parent training component.

Maternal depression

Sanders and McFarland (2000) took 47 families with a depressed mother and a child with conduct disorder. They were allocated to either 12 sessions of individual standard behavioural parent training, or the same intervention but including cognitive therapy elements for depression. Both interventions reduced maternal depression and improved child behaviour, but the effects on maternal depression were stronger for the cognitive condition, with 72% as opposed to 35% moving into the nonclinical range; there was no difference in child behaviour improvement.

Partner discord

Griest et al. (1982) randomly assigned 17 families to basic parent training or basic plus an adjunctive treatment that included work on personal and marital adjustment and extrafamilial relationships. Greater changes were seen for the adjunctive treatment in child compliance and deviant behaviour, and for several specific parental behaviours. In an elegantly designed study, Dadds et al. (1987) compared the addition of partner communication and support to basic individual parent training in 12 maritally discordant families and 12 non-discordant families, all of whom had conduct problem children. Each condition received the same amount of therapist contact. The adjunctive treatment led to substantially enhanced gains at 6-month follow-up in the maritally discordant families but not in the non-discordant families. This suggests that intervention should be tailored to the presenting problem, and that a 'one-size fits all' preventive approach may not be efficient.

Adult social skills

Webster-Stratton noted that parents' own difficulties in their partner relationship was one of the most potent predictors of failure to improve parenting, so devised her 'advanced' programme to address adult relationship skills (Webster-Stratton, 1994). She studied the outcome of her basic 12-week programme in comparison to the basic plus the advanced 14-week programme. Whilst observed partner communication and child generated solutions to hypothetical social problems improved more in the advanced group, directly observed parenting behaviour and all measures of behaviour improved equally in both groups.

Puckering et al. (1994) found a group intervention that provided mother support improved self-esteem, depression and social isolation, but not parenting style (Cox et al., 1990). They therefore developed an additional parenting skills component and named the programme Mellow Parenting. It was specifically devised to help highly disadvantaged mothers. The programme runs for a whole day a week over 16 weeks, and has three components. In the morning, a psychotherapeutic group is run for the mothers on their own that addresses past and current relationships and present feelings and encourages members to reflect on how these link to being a parent. At lunch, mothers and children eat together, then the mothers are asked to become involved with their children in an activity such as cooking or arts and crafts, and may be helped by staff. In the afternoon, mothers review videotapes of themselves with their children in everyday situations at home and work on specific parenting skills. Outcome using direct observation and questionnaires showed large improvements in reducing negative affect, promoting child autonomy and increasing maternal sensitivity (Puckering et al., 1994); 83% of the families on the local Child Protection Register were subsequently deregistered because their children were no longer judged to be at risk of abuse.

Social isolation

Dadds and McHugh (1992) offered a group parent management training programme to 22 lone parents recruited as volunteers but with substantial child behaviour problems. One group received a basic eight-week programme, called Child Management Training. The other group received the same eight-week management training course, but were asked to recruit an *ally* who was present at the first meeting, whose role was to

• be available to offer support when needed;
• communicate regularly with the parent and listen to him or her;
• be involved in problem-solving and solution implementation.

This arm of the trial was named child management training plus ally support training. The results showed that parents in the combined condition did indeed use their allies to offer support, listen to them and help in problem-solving. However, although both groups made large improvements in child behaviour, the gains of the ally support group were no greater. This may be because although the parents carried out the support procedures, measures of *perceived* support did not increase. Whichever treatment was received, those parents who perceived they received substantial support from friends showed considerably greater improvement in child outcome. This confirms the importance of support as a predictor, but suggests it is not easy to increase substantially in brief programmes. Equally, lack of support may well also be an indicator of less ability to create and maintain good relationships of all kinds.

Adding other interventions

Child social skills training

There are several reasons to compare child social skills training with parent training. Firstly, as the referred patients are children, trying to alter their behaviour directly is logical. Secondly, it has shown to be reliably effective in reducing antisocial behaviour in adolescents (Lochman et al., 2000), although initial trials showed it to be less effective with younger children, say under six (Denham and Almeida, 1987; Lochman et al., 1993). Thirdly, some parents are either unable to change their parenting style, or are unwilling to attend for sessions, yet may be prepared to put their children forward for treatment because they believe something is 'wrong' with them. Fourthly, although parent training improves children's relationships with their parents, it does not reliability improve their behaviour at school, nor with their peers.

Kazdin et al. (1987) compared a programme of combined individual parent management training plus individual child problem-solving skills training versus general discussion sessions of comparable duration in a sample of 40 7 to 12-year-olds who were psychiatric inpatients because of antisocial behaviour. Results showed good improvements in the combined treatment group over controls not only on parent report (es 1.5 standard deviations) but also on teacher report (es 1.0 standard deviation). No direct observations were made. There was no significant loss of effectiveness at one-year follow-up. A subsequent paper (Kazdin et al., 1992) teased out the effectiveness of each component by comparing parent training alone, child social skills training alone, and both combined. All groups improved substantially, with improvements seen not only by parents at home, but also by teachers at school and self-reported offending by the young people. However, the combined treatment had greater effectiveness on nearly all measures, notably 0.5 to 1.1 standard deviations greater effect than parent training alone on antisocial behaviour.

Webster-Stratton and Hammond (1997) used a group format with video-tapes to compare parent training only with child training only, both parent training plus child training, and a waiting-list control group: 97 children aged 4 to 8 years specifically referred to a parenting clinic were studied with a thorough set of measures including direct observation at home, and observation of interaction with a friend. The intervention was relatively long (22 weekly sessions of two hours) and attendance was excellent, with all cases attending at least half the sessions and most attending nearly all. There were no drop-outs. There were several important findings. Firstly, on parent questionnaire, children in all three intervention conditions did considerably better than waiting-list controls who did not improve significantly. The fact that *child training alone* led to improvements in child behaviour is important practically because there will always be some parents who are unable or unwilling to attend for intervention. Secondly, all interventions had an effect in reducing observed directive parenting behaviour. From a theoretical standpoint, it is interesting that child training led to less coercive parenting behaviour, confirming the hypothesis that for children with clinically significant antisocial behaviour (as for non-clinical children) child as well as parent factors are involved in driving parenting style; it shows that the coercive cycle of negative parenting and child defiance can be interrupted from either end. Thirdly, parent training led to greater changes in parent-reported child behaviour problems than child training, whereas child training led to better improvements in the ratio of positive to negative strategies used by children when interacting with a friend on direct observation, and on laboratory tests of social problem-solving. Fourthly, the combined parent-plus-child intervention led to similar effect sizes as one would predict from either intervention alone in the domain in which they were most effective, but did not act synergistically. Thus parent-rated child behaviour was no more improved in the combined condition than for child training alone, and observed child-peer behaviour was no more improved in the combined condition than with parent training alone. The exception was observed antisocial behaviour in the home at one-year follow-up, where the combined condition had a greater effect than either alone. Unfortunately although in all intervention conditions there was a good effect compared to controls for observed reduction in child behaviour at home (es 0.7 to 0.8, total deviant behaviour reduced to half original levels whereas controls did not change), the variance was large (standard deviations greater than means in all cases) so none was significant.

Fifthly, all gains were maintained at one-year follow-up, suggesting that the reduction in antisocial behaviour is lasting. Unfortunately further follow-up to test longer term persistence of benefits will not be possible from this study as the control group were treated after the waiting period for ethical reasons. Sixthly, no intervention made any difference to teacher-rated child behaviour in either the short or longer term. Partly this was because some of the children had no significant problems at school, but nonetheless it suggests that child behaviour may be fairly context specific. This supports an interactional framework, whereby the contingencies and expectations in a situation influence child behaviour. Given that child behaviour at school is also a major predictor of later child antisocial behaviour, and that classroom disruption is a major issue for teachers and because of its impact on other pupils, findings such as this have fuelled the search for interventions that include a teacher element.

Teacher programmes

Barkley et al. (2000) screened 3,100 5-year-old children in kindergarten and selected the top 9.3% with ADHD and conduct symptoms. They were allocated to group parent training only, special treatment classroom only, combined parent training and classroom treatment, or to no-treatment control. The parent training used Barkley's protocol (Barkley, 1997) and lasted 10 weeks in the autumn term, followed by monthly boosters; it was held at a medical centre. The special treatment classroom children spent a year at another school in a class that consisted of about 15 other similarly selected disruptive children. Teachers were highly trained and supervised in behaviour management techniques, and also were trained to deliver an accelerated curriculum aimed to advance academic skills; close supervision was provided. Children allocated to either of the classroom intervention conditions effectively received the full planned intervention in that context, but of those allocated to a condition with parent training, take-up was low: a third of the parents did not attend at all, and only 42% attended five sessions or more. Crucially, the results of this study that targeted a whole high-risk population were analysed on an intention-to-treat basis. The outcomes showed no difference on parent-rated measures for any condition, and no difference on observed parent–child interaction or observed child attending ability. There were improvements in the classroom conditions on some teacher-rated measures, for example on the Teacher Report Form (Achenbach, 1991) aggression and attention subscales, but not on the delinquency subscale or any of the internalizing subscales; some other scales measuring rather similar behaviours also showed no change. Direct observation of classroom behaviour showed reasonable (0.3 to 0.5 standard deviations) improvements in externalizing behaviour. The authors attribute the failure of the parenting programme to low attendance at the parenting group, but do not give a dose-response curve or analyse the results of those parents who attended say half or more sessions. The classroom intervention had useful effects on some but not other measures. There were no cross-context or synergistic effects.

Adding both child social skills and classroom intervention

The FastTrack project (Conduct Problems Prevention Research Group, 1999) is a 'state of the art' multimodal intervention study. Five-year-olds in kindergarten were screened and the top 10% with antisocial behaviour selected; 891 children were allocated to a multimodal intervention or to no intervention. The intervention included:

- A universal element given to all pupils in the classroom that consisted of two or three lessons a week of recognizing emotions, friendship skills, self-control skills, social problem-solving skills, plus classroom management consultation for the teachers.
- Parent training for two hours a week over 22 weeks for which the parents were paid $15 per session; for half-an-hour a reading tutor worked with the child on reading skills while parents watched.
- Child social skills group for one hour a week for 22 weeks.
- Child reading skills for three half-hour sessions a week with a special tutor.
- Home visits fortnightly alternating with telephone calls to develop a close relationship with the parents and promote generalization of parenting skills.

- A peer friendship promotion programme that paired the index child with another, low-risk child from the class for half-an-hour a week of constructive play time together.

Parental participation was relatively high, 72% received more than half of the sessions, and 81% received at least half the home visits. Given this massive input of resources, and thorough coverage of theoretical risk factors, the outcomes were very modest. *Antisocial behaviour* was assessed on eight measures: on all but one, there was no significant change; the mean effect size across all was 0.11 standard deviations. *Social behaviour* – only two of the five social behaviour measures changed significantly, with a mean effect size across all of 0.18 standard deviations. *Social cognition tests* showed gains on four out of five measures, mean es 0.28. *Reading skills:* reading attainment scores showed no improvement, although a reading process test ('word attack') did, and grades for language arts improved; mean effect size for all three was 0.33. *Parental behaviour:* harsh discipline did not change on questionnaire or observation, although it did on a hypothetical test of responses to vignettes; appropriate and consistent discipline did not improve according to parental report or event recorded observation, though did on coder impression of the observation. Warmth increased on direct observation but not according to parental report. Thus of the eight measures of parenting behaviour, three changed significantly; the mean effect size for all eight was 0.17 standard deviations. The intervention is ongoing and the hope must be that the children will show bigger changes later, although such a comprehensive, prolonged and intensive intervention is likely to be too expensive to replicate.

Implications for practitioners

Children with antisocial behaviour cost society a great deal of money – an economic analysis found that those with conduct disorder aged 10 cost ten times as much as controls by age 27 (Scott et al., 2001a). Therefore there is a strong financial incentive to invest in these children's futures, as well as a humanitarian one. In the US and the UK there is considerable governmental interest in early prevention. However, to stand a chance of being effective, several characteristics need to be in place. In addition to choosing empirically-supported interventions (which is far from always the case), staff need to be supervised to deliver them to a high standard, otherwise efficacy is lost (Henggeler et al., 1998). Management needs to be good, with reasonable staff morale and training. A total population has to be targeted, not just those who are motivated to turn up; an assertive outreach strategy needs to be pursued to reach the most needy families. Currently, group parent training is more cost-effective than individual work. Scott et al. (2001b) found that a 12-week programme cost £571 per child, no more than standard individual treatment for six sessions.

Given that say 5% children have conduct disorder with impairment (Meltzer et al., 2000), and up to 20% have DSM IV oppositional-defiant disorder (Kazdin, 1995), parenting programmes could not possibly be delivered by mental health professionals to most of the population who would benefit. A change in the culture around parenting is necessary, plus a stepped approach to intervention. The broadcast programmes of Sanders and colleagues suggest that this might be achieved, backed up by a carefully graded range of services, starting with self-administered programmes and only working up to intensive approaches for those who do not respond. Schools will need to focus more on children's behavioural and social development and implement approaches shown to work. If this occurs and the culture changes towards more informed and effective parenting, there is a prospect of making a considerable reduction in children's misery and of helping them to achieve a balanced way of life integrated with their family, friends and school.

Conclusions

Treatments for conduct disorder have come a long way. They are now more responsive to parents' own views, and can address contextual and mental health issues that impair 'good enough' parenting. Scores of careful studies attest that programmes lead to improvements in the way parents relate to their children *and* to reduced antisocial behaviour in the children, thus giving them better chances for successful adjustment. Combining parenting programmes with child social skills training appears to increase the benefits outside the home. However, problems remain in making programmes acceptable to the most needy parents, and population-based prevention programmes have so far shown only modest benefits.

Unanswered questions

Whilst the effectiveness of parent training in referred cases is firmly established, the precise mode of action is not. From the evidence reviewed above, it seems likely that humane, empathetic interpersonal skills are necessary to engage and retain parents, but good inculcation of behavioural skills is necessary to bring about changes in parenting style and child behaviour. Studies suggest that parental mood, beliefs about the child, expressed emotion towards the child, and behaviour all change. Which is the active ingredient, or are changes in all necessary? Which aspects of parenting are most crucial: sensitive responding and communication, encouragement of prosocial behaviour, setting of clear boundaries, or effective punishment for misbehaviour? Does child attachment status become more secure as parenting is improved? Is the child's capacity for empathy increased, and is the likelihood of developing antisocial personality reduced? One hopes that future studies may answer these questions.

Further reading

Hill J, Maughan B (2001) Conduct Disorders in Childhood and Adolescence. Cambridge: Cambridge University Press.

Kazdin AE, Wassell G (2000) Therapeutic changes in children, parents, and families resulting from treatment of children with conduct problems. Journal of the American Academy of Child and Adolescent Psychiatry 39: 414–20.

Scott S, Spender Q, Doolan M, Jacobs B, Aspland H (2001) Multicentre controlled trial of parenting groups for child antisocial behaviour in clinical practice. British Medical Journal 323: 194–7.

References

Achenbach TM (1991) Manual for the Child Behavior Checklist/4-18 and 1991 Profile. Vermont: Department of Psychiatry, University of Vermont.

Bank L, Duncan T, Patterson GR, Reid J (1993) Parent and teacher ratings in the assessment and prediction of antisocial and delinquent behaviours. Journal of Personality 61(4): 693–709.

Barkley R (1997) Defiant Children: A Clinician's Manual for Assessment and Parent Training. 2 edn. New York: Guilford Press.

Barkley RA, Shelton TL, Crosswait C, Moorehouse M, Fletcher K, Barrett S, Jenkins L, Metevia L (2000) Multi-method pyscho-educational intervention for preschool children with disruptive behaviour: preliminary results at post-treatment. Journal of Child Psychology and Psychiatry 41(3): 319–32.

Barlow J (1999) Systematic Review of the Effectiveness of Parent-Training Programmes in Improving Behaviour Problems in Children Aged 3–10 Years. A Review of the Literature on Parent-training Programmes and Child Behaviour Outcome Measures. Oxford: Health Services Research Unit, University of Oxford.

Belsky J, Hsieh K-H, Crnic K (1998) Mothering, fathering, and infant negativity as antecedents of boys' externalizing problems and inhibition at age 3 years: differential susceptibility to rearing experience? Development and Psychopathology 10(2): 301–19.

Bernal ME, Klinnert MD, Schultz LA (1980) Outcome evaluation of behavioural parent-training and client-centered parent counselling for children with conduct problems. Journal of Applied Behaviour Analysis 13(4): 677–91.

Blechman EA (1998) Parent training in moral context: pro-social family therapy. In Breismeister JM (ed.) Handbook of Parent Training: Parents as Co-therapists for Children's Behavior Problems. 2 edn. New York: Wiley, pp. 508–48.

Bohman M (1996) Predisposition to criminality: Swedish adoption studies in retrospect. In Bock G, Goode J (eds) Genetics of Criminal and Antisocial Behaviour – Ciba Foundation Symposium 194. Chichester: Wiley, pp. 99–114.

Brunk M, Henggeler SW, Whelan JP (1987) A comparison of multisystemic therapy and parent training in the brief treatment of child abuse and neglect. Journal of Consulting and Clinical Psychology 55: 311–18.

Cadoret RJ, Yates WR, Troughton E, Woodworth G (1995) Genetic environmental interaction in the genesis of aggressivity and conduct disorders. Archives of General Psychiatry 52(11): 916–24.

Chamberlain P, Rosicky JG (1995) The effectiveness of family therapy in the treatment of adolescents with conduct disorders and delinquency. Journal of Marital and Family Therapy 21(4): 441–59.

Cohen J (1988) Statistical Power Analysis for the Behavioral Sciences. Hillsdale: Erlbaum.

Conduct Problems Prevention Research Group (1992) A developmental and clinical model for prevention of conduct disorder. Development and Psychopathology 4: 509–27.

Conduct Problems Prevention Research Group (1999) Initial impact of the fast track prevention trial for conduct problems: 1. The high-risk sample. Journal of Consulting and Clinical Psychology 67(5): 631–47.

Cox AD, Puckering C, Pound A, Mills M, Owen AL (1990) The Evaluation of a Home Visiting and Befriending Scheme. London: NewPin.

Cox WD, Matthews CO (1977) Parent group-education: what does it do for the children? Journal of School Psychology 15: 358–61.

Cunningham CE, Bremner R, Boyle M (1995) Large group community-based parenting programmes for families of preschoolers at risk for disruptive behaviour disorders: utilization, cost effectiveness, and outcome. Journal of Child Psychology and Psychiatry 36(7): 1141–59.

Dadds MR, McHugh TA (1992) Social support and treatment outcome in behavioral family therapy for child conduct problems. Journal of Consulting and Clinical Psychology 60(2): 252–9.

Dadds MR, Schwartz S, Sanders MR (1987) Marital discord and treatment outcome in behavioral treatment of child conduct disorders. Journal of Consulting and Clinical Psychology 55(3): 396–403.

Davis H, Spurr P (1998) Parent counselling: an evaluation of a community child mental health service. Journal of Child Psychology and Psychiatry 39: 365–76.

Deater-Deckard K, Dodge KA, Bates JE, Pettit GS (1996) Physical discipline among African American and European American mothers: links to children's externalizing behaviors. Developmental Psychology 32(6): 1065–72.

Denham SA, Almeida MC (1987) Children's social problem-solving skills, behavioral adjustment, and interventions: a meta-analysis evaluating theory and practice. Journal of Applied Developmental Psychology 8(4): 391–409.

Dishion T, Andrews D (1995) Preventing escalation in problem behaviors with high-risk young adolescents: immediate and 1-year outcomes. Journal of Consulting and Clinical Psychology 63: 538–48.

Dodge K, Schwartz D (1997) Social information processing mechanisms in aggressive behavior. In: Stoff D, Breiling J, Maser J (eds) Handbook of Antisocial Behavior. New York: Wiley, pp. 171–80.

Dowdney L, Skuse D (1993) Parenting provided by adults with mental retardation. Journal of Child Psychology and Psychiatry and Allied Disciplines 34(1): 25–47.

Dumas JE, Wahler RG (1983) Predictors of treatment outcome in parent training: mother insularity and socio-economic disadvantage. Behavioural Assessment 5(4): 301–13.

Eyberg SM, Robinson EA (1982) Parent-child interaction training: effects on family functioning. Journal of Clinical Child Psychology 11: 130–7.

Fergusson DM, Lynskey MT (1997) Early reading difficulties and later conduct problems. Journal of Child Psychology and Psychiatry and Allied Disciplines 38(8): 899–907.

Fergusson DM, Woodward LJ, Horwood LJ (1999) Childhood peer relationship problems and young people's involvement with deviant peers in adolescence. Journal of Abnormal Child Psychology 27(5): 357–69.

Forehand R, Long N (1988) Outpatient treatment of the acting out child: procedures, long term follow-up data, and clinical problems. Journal of Advanced Behavioural Research Therapy 10: 129–77.

Forehand RL, McMahon RJ (1981) Helping the Noncompliant Child: A Clinician's Guide to Parent Training. London: Guilford Press.

Forehand R, Sturgis ET, McMahon RJ, Aguar D, Green K, Wells KC, Breiner J (1979) Parent behavioral training to modify child noncompliance: treatment generalization across time and from home to school. Journal of Behavior Modification 3(1): 3–25.

Forehand R, Wells KC, Griest DL (1980) An examination of the social validity of a parent training program. Journal of Behavior Therapy 11: 488–502.

Frankel F, Myatt R, Cantwell DP, Feinberg DT (1997) Parent-assisted transfer of children's social skills training: effects on children with and without attention-deficit hyperactivity disorder. Journal of the American Academy of Child and Adolescent Psychiatry 36(8): 1056–64.

Frasier F, Matthes WA (1975) Parent education: a comparison of Adlerian and behavioral approaches. Elementary School Guidance and Counseling 10: 31–8.

Freeman C (1975) Adlerian mother study groups and traditional mother discussion groups: effects on attitudes and behavior. Journal of Individual Psychology 31: 37–50.

Gowers S, Bailey-Rogers SJ, Shore A, Levine W (2000) The Health of the Nation Outcome Scales for Child and Adolescent Mental Health. Child Psychology and Psychiatry Review 5(2): 50–6.

Griest DL, Forehand R, Rogers T, Breiner J, Furey W, Williams CA (1982) Effects of parent-enhancement therapy on the treatment of outcome and generalization. Behavior Research and Therapy 20(5): 429–36.

Henggeler SW, Schoenwald SK, Borduin CM, Rowland MD, Cunningham PB (1998) Multisystemic Treatment of Antisocial Behavior in Children and Adolescents. New York: Guilford Press.

Herbert M (1987) Behavioural Treatment of Children with Problems: A Practice Manual. 2 edn. London: Academic Press.

Hinshaw S (1992) Externalizing behaviour problems and academic under-achievement in childhood and adolescence: causal relationships and underlying mechanisms. Psychological Bulletin 111(1): 127–55.

Hoag MJ, Burlingame GM (1997) Evaluating the effectiveness of child and adolescent group treatment: a meta-analytic review. Journal of Clinical Child Psychology 26(3): 234–46.

Horn WF, Ialongo N, Popovich S, Peradotto D (1987) Behavioral parent training and cognitive-behavioral self-control therapy with ADD-H children: comparative and combined effects. Journal of Clinical Child Psychology 16(1): 57–68.

Humphries L, Forehand R, McMahon R, Roberts M (1978) Parent behavioral training to modify child noncompliance: effects on untreated siblings. Journal of Behavior Therapy and Experimental Psychiatry 9: 235–8.

Jacobson NS, Truax P (1991) Clinical significance: a statistical approach to defining meaningful change in psychotherapy research. Journal of Consulting and Clinical Psychology 59(1): 12–19.

Kazdin AE (1995) Conduct disorder. In Verhulst FCK (ed.) The Epidemiology of Child and Adolescent Psychopathology. New York: Oxford University Press, pp. 258–90.

Kazdin AE (2001) Treatment of conduct disorders. In Hill J, Maugham B (eds) Conduct Disorders in Childhood and Adolescence. Cambridge Child and Adolescent Psychiatry. New York: Cambridge University Press, pp. 408–48.

Kazdin AE, Esveldt-Dawson K, French NH, Unis AS (1987) Effects of parent management training and problem-solving skills training combined in the treatment of antisocial child behavior. Journal of the American Academy of Child and Adolescent Psychiatry 26: 416–24.

Kazdin A, Siegel T, Bass D (1992) Cognitive problem-solving skills training and parent management training in the treatment of antisocial behavior in children. Journal of Consulting and Clinical Psychology 60: 733–47.

Kendall PC (1998) Empirically supported psychological therapies. Journal of Consulting and Clinical Psychology 66(1): 3–6.

Lochman J, Wells K (1996) A social-cognitive intervention with aggressive children: prevention effects and contextual implementation issues. In Peters R, McMahon R (eds) Preventing Childhood Disorders, Substance Abuse and Delinquency. Thousand Oaks CA: Sage Publications, pp. 111–43.

Lochman JE, Coie JD, Underwood MK, Terry R (1993) Effectiveness of a social relations intervention program for aggressive and nonaggressive, rejected children. Journal of Consulting and Clinical Psychology 61(6): 1053–8.

Lochman JE, Whidby JM, FitzGerald DP (2000) Cognitive-behavioral assessment and treatment with aggressive children. In Kendall PC (ed.) Child and Adolescent Therapy. Cognitive-behavioral Procedures. 2 edn. New York: Guilford Press, pp. 31–87.

Main M (1996) Introduction to the special section on attachment and psychopathology: overview of the field of attachment. Journal of Consulting and Clinical Psychology 64(2): 237–43.

McMahon RJ, Forehand R, Griest DL (1981) Effects of knowledge of social learning principles on enhancing treatment outcome and generalization in a parent training program. Journal of Consulting and Clinical Psychology 49(4): 526–32.

McNeil CB, Eyberg S, Eisenstadt TH, Newcomb K, Funderburk B (1991) Parent-child interaction therapy with behavior problem children: generalization of treatment effects to the school setting. Journal of Clinical Child Psychology 20(2): 140–51.

Meltzer H, Gatward R, Goodman R, Ford T (2000) The Mental Health of Children and Adolescents in Great Britain. London: Office of National Statistics.

Moffitt T (1993) Adolescence-limited and life-course persistant antisocial behaviour: a developmental taxonomy. Psychology Review 100: 674–701.

Murray L, Cooper PJ (1997) Postpartum Depression and Child Development. New York: Guilford Press.

Nicol AR, Smith J, Kay B, Hall D, Barlow J, Williams B (1988) A focused casework approach to the treatment of child abuse: a controlled comparison. Journal of Child Psychology and Psychiatry 29(5): 703–11.

Patterson GR (1974) Interventions for boys with conduct problems: multiple settings, treatments and criteria. Journal of Consulting and Clinical Psychology 42: 471–81.

Patterson GR, Chamberlain P, Reid JB (1982) A comparative evaluation of a parent-training program. Behavior Therapy 13: 638–50.

Patterson GR, Reid JB, Dishion TJ (1992) Antisocial Boys. Eugene OR: Castalia.

Peed S, Roberts M, Forehand R (1977) Evaluation of the effectiveness of a standardized parent-training programme in altering the interaction of mothers and their noncompliant children. Behavior Modification 1(3): 323–50.

Pettit GS, Bates JE, Dodge KA (1997) Supportive parenting, ecological context, and children's adjustment: a seven-year longitudinal study. Child Development 68(5): 908–23.

Pfiffner LJ, Jouriles EN, Brown MM, Etscheidt MA (1990) Effects of problem-solving therapy on outcomes of parent training for single-parent families. Child and Family Behavior Therapy 12(1): 1–11.

Pinsker M, Geoffrey K (1981) A comparison of parent-effectiveness training and behavior modification training. Family Relations 30: 61–8.

Poulin F, Dishion TJ, Haas E (1999) The peer influence paradox: friendship quality and deviancy training within male adolescent friendships. Merrill-Palmer Quarterly 45(1): 42–61.

Puckering C, Rogers J, Mills M, Cox AD, Mattsson-Graff M (1994) Process and evaluation of a group intervention for mothers with parenting difficulties. Child Abuse Review 3: 299–310.

Quinton D, Rutter M (1988) Parenting Breakdown: The Making and Breaking of Inter-generational Links. Aldershot: Avebury.

Rogers CR (1961) On Becoming a Person. London: Constable.

Rushton A, Dance C, Quinton D (2000) Findings from a UK based study of late permanent placements. Adoption Quarterly 3(3): 51–72.

Rutter M (1995) Psychosocial Disturbances in Young People: Challenges for Prevention. New York: Cambridge University Press.

Rutter M, Giller H, Hagell A (1998) Antisocial Behavior by Young People. New York: Cambridge University Press.

Sanders MR (1999) Triple P-Positive Parenting Program: towards an empirically validated multilevel parenting and family support strategy for the prevention of behavior and emotional problems in children. Journal of Clinical Child and Family Psychology Review 2(2): 71–89.

Sanders MR, Markie-Dadds C, Tully LA, Bor W (2000) The Triple P-Positive Parenting Program: a comparison of enhanced, standard and self-directed behavioral family intervention for parents of children with early onset conduct problems. Journal of Consulting and Clinical Psychology 68: 624–40.

Sanders MR, McFarland MT (2000) Treatment of depressed mothers with disruptive children: a controlled evaluation of cognitive behavioral family intervention. Behavior Therapy 31: 89–112.

Sanders MR, Montgomery DT, Brechman-Toussaint ML (2000) The mass media and the prevention of child behavior problems: the evaluation of a television series to promote positive outcomes for parents and their children. Journal of Child Psychology and Psychiatry and Allied Disciplines 41: 939–48.

Scott S (1994) Mental retardation. In Rutter M, Taylor E, Hersov L (eds) Child and Adolescent Psychiatry: Modern Approaches. 3 edn. Oxford: Blackwell, pp. 616–46.

Scott S (2000) Conduct disorders in childhood and adolescence. In Gelder MG, Lopez-Ibor JJ, Andreason NC (eds) New Oxford Textbook of Psychiatry. Oxford: Oxford University Press.

Scott S (2001) Deciding whether interventions for antisocial behaviour work: principles of outcome assessment and practice in a multicentre trial. European Child and Adolescent Psychiatry 10(1): 59–70.

Scott S, Sylva K (2002) The 'Spokes' Project: Supporting Parents on Kids' Education. London: Department of Health.

Scott S, Knapp M, Henderson J, Maughan B (2001a) Financial cost of social exclusion: follow up study of antisocial children into adulthood. British Medical Journal 323: 191–4.

Scott S, Spender Q, Doolan M, Jacobs B, Aspland H (2001b) Multicentre controlled trail of parenting groups for child antisocial behaviour in clinical practice. British Medical Journal 323: 194–7.

Serketich WJ, Dumas JE (1996) The effectiveness of behavioral parent training to modify antisocial behavior in children: a meta-analysis. Journal of Behavior Therapy 27: 171–86.

Sheeber LB, Johnson JH (1994) Evaluation of a temperament-focused, parent-training programme. Journal of Clinical Child Psychology 23(3): 249–59.

Silberg J, Meyer J, Pickles A, Simonoff E, Eaves L, Hewitt J, Maes H, Rutter M (1996) Heterogeneity among juvenile antisocial behaviours: findings from the Virginia Twin Study of Adolescent Behavioral Development. In Bock G, Goode J (eds) Genetics of Criminal and Antisocial Behaviour. CIBA Symposium No. 194. Chichester and New York: Wiley, pp. 76–86.

Skinner BF (1953) Science and Human Behaviour. New York: Macmillan.

Smith C (1996) Developing Parenting Programmes. London: National Children's Bureau.

Sutton C (1992) Training parents to manage difficult children: a comparison of methods. Journal of Behavioural Psychotherapy 20: 115–39.

Sutton C (1995) Parent training by telephone: a partial replication! Behavioural and Cognitive Psychotherapy 23: 1–24.

Taylor E, Chadwick O, Heptinstall E, Danckaerts M (1996) Hyperactivity and conduct problems as risk factors for adolescent development. Journal of the American Academy of Child and Adolescent Psychiatry 35: 1213–26.

Taylor TK, Schmidt F, Pepler D, Hodgins C (1998) A comparison of eclectic treatment with Webster-Stratton's parents and children series in a children's mental health center: a randomized controlled trial. Journal of Behavior Therapy 29: 221–40.

Tremblay RE (2000) The development of aggressive brain behaviour during childhood: what have we learned in the past century? International Journal of Behavioural Development 24: 129–41.

Wahler RG, Dumas JE (1989) Attentional problems in dysfunctional mother-child interactions: an interbehavioral model. Psychological Bulletin 105(1): 116–30.

Wahler RG, Cartor PG, Fleischman J, Lambert W (1993) The impact of synthesis teaching and parent training with mothers of conduct-disordered children. Journal of Abnormal Child Psychology 21(4): 425–40.

Webster-Stratton C (1984) A randomized trial of two parenting training programs for families with conduct disordered children. Journal of Consulting and Clinical Psychology 52(4): 666–78.

Webster-Stratton C (1994) Advancing videotape parent training: a comparison study. Journal of Consulting and Clinical Psychology 62(3): 583–93.

Webster-Stratton C, Hammond M (1997) Treating children with early-onset conduct problems: a comparison of child and parent training interventions. Journal of Consulting and Clinical Psychology 65(1): 93–109.

Webster-Stratton C, Hammond M (1999) Marital conflict management skills, parenting style, and early-onset conduct problems: processes and pathways. Journal of Child Psychology and Psychiatry and Allied Disciplines 40(6): 917–27.

Webster-Stratton C, Hancock L (1998) Training for parents of young children with conduct problems: content, methods and therapeutic processes. Handbook of Parent Training 98–152.

Webster-Stratton C, Kolpacoff M, Hollinsworth T (1988) Self-administered videotape therapy for families with conduct-problem children: comparison with two cost-effective treatments and a control group. Journal of Consulting and Clinical Psychology 56(4): 558–66.

Webster-Stratton C, Hollinsworth T, Kolpacoff M (1989) The long-term effectiveness and clinical significance of three cost-effective training programs for families with conduct-problem children. Journal of Consulting and Clinical Psychology 57(4): 550–3.

Weisz JR, Donenberg GR, Han SS (1995) Bridging the gap between laboratory and clinic in child and adolescent psychotherapy. Journal of Consulting and Clinical Psychology 63(5): 688–701.

Wells KC, Griest DL, Forehand R (1980) The use of a self-control package to enhance temporal generality of a parent training program. Journal of Behavioral Research and Therapy 18: 347–53.

Woodward L, Dowdney L, Taylor E (1997) Child and family factors influencing the clinical referral of children with hyperactivity: a research note. Journal of Child Psychology and Psychiatry 38: 479–85.

CHAPTER 4

Adopted children's behaviour and development in childhood and adolescence

DAVID HOWE

Introduction

Psychologists and other social scientists have long had an interest in the behaviour and development of adopted children. As well as clinical concerns, developmental scientists have also recognized that the adopted child's situation is akin to a 'natural experiment' in which the effects of genes and environment on children's progress – nature and nurture – can be examined. Most children are raised by their biological parents. This makes it difficult to determine whether a child's characteristics have been acquired genetically or experientially. However, in the case of a child adopted at birth, it is possible to examine the separate effects of genes and environment. On the one hand, to the extent that adopted children are like their biological parents, with whom they have never lived, then those traits are likely to have been inherited. And on the other, characteristics that correlate with those possessed by their adoptive parents indicate the power of environmental experiences to shape development.

Current evidence based on adoption and twin studies increases the weight given to the effect of genes on children's psychosocial development, although the preferred view sees a complex interplay between heredity and environment (Plomin, 1994). For example, in the case of cognitive ability, genetic inheritance appears to play the major role in children's performance, although the environment modifies actual scores, either up or down. As many baby-adopted children move from environments of poor to good quality stimulation, their IQ scores tend to be higher than those of either their birth mothers or fathers. Even so, their IQs still correlate with those of their biological parents and not those of their adopters. New adoptive environments appear to allow children's genetic potential to be reached.

However, the majority of children placed for adoption today are not babies. Prior to being adopted, older children will have spent one or more years living with their biological parents or other carers. The early years experience of these children is typically one of abuse, neglect, deprivation, rejection or serial caregiving. These experiences adversely affect aspects of their development and behaviour. They arrive in their adoptive homes at an older age, often with a history of maltreatment, and generally with one or more problem behaviours. Older placed children therefore provide researchers with the opportunity to examine the extent to which children are able to recover from early life adversity and impaired development when placed in more advantaged environments.

If clinicians are to make appropriate and sensitive diagnoses, they need to appreciate these several dimensions to the adopted child's history and character. For example, in the case of an older placed child, low IQ and a difficult temperament might be compounded by a history of sexual abuse. Added to these factors will be a number of post-placement experiences, including the ability of the adoptive parents to deal with difficult behaviours arising out of the child's earlier caregiving experiences. And the fact of being adopted itself might also be thought of as an extra risk factor, implying as it does that one's birth parents either would not (cases of rejection), could not (cases of incompetence), or should not (cases of maltreatment) look after one.

The research evidence will now be considered in more detail (also see Howe, 1998). We shall first examine the behaviour and development of children adopted as babies before going on to look at the outcomes of those placed at older ages.

Children adopted as babies

Most researchers in the field define a case as a 'baby adoption' when the child is placed before the age of 6 months, although occasionally the cutoff point rises to 1 year. The younger the child is at the age of placement, the less influential the original caregiving environment is likely to be on the child's development. Historically, in the UK, the peak year for baby adoptions was 1968 when around 12,000 babies were placed with non-related adoptive parents. The majority of these children joined their new carers before the age of 3 months. The figures today are much lower, numbering well below 1,000 for children adopted before the age of one.

The outcome news for children placed as babies is generally very good. Developmentally speaking they compare well with children raised in families matched for adoptive parents' socioeconomic status. In terms of physical and cognitive ability, they show very little difference from their matched peers. The only impairment seems to be that children adopted as babies run a slightly higher risk of suffering poor peer relationships, particularly in late childhood and adolescence. Young men, in particular, find greater difficulty in conducting themselves effectively in peer and intimate relationships. However, there are those who counsel caution in interpreting even this risk. It is suggested that much of the variance in poor relationships is explained by a relatively small number of baby placed children who do show disturbed behaviour, particularly in the conduct and quality of their relationships with peers. This leaves the majority of baby adopted children functioning well within the normal range of interpersonal conduct (Seglow et al., 1972; Howe, 1997).

More difficult to quantify are the clinical consequences of adopted children inheriting characteristics that place them at increased risk of developing mental health and behavioural problems. For example, there is a significant genetic component present in those who suffer schizophrenia. Adopted children of schizophrenic biological parents are more likely to develop schizophrenia than adopted children whose biological parents did not have the illness (Heston, 1966; Kety et al., 1978; Tienari et al., 1990). However, for children at genetic risk of developing schizophrenia, adoption by non-schizophrenic parents appears to act as a protective buffer. The rate of developing schizophrenia for children born to and who live with a schizophrenic parent is about 10%. This figure falls to 3% if the vulnerable child is placed with adoptive parents, a rate still three times greater than that of the general population (1% risk) but considerably less than if the child had remained with his or her biological parents. Similar protective effects are found for depression, crime and alcoholism.

Genetic vulnerability may therefore explain some or all of the observation that children adopted as babies are generally two to three times more likely to be referred to the child psychiatric and psychological services than the general population (Humphrey and Ounsted, 1963; Howe and Hinings, 1987). Fergusson et al. (1995) compared 16-year-olds who had been raised in either biological two-parent families, single parent families, or two-parent adoptive families. The children raised by adoptive parents enjoyed the highest social and material standards whereas those in single-parent households suffered the lowest. Their investigations found no difference between the three groups in terms of depression, anxiety and the mood disorders. However, there were significant differences in the rates of 'externalizing problem behaviours'. The rates of conduct and oppositional disorders, self-reported offending, and daily cigarette smoking were highest for adolescent children of single parents and lowest for two-parent families, with adopted children falling in between. In a review of the literature, Ingersoll (1997) also found that adopted children are referred to mental health professionals at higher than expected rates, presenting problems mainly of the externalizing kind. Studies by Horn et al. (1975), Smith et al. (1982) and Cadoret (1990) observed that the birth mothers of adopted children showed increased rates of difficult and anti-social behaviours. Genetic explanations therefore offer a potentially good account of why adopted children appear to be at a modestly increased risk of developing problem behaviours (for example, by inheriting a high threshold for stimulation or a difficult temperament etc.).

However, other factors have also been examined by way of explanation. It has been argued that adoptive parents are more likely to refer their children for psychiatric help when their behaviour becomes difficult. In a more elaborate explanation, Brodzinsky (1987, 1990) has developed a 'stress and coping model of adoption adjustment' in which he suggests that there are extra psychosocial and developmental tasks associated with being adopted, for both children and parents, and that these increase the risk of impaired development. He believes that there is a 'psychological risk factor' in being adopted. Most children and their parents cope well with these risks but a few show vulnerability. Loss plays a central part in adoption, for both children and their parents. Infertile parents have to adjust to the 'loss' of the child they never had. Children have to think about the loss of their biological parents and ponder why they were 'given up' for adoption.

Most adopted children say that they think about their birth parents while growing up, wondering what they might be like and whether they look like them (Howe and Feast, 2000). These extra psychosocial tasks might increase the stress experienced by children and parents, which, if not coped with well, might increase the risk of children developing problem behaviours. At such heightened and sensitive times, children might be more likely to be referred for psychological help and counselling. Indeed, Verhulst (2000) argues that adopted children's increased display of problem behaviour during adolescence is exacerbated by their growing awareness and concerns about their biological parentage. 'Their increased cognitive abilities', he says, 'enable them to reflect on the meaning of being adopted . . . Their sense of loss of having once been abandoned, and their awareness of the lack of genealogical connectedness are evaluated in adolescence in terms of their developing identity' (p. 41).

In summary, the development of children adopted as babies is seen as a product of genetic inheritance; the psychosocial environment generated by the adoptive parents; and the psychological meaning, interpretation and experience of being either an adopted child or adoptive parent.

Adopted children appear at slightly increased risk of experiencing difficulties or deficits in at least one of these domains. Much of this risk is
accounted for by a small minority of baby adopted children who do develop mental health and behavioural problems, leaving the majority to
progress through their childhood in good psychological order. And
although the origins of a particular difficulty might be understood independently of children's adoptive status, in practice, being adopted often
becomes a meaningful factor in many children's minds and in their interactions with their adoptive parents, matters which clinicians need to
understand in making their diagnoses and carrying out their treatments
(also see Howe and Feast, 2000). For example, 14-year-old, adopted
Jessica reflected:

> I get on OK with my mum and dad. I kind of know it's not their fault. But I
> keep thinking that there's supposed to be a natural, loving bond thing
> between a mum and daughter. And there is. But I've got this other mum
> that for a few years now I've been thinking of, off and on. Why did she give
> me up and have me adopted? I know I've been told that she was in her late
> teens and her own parents were not supporting her, but it does make me
> feel rejected, that I was, like, not wanted. I keep thinking I mustn't have
> been good enough in some way, which makes me feel a bit hurt and
> annoyed. And I wanted to know things that my mum and dad didn't know.
> Like what was I like in those first few months after I was born? Who do I
> look like? Why did she give me away? At the moment I kind of can't get these
> thoughts out of my mind.

Children adopted at older ages

Up until the 1980s, it was comparatively rare for children much beyond the
age of 12 months to be placed for adoption. However, with big reductions
in the number of babies available for adoption (the result of improved con-
traception, unmarried mothers experiencing less social stigma and
improved benefits for single parents) and a growing belief that children in
the public care system should have the chance to experience normal family life, there was a gradual increase in the number of older children being
placed for adoption. There was much optimism that adoptive parents
could cope with these children and that no child was 'unadoptable'. In
practice, the majority of these children have experienced adversity or deprivation in their early years, hence their classification as 'children in need'.
Not surprisingly, they often arrive in their adoptive homes with a range of
developmental impairments and behavioural problems.

The increase in the number of older children with histories of adversity placed for adoption provided scientists and researchers with the

opportunity to test out two competing theories of child development. The first suggests that early life deprivation and maltreatment has long lasting negative effects on children's personality, development and behaviour (for example Bowlby, 1951). The second believes that children who have suffered poor care and major setbacks can nevertheless, with sound parenting, make good if not full developmental recoveries and that early experiences do not set children on an invariant life path (for example, Clarke and Clarke, 1976, 2000). By 1976, Clarke and Clarke (2000) had concluded 'that there is no known adversity from which at least some children had not recovered if moved to something better and that the whole life path is important, including the early years' (p. 19). Research evidence tells us that the developmental pathways taken by older placed adopted children are often tortuous and complicated. Understanding their needs and difficulties therefore tends to demand a subtle and flexible state of mind on the part of the clinician.

As we shall see, a transactional model is generally preferred in which the child's past and present are seen to interact in complex ways. There is no single factor that leads to a single main effect. Many variables, including genetic factors as well as early life experiences, continue to interact across the lifespan. This means that clinical assessments have to take into account the quality of the child's early caregiving as well as the characteristics of their present psychosocial environment. There is not a particular syndrome for older placed adopted children, although it is recognized that they are at increased risk of a range of developmental and behavioural difficulties. For example, a child who has suffered severe neglect and deprivation might present her adoptive parents and indeed peers and teachers, with a very different array of behaviours to those shown by a child who has been physically abused. Parents, peers and teachers who recognize that these contrasting behaviours need to be handled in *different* ways might find that the neglected child and the abused child achieve the same happy outcome (equifinality) – that unequals have to be treated unequally if the same end point is to be reached. However, treating both children the same might produce different behavioural outcomes, with one child showing improvement and the other not, or both children continuing to display difficult behaviour but of a different and contrasting kind.

As the developmental outcomes are more varied for older placed children and more likely to show impairment, the research findings for this group will be considered in more detail than those for children adopted as babies. The following four headings will be used to order the presentation of the findings: disruption rates; physical development; cognitive competence; and social, emotional and behavioural adjustment.

Disruption rates

It has long been recognized that, compared with children adopted as babies, older placed children are at increased risk of their placements breaking down. As a rough rule of thumb, increasing age at placement increases the risk of the adoption disrupting. Observers intent on putting a positive spin on the outcomes of older placed children sometimes omit those whose adoptions broke down, thus giving late placements a slightly rosier glow than they might otherwise receive.

A range of disruption rates is reported in the research literature. For example, Barth and Berry (1988) reported a disruption rate of 10% for children placed before the age of 10, most breaking down within the first 18 months. The breakdown figures rose to 22% and 26% for children adopted aged 12 to 14 years and 15 to 17 years respectively. Their sample included a large number of children adopted by their foster carers, a group of adopters associated with lower breakdown rates. Disruption rates were higher in all three age groups for children not adopted by their foster carers. Thoburn (1991) found higher rates of breakdown with 21% ceasing within 18 to 78 months, again with the finding that rates were lowest for the youngest and highest for the oldest children at the time of placement. A prospective study of boys placed after the age of five described a 19% disruption rate (Quinton et al., 1998). The aggressive behaviour of the boys was one of the main reasons given by adopters for the breakdown. Reviewing a number of studies, Borland et al. (1991) suggested that disruption rates for children placed before the age of 10 ran at around 10% whereas those placed after the age of 10 varied from between 15% and 50%. Turning these figures around, however, reminds us that the majority of older placed children, many with very disturbed histories, nevertheless remain in placement until the age of their majority.

Physical development

Here the evidence is generally very encouraging. Children's ability to recover from early physical neglect and malnutrition appears to be extraordinarily good when they are placed with adopters who provide a nutritious diet and a warm family life (Martorell et al., 1994). Good health is quickly restored, height and weight potentials are reached and normal physical milestones are achieved. The various studies that are currently tracking Romanian orphanage children adopted in the UK, Canada and the US are providing us with some powerful evidence not just about children's ability to recover physically but also psychologically. For example, Rutter et al. (1998) report substantial physical catch-up by the age of

4 years in terms of weight, height and head circumference for a sample of 111 Romanian orphans who entered England before the age of 2 years, the majority in a physically very poor condition.

Cognitive development

A similar picture emerges for the ability of older placed children to recover cognitive competence, many realizing their full potential (for example, Duyme et al., 1999). The studies by Hodges and Tizard (1989a, 1989b) looked at children who had spent the first 2 to 7 years of their life in a residential institution, some of whom were later adopted, some who returned home to their biological families, and some who remained in institutional care. The children adopted before the age of four continued to perform better (mean IQ 114) than those restored to their biological parents (mean IQ 96) and those who had remained in institutional care (mean IQ 96).

The various studies of Romanian orphanage children also report considerable cognitive developmental catch-up, although those placed after the age of 6 months perform slightly less well than those placed at younger ages. Ames (1997), studying Canadian placed Romanian children, tested the children's IQ at age 4.5 years. The mean of those placed between 8 and 68 months was 90 compared to 98 for those adopted before the age of 4 months. A comparison group of 30 adopted Canadian children scored 109. The UK study of Romanian children also reported a huge intellectual catch-up, but again different rates were observed depending on the length that children had been in institutional care (O'Connor et al., 2000). By the age of 4 years, children placed after the age of 6 months scored a mean of 90, well within the normal range, compared with means of 102 for those placed before 6 months, and 109 for a comparison group of within-UK adopted children. Rutter et al. (2000) conclude that 'the total duration of privation during the first 2 years of life is more important as a predictor of cognitive outcome than is the extent to which the privation involved subnutrition. The inference, therefore, is that psychological privation constituted an important part of the risk experiences prior to coming to the UK' (p. 129).

Social, emotional and behavioural development

Although older age at placement is associated with increasing rates of adoption breakdown and displays of problem behaviour, it is not older age as such that appears to be the risk. Rather, older placed children generally have experienced longer exposure to abuse, neglect and rejection and it is these that make later psychosocial adjustment more difficult.

Research findings broadly suggest that children with histories of mal-treatment, multiple placements and severe deprivation are at much greater risk of impaired socioemotional development and problem behaviour. Nevertheless, despite this increased risk, it remains impressive that a significant proportion, often a majority, of older placed children show good recovery and clearly benefit from being adopted.

Certainly compared with children who remain in or who are restored to biological families where they might expect to experience adversity, older placed children are at decreased risk of developing psychosocial difficulties. For example, Tizard (1977) found that institutional children restored to their birth families compared with those who had been adopted were more tense, twitchy and unhappy. However, institutional children, whether adopted or restored, tended to be less popular and more aggressive and quarrelsome with their peers, as well as being more attention-seeking with teachers and resentful when corrected, than other working-class children who had been continuously cared for by their biological families (Tizard, 1977). By the time they reached 16 years, the restored and adopted children continued to be at greater risk of showing a range of problem behaviours including restlessness, anxiety and aggression, although the rates were higher for those restored to their birth families. Indeed, the restored children were much more likely to be referred to a psychologist or psychiatrist, suggesting that adoption afforded a degree of protection and that a measure of recovery had taken placed for many of the adopted children (Hodges and Tizard, 1989a, 1989b; also see Chisholm, 1998).

In their prospective study of boys placed after the age of five, Quinton et al. (1998) report that the majority had experienced neglect and/or abuse prior to being adopted. About half of the children had a parent who had suffered a psychiatric illness or experienced marital conflict. At the time of placement, the majority of the boys showed a variety of conduct and emotional problems often manifested in difficult relations with their peers. By the end of the first year in their placement, the mean number of problems had halved, although restlessness and overactivity tended to remain high. Eight years after their placement, 19% of the adoptions had broken down. Children who had actively been *rejected* by their birth parents were the group most likely to experience placement breakdown, especially when accompanied by overactive behaviour (Rushton et al., 2000). Of the remainder, about half were said by their adoptive parents to be making good progress. The other half were described as still difficult, many showing a variety of problem behaviours including restlessness, stealing, aggression and poor concentration.

Howe (1997) also found that older placed children were much more likely to develop problem behaviours in adolescence than baby placed children. However, he also noted that older placed adopted children who had not suffered neglect or maltreatment during their first year or so of life appeared significantly less at risk of displaying problem behaviours. He concluded that reasonably good care in the first year offered protection against later maladjustment, even when later life events took a turn for the worst leading to eventual adoption.

The above findings are in line with the observations of Versluis-den Bieman and Verhulst (1995) who found that antisocial behaviours and maladjustment, particularly during adolescence, appear to rise at a higher rate amongst older placed adopted children than socioeconomic controls (for the adoptive families' status). Indeed, most studies of older placed adopted children suggest that they are at particular risk of developing externalizing, oppositional and antisocial problem behaviours. These tend adversely to affect their social relationships with parents at home and peers at school. Although shown at less frequent rates than for children who remain in situations of adversity, older placed children are more likely to show one or more of the following behaviours and personality traits: anxiety, insecurity, attention-seeking and demanding behaviours, restlessness, poor concentration, unpopularity with peers, lying, aggression, oppositional behaviour, conduct disorders and criminal behaviour. However, in contrast, adopted children are more likely than children who remain in adversity to show significant improvement on all these fronts by early adulthood.

In a Dutch longitudinal study of internationally adopted children, Verhulst (2000) found that although older age at placement was significantly associated with an increased risk for later maladjustment, early adversity was the more powerful predictor. 'Children who have experienced early negative environmental influences . . . run a greater risk for developing problem behaviors than children with relatively favorable backgrounds' (Verhulst, 2000, p. 35). Children who had suffered abuse were particularly at risk of later maladjustment. Again, this is a reminder that the type of adversity suffered by a child prior to adoption appears to predict not only the extent to which the child is able to recover from early developmental setbacks but also the kind of maladjustment shown later, particularly in adolescence.

Howe (1996) found that many adopters who had experienced major relationship problems with their adopted children in adolescence described significant improvements by the time their children had reached young adulthood. Thoburn (2001) suspects that many 'adopted young people move towards emotional maturity at a slower pace than those who have not been adopted – not surprisingly with at least two extra hurdles to surmount: that of loss and separation, and that of making sense of their adoptive identity' (p. 1844).

Thus, studies generally show that children adopted after the age of 6 months compared to baby placed children show higher rates of anxiety, feelings of insecurity and antisocial 'externalizing' problem behaviour, particularly during adolescence (Haugaard et al., 1999; Humphrey and Ounsted, 1963; Kotsopoulos et al., 1993) but that these rates are much lower than for children who remain in birth families where there is neglect, abuse or rejection. Adoption therefore appears to confer some protection against maladjustment. Early adversity does not necessarily predict problem behaviour, although a degree of elevated risk remains suggesting a complex interaction between older placed children's continuing vulnerability and the protective potential provided by adoption.

A transactional model of older placed adopted children's development

The risk factors we have considered so far have all been present prior to the children's placement. However, a number of post-placement factors have also been found to affect children's development. These post-adoption elements interact with the characteristics that children bring to their new family. A number have been investigated.

Older children placed transracially appear to be at no higher risk of problem behaviours than children in matched same-race placements, although there is the suggestion that their self-identity development is at increased risk of impairment (see, for example, Thoburn et al., 2000). The sibling composition of the adoptive family has been examined to see whether it affects outcomes, but the findings appear inconclusive (see, for example, Barth and Berry, 1990; Festinger, 1986; Howe, 1997). The research evidence on the benefits of children having contact with their birth parents and siblings is still emerging. Again, the picture appears to be complex. Grotevant and McRoy (1998) suggest that many children do benefit from contact but it is important for placement workers not to operate these findings as a blanket formula. Older placed children who have experienced rejection, abuse and trauma at the hands of their carer might well remain in a state of disorganization if contact with a frightening caregiver is maintained. Having said this, the way adopters handle and present their own and their child's psychological relationship with their birth family does appear to be important. Adopters need to understand that their children will have complex and mixed feelings about their birth parents. Being judgemental about the birth family appears to harm relationships between adopters and their children.

The emerging consensus is that the developmental outcomes achieved by older placed adopted children are best understood in terms of a transactional model. A child's 'movement along a particular developmental pathway is determined by the transactions that occur between the child and his or her environment. In a transactional model, the child and the environment co-determine a child's developmental progress' (Stovall and Dozier, 1998, p. 66). Children bring to their adoptions their own unique histories, and the mental states and their associated behavioural and relationship styles formed in their earlier caregiving environments. Many of these mental states and adaptive strategies will have been forged in situations of abuse, neglect and rejection (Howe et al., 1999). Stovall and Dozier (1998) believe that although these strategies will have helped children survive in very difficult environments, they can mean that children are ill-equipped to take advantage of good quality, loving and responsive substitute care. In particular, many children seem unable to elicit or respond to sensitive care and protective parenting. Not only are children affected by their environment, the social environment is affected by children and their needs and behaviours.

This model helps explain the different behavioural and developmental pathways taken by older placed children. Each child's pathway depends on the type of abuse, neglect and rejection suffered and the particular reactions of the adoptive parents to the behavioural consequences of that abuse, neglect or rejection. For example, an abused and rejected child might have developed an avoidant attachment. In the new placement, such a child might behave in an emotionally self-sufficient manner believing that caregivers are not available at times of need and distress. Faced with such a child, an adoptive mother might feel not needed or wanted. She might therefore either back off, deactivate her caregiving or ignore the child. In contrast, a parent who manages not to be drawn into the child's relationship logic and instead behaves in a consistent and persistently responsive, caring and protective manner might allow the child to feel safe and less anxious whenever care and protection are needed.

A robust version of the transactional model has been developed by Clarke and Clarke (2000). For several decades they have argued against the power of early life events significantly to determine children's development and life chances. In their book *Early Experience and the Life Path* (2000) they marshal a good deal of research evidence to make the point that children show considerable resilience and a remarkable ability to extract from new environments experiences that aid developmental recovery. They identify a 'self-righting tendency' in all children, which promotes recovery once new and better environments are met. It was observed that the effects of early adversity appear to fade over time once children enjoy new and improved circumstances (for example, see the classic study by Lewis, 1954).

Clarke and Clarke (2000) concentrate on the research that recognizes that older placed adopted children generally fare much better than children who remain in environments of adversity similar to those out of which the adopted children were removed. Seen this way the level of recovery shown by older placed adopted children is impressive. However, it should be recognized that they are still at increased risk of a range of problem behaviours and developmental impairments. Clarke and Clarke do not see these maladjustments as some inbuilt limitation laid down in early childhood on the potential of the older placed child fully to recover from early privation and deprivation. Rather, they see a less than full recovery as a failure of the social environment to provide sufficient of the right kinds of stimulation and experience.

However, in the light of Rutter et al.'s (1998) recent adopted Romanian orphanage children studies, the Clarkes have slightly modified their thesis, acknowledging that extreme disadvantage in the early years may have some long-lasting effects.

> Following conditions of severe global privation, those babies rescued before the age of six months made, on average, spectacular gains in development by age four, maintained at age six. The children adopted after the age of six months also made massive average gains, though not as great, from an initially lower level . . . the difference between before and after six months must have reflected lengthier institutional privation, suggesting a sensitive (but not critical) period in their lives. But this sensitive period was not universal; some children did well or very well cognitively, even though adopted after (and sometimes long after) six months, both at age four and six follow-up. (Clarke and Clarke, 2000, pp. 97–8)

In their conclusion, the authors cite Schaffer's (2000) review paper in which he reassesses the influence of children's early years experience on their development. Schaffer sees the effects of early experience as complex with an ever greater number of factors over and above early experience itself also affecting a child's final developmental outcome (cited in Clarke and Clarke, 2000, p. 103).

Thus, although good post-adoption experiences are hugely beneficial, with the effects of early adversity fading over time, some effects, particularly those to do with relationship (socioemotional) difficulties, do seem more long lasting. They suggest that early emotional trauma and severe neglect might continue to have some deep adverse affect on aspects of children's and adults' emotional processing capacities. These impairments, possibly organic and hard-wired during the early years, are much more difficult to treat (see Schore, 1996).

The message for clinicians working with older placed adopted children is to see them as a highly differentiated group. Assessments have to be aware of how the different developmental sequelae associated with particular pre-placement adversities (for example, sexual abuse, rejection, neglect) in turn interact with and are affected by particular post-placement experiences, the most important of which is likely to be the parenting and relationship style provided by the adopters. As an example of this way of thinking, brief consideration will be given to particular disorders often associated with older placed adopted children and ones that typically present adopters with a lot of difficulty.

Disorders of attachment

Since the early 1990s, there has been an increase in the number of adopted children said by their parents to be showing very difficult and challenging behaviours. Clinicians who specialize in this field suggest they are typical of children who have a disorder of attachment, sometimes known as 'reactive attachment disorder'. Both DSM-IV and ICD-10 describe the criteria for two types of attachment disorder: inhibited and disinhibited. Young children showing inhibited attachment disorders resist being comforted and have contradictory, ambivalent and inhibited responses towards their carer. Those with the disinhibited type are indiscriminately oversociable, fail to develop selective attachments, lack selectivity in people from whom they seek comfort and are unable to modulate their social interactions with unfamiliar persons (Zeanah, 1996).

More generally, children diagnosed with a disorder of attachment have symptoms that include a range of social, emotional, behavioural and developmental dysfunctions including several of the following: bossiness, poor peer relationships, the need to be in control rather than be controlled, indiscriminate affectionate behaviour with strangers (disinhibited), lack of affection with carers, high levels of anger and rage, restlessness, 'crazy' lying, stealing from carers, self-endangerment, recklessness, accident proneness, precocious competence in self-protection, preoccupation with fire and violence, cruelty to animals, lack of cause-and-effect thinking, gorging, hoarding food, self-neglect, very poor personal hygiene (particularly in teens), and urinating in inappropriate places. No one child will show all of these symptoms but highly characteristic is an avoidance of intimacy and extreme attempts to control close relationships coercively. The child acts as if being cared for is frightening and potentially dangerous. As a consequence they tend to prefer to be in control, usually in a hostile manner, becoming anxious and aggressive if they find themselves in a dependent, vulnerable position. Some children weave into this profile elements of 'parentified' (compulsive caregiving) behaviour, depression, and states of profound helplessness (Liotti, 1999, talks about these mental state switches as a form of 'dissociation').

Although these symptoms might present at any time after the child has been adopted, they are likely to be at their most severe during mid-to-late childhood and early adolescence. The clinical evidence suggests that certain preplacement experiences, particularly if met before the age of two, act as major risk factors for the development of an attachment disorder. These include a variety of traumatic and adverse caregiving experiences including extreme combinations of physical/sexual abuse and neglect, chronic maternal depression, severe neglect, serious misuse of drugs/alcohol by parents, primary caregivers who have experienced serious childhood traumas that remain unresolved and frequent and multiple moves between different carers. Theorists explain that one way of understanding these behaviours is to see them as a desperate strategy in which children try to increase feelings of safety in a world that is unpredictably frightening, both physically and psychologically. They try to take control of the self, other people and the environment – hence the classification of 'controlling' attachment (Solomon and George, 1999; Howe et al., 1999). Recent policies that have encouraged the adoption of many of these older, traumatized children appear to have resulted in more adopters than in the past running into major parenting difficulties. The case of 13-year-old James is highly typical of the many adopted children displaying a disorder of attachment and who present themselves in a variety of clinical and child welfare settings:

> Along with his baby brother, three year old James was placed in local authority care after a prolonged history of severe neglect and some physical abuse. Their mother was a drug addict who regularly left both boys on their own in cots for anything up to 36 hours. Earlier referrals had involved allegations of physical abuse (though not proved) and maternal rejection. When James was finally removed, he was first taken to hospital where he was found to be dirty, grossly underweight, quiet and unsmiling, and slightly bruised around his arms and back. Three weeks later he was transferred to a foster home before finally being adopted aged three and a half.

> On joining them, his adoptive parents said it was as if James had 'emotionally switched off.' For a number of months he rocked, head-banged, and ate voraciously. In fact, food remained an important issue for James for much of his childhood. He always wanted to know when was the next meal. His parents said that even after a huge dinner he would crawl around the floor picking up crumbs. He remained enuretic until he was aged six. He did not smile much and this continued to disappoint his parents. His adoptive mother said she spent years giving James cuddles, love and kisses 'in the hope that I could compensate for those first years of nothing, those years without food or love.'

> Matters seemed to be going tolerably well until James reached ten. He began to interact more with his parents and his brother, a younger boy who had

been adopted a couple of years after James had been placed. The school said that James was bright, but had poor concentration, although they felt he was making good progress relating with peers after a difficult start.

However, just before his eleventh birthday, James's behaviour deteriorated. He began to argue with his mother over every little thing. He developed an interest in weapons and began to make large, home-made knives that he sharpened to a lethal degree, hiding them at the back of one of his bedroom drawers. When tackled by his mother about these knives, James said that one night when his parents were asleep, he was going to take a knife and cut their throats. He laughed as he said it.

The quarrels with his mother became even more aggressive, even though they were triggered by the littlest of things such as blaming her for stealing his money, which she knew he had spent on CDs or a wristwatch. James constantly lost things, never remembering where he had left them. Lying and deceit became automatic. His mother began to feel frightened of him. At first, her husband felt she was either exaggerating the problems or was even partly to blame herself. When he got home from work, James could be particularly attentive and friendly. Tensions began to develop between James's parents. However, as his mother began to increase her distance from James, her husband began to be on the receiving end of more and more of James' difficult behaviour. James began to steal money from his parents and brother. Later on, he stole and sold the family's computer, video, camera and several mobile phones. He set fire to his school's large waste paper bins, causing considerable damage. It was not unusual for James to stay out all night, sleep in his day clothes and not wash for weeks. He said he liked the smell of his unwashed hair: 'It makes me feel better,' he once said.

Although most of the time, he was loud, hostile and even violent, particularly towards caring adult females (his mother, women teachers), he could suddenly switch between a variety of other mental states, including feeling very affectionate and needy, desperately sad and even suicidal, and frightened and confused. His mother sensed his desperate mental condition, but felt helpless as well as frightened. By his thirteenth birthday, his parents said he was 'hell to live with' and were on the brink of giving up. He began to smoke cannabis, shoplift, and develop a 'couldn't-care-less' attitude to all those he either hurt, let down, stole from, deceived, 'ripped off', or borrowed from and never returned. 'They're suckers' he said, acting as if the world owed him a living. One afternoon, while he should have been at school, his mother found him in bed with a girl. His rages became increasingly violent. He trashed his bedroom, regularly punched his fist through doors and windows, and got into fights at school (in which, after 'winding-up' someone, he would generally come off worse). From the age of twelve, James had been seen by a number of mental health specialists, including two psychologists and a psychiatrist, the latter concluding that it was not possible to work with James, saying he would have to close the case.

Of course, in line with the thinking of Clarke and Clarke (2000), many of these abused and neglected children do well when placed for adoption. Nevertheless, a transactional model would predict that the major deficits and disturbed states of mind that these children bring to the relationship with their adopters are likely to increase the levels of stress between children and their parents along the lines suggested by Stovall and Dozier (1998). Typical of many of these cases at clinical presentation is a child who avoids being cared for, behaving as if the adoptive parent (usually the mother) is both a potential source of neglect and danger and unable to provide care and protection (which is frightening). Overwhelmed by these feelings, the child tries to remain in control by being bossy, angry, rageful, aggressive or seductive. In response, carers are in danger of feeling helpless and angry when faced with so much aggression, confusion, need and mental fragmentation. In extreme cases, adopters might feel like abdicating the role of caregiver, no longer willing or able to provide their child with care and protection ('I give up; she's on her own; I feel helpless, utterly exhausted and depressed').

However, children with these extreme disorders clearly illustrate the complex interplay between the impact of early life experiences and the ability of the child's current environment to bring about changes and achieve developmental recovery. Trauma, abuse and neglect in a child's early years have the capacity to produce dissociated mental states, disturbed relationships and behaviours, and disorganized/disordered attachments. Behaviours shown by these children are generally described as 'controlling' in which children appear to find it difficult to let carers, including adopters, carry out their role as providers of care, love, intimacy and protection. Many parents, without support and expert help, find themselves caught up in the child's perverted rationale of how relationships work. Eventually the adopters give up. The placement either staggers on unhappily, breaks down, or the child, if old enough, is ejected prematurely into some form of independent living, with or without financial support from the adopters.

Fortunately, clinical experience and research evidence is beginning to help us understand these children. We are also starting to see the emergence of therapeutic interventions and support packages designed specifically with these older placed adopted children in mind. They are premised on the belief that recovery is possible, although in the case of these children it is likely to be extremely difficult and challenging. Severe adversity in early childhood produces imbalanced states of mind that are poor at processing cognitive and emotional information. These mental states and the behaviours that they produce tend to generate long negative chain reactions in which transactions spiral rapidly downwards with one bad psychosocial reaction leading to another. Therapies are designed to interrupt these reactions by introducing positive responses and planned discontinuities. Even gross deprivations that have resulted in a range of physical, cognitive and socioemotional deficits can be overcome with strong and prolonged interventions. Most treatments recognize that these children have attempted to survive by developing a variety of controlling strategies based on aggression, hostility, manipulation and seduction. When these strategies break down, as they regularly do, children feel either frightened and helpless, or sad and depressed.

Initial treatments often focus on helping children to feel safe when they let go of being in control. Treatment generally involves a number of phases that include:

- regaining a sense of safety;
- providing corrective emotional experiences;
- building self-efficacy;
- remembering and mourning;
- promoting cognitive restructuring and reconceptualization of emotional experiences and 'disconfirming';
- negative insecure working models of the self and others, and
- developing positive self-esteem (Herman, 1992; Pearce and Pezzot-Pearce, 1994; Levy and Orlans, 1998).

As a result of early neglect and trauma, many children have a very poor understanding of how their minds and bodies work (for example, children can seem unsure about whether they are full or hungry, hot or cold). They are therefore unable to regulate heightened states of arousal. This results in confusion, fear, aggression, impulsive behaviour and inappropriate responses. Therapies, many of which directly involve the adoptive parents, concentrate on helping children to explore, recognize, understand and control their cognitive and emotional experiences. As many children initially are unable to express their thoughts and feelings verbally, children are often helped to explore their mental states through play, drawing or music.

It is not until they can learn to let go and feel safe in their relationship with their new carers that many adopted children begin to understand the social nature of emotions. Children's ability to 'mentalize' and develop empathy, social understanding and 'metacognition' can be achieved only in relationships that are attuned and reciprocal (Fonagy and Target, 1997). Adopters and children need to achieve a normal caregiving/care-seeking relationship. Only then can 'controlling' children and attachment disordered children begin to recognize and understand the self and others as intentional, mind-driven beings. And only when children begin to understand the relationship between thoughts, feelings and behaviour in the self and others can they begin to develop social competence.

The effects of past traumatic experiences are powerfully present in the minds of many older placed adopted children. However, they can be helped to develop an integrated sense of self in the context of a well-informed and highly supported adoptive family. Recovery, although prolonged and difficult, is possible.

I have dwelt on children with disorders of attachment at some length deliberately. The push towards the adoption of increasing numbers of children who have experienced severe abuse, neglect and rejection, often accompanied by multiple placements, will mean that many more adopters will be faced with caring for very disturbed and traumatized children. It must be remembered that the development and impairments of children who have suffered abuse and rejection appear to be very different from those who have suffered severe deprivation (the case with the Romanian orphanage children). Children with different caregiving histories arrive in their placements with very different mental health needs and problems and thus may well set in train very different transactional effects. Adopted children who have suffered the double insult of abuse and neglect (danger and deprivation) are likely to make the greatest demands on a range of social, therapeutic, mental health and voluntary support services. If support and interventions are to be effective, specialist expertise and understanding are essential.

Conclusion

Adoption and foster care offer powerful experiences capable of breaking the transmission of adversity and maltreatment across the generations. Certainly the evidence supports the effectiveness of substitute care, although it must be remembered that even in situations where children remain in environments of abuse and neglect, a sizeable proportion will escape being developmentally impaired. So, although family disadvantage significantly increases the risk of behavioural problems and psycho-pathology, many children of distressed families nevertheless emerge into adulthood in reasonably good psychological health. For example, Kaufman and Zigler (1989) calculated that the risk of a child being abused if the parents themselves had suffered abuse in childhood, although much higher than non-abused populations, is nevertheless often significantly less than 100% and in some studies reaches as low as 30% (see also Sadowski et al., 1999).

The presence of these developmental discontinuities adds a moral dilemma to the equation that suggests that children adopted out of adversity generally fare much better than those who remain. Psychologists and psychiatrists, social workers and court child welfare officers often have to make recommendations about whether or not a child should be permanently removed from his or her birth family and placed for adoption. In the more extreme cases of abuse and neglect the decision can be reasonably clear cut. However, shifts in policy are seeing an increasing number of older children being put forward for adoption in cases where the parenting is certainly poor but not obviously dangerous. In less stark cases, and given the complex interaction of risk and protective factors, confidence in the long-term outcome decreases. A significant proportion of children in situations of moderate adversity are likely to have improved developmental prospects if adopted. The moral difficulty lies in the inexactness of the science, particularly when experts are asked to predict the risks and benefits should the child either remain with incompetent birth parents or be placed for adoption, recognizing that adoption itself is not an entirely risk-free developmental option.

Some commentators, including Morgan (1998) and Clarke and Clarke (2000) believe that the evidence for significantly increasing the number of older children placed for adoption is overwhelming. My own view is that the answer probably lies somewhere in between the strong views of people such as Morgan, Clarke and Clarke and the failure of some child protection practitioners to recognize the long-term developmental damage exacted on children who remain in caregiving environments where there is maltreatment.

Current policy is likely to see an increase in the number of older children with histories of abuse, neglect and rejection being placed for adoption. Undoubtedly, this will lead to an increase in the number of adopted children referred to the child psychological, psychiatric and post-adoption services suffering disorders of attachment, ADHD, post-traumatic stress disorder and dissociation. Treatment is likely to be most effective to the extent that the clinician appreciates

- the continuing influence on the child's current psychological state of early trauma and neglect;
- transactionally how this affects the quality and character of the caregiving provided by the adopters; and
- the psychological demands that being adopted places on both children and their adoptive parents in terms of loss, rejection, identity, and self-worth.

Recommended reading

Adoption Quarterly New York: The Haworth Press.
Howe D (1998) Patterns of Adoption: Nature, Nurture and Psychosocial Development. Oxford: Blackwell Science.

Sellick C, Thoburn J (1996) What Works in Family Placement. London: Barnardos.
Triseliotis J, Shireman J, Hundelby M (1997) Adoption: Theory, Policy and Practice. London: Cassell.

References

Ames EW (1997) The Development of Romanian Orphanage Children Adopted to Canada. Final Report to Human Resources Development, Canada.

Barth R, Berry M (1988) Adoption and Disruption: Rates, Risks and Responses. New York: Aldine de Gruyter.

Borland M, O'Hara G, Triseliotis J (1991) Placement outcomes for children with special needs. Adoption and Fostering 15(2): 18–28.

Bowlby J (1951) Maternal Care and Mental Health. Geneva: World Health Organisation.

Brodzinsky DM (1987) Adjustment to adoption: a psychosocial perspective. Clinical Psychological Review 7: 25–47.

Brodzinsky D (1990) A stress and coping model of adoption adjustment. In Brodzinsky D, Schechter M (eds) The Psychology of Adoption. New York: Oxford University Press.

Cadoret R (1990) Biologic perspectives on adoptee adjustment. In Brodzinsky D, Schechter M (eds) The Psychology of Adoption. New York: Oxford University Press, pp. 25–41.

Chisholm K (1998) A three-year follow-up of attachment and indiscriminate friendliness in children adopted from Romanian orphanages. Child Develpoment 69: 1092–106.

Clarke A, Clarke A (eds) (1976) Early Experience: Myth and Evidence. London: Open Books.

Clarke A, Clarke A (2000) Early Experience and the Life Path. London: Jessica Kingsley.

Duyme M, Dumaret A-L, Tomkiewicz S (1999) How can we boost IQs of 'dull children'? A late adoption study. Proceedings of the National Academy of Science 96: 8790–4.

Fergusson DM, Linskey M, Horwood LJ (1995) The adolescent outcomes of adoption: a 16 year longitudinal study. Journal of Child Psychology and Psychiatry 36(4): 597–616.

Festinger T (1986) Necessary Risk: A Study of Adoptions and Disrupted Adoptive Placements. Washington: Child Welfare League of America.

Fonagy P, Target M (1997) Attachment and reflective function: their role in self-organization. Development and Psychopathology 9, pp. 679–700.

Grotevant H, McRoy R (1998) Openness in Adoption. New York: Sage.

Haugaard J, Wojslawowicz J, Palmer M (1999) Outcomes in adolescent and older-child adoptions. Adoption Quarterly 3(1): 61–70.

Herman JL (1992) Trauma and Recovery. New York: Basic Books.

Heston L (1966) Psychiatric disorders in foster home-reared children of schizophrenic mothers. Bristish Journal of Psychiatry 112: 819–25.

Hodges J, Tizard B (1989a) IQ and behavioural adjustment of ex-institutional adolescents. Journal of Child Psychology and Psychiatry 1: 77–98.

Hodges J, Tizard B (1989b) Social and family relationships of ex-institutional adolescents. Journal of Child Psychology and Psychiatry 1: 99–122.

Horn J, Green M, Carney R, Erikson M (1975) Bias against genetic hypothesis in adoption studies. Archives of General Psychiatry 32: 1365–7.

Howe D (1996) Adopters' relationships with their adopted children from adolescence to early adulthood. Adoption and Fostering 20(3): 35–43.

Howe D (1997) Parent reported problems in 211 adopted children: some risk and protective factors. Journal of Child Psychology and Psychiatry 37: 401–12.

Howe D (1998) Patterns of Adoption: Nature, Nurture and Psychosocial Development. Oxford: Blackwell Science.

Howe D, Feast J (2000) Adoption, Search, Reunion. London: The Children's Society.

Howe D, Hinings D (1987) Adopted children referred to a child and family centre. Adoption and Fostering 11(3): 44–7.

Howe D, Brandon M, Hinings D, Schofield G (1999) Attachment Theory, Child Maltreatment and Family Support: A Practice and Assessment Model. Basingstoke: Palgrave/Macmillan Press.

Humphrey M, Ounsted C (1963) Adoptive families referred for psychiatric advice: I the children. British Journal of Psychiatry 109: 599–608.

Ingersoll B (1997) Psychiatric disorders among adopted children: a review and commentary. Adoption Quarterly 1 (1): 57–73.

Kaufman J, Zigler E (1989) The intergenerational transmission of child abuse. In Cicchetti D, Carlson V (eds) Child Maltreatment: Theory and Research in the Causes of Child Abuse and Neglect. Cambridge: Cambridge University Press.

Kety S, Rosenthal D, Wender P, Schulsinger F, Jacobson B (1978) The biologic and adoptive families of adopted individuals who became schizophrenic: prevalence of mental illness and other characteristics. In Wynne LC, Cromveel R, Mathysse S (eds) The Nature of Schizophrenia. New York: Wiley.

Kotsopoulos MD, Walker SW, Copping W, Cote A, Chryssoula S (1993) A psychiatric follow-up study of adoptees. Canadian Journal of Psychiatry 38(6): 391–6.

Levy TM, Orlans M (1998) Attachment Trauma and Healing: Understanding and Treating Attachment Disorder in Children and Families. Washington DC: Child Welfare League of America Press.

Lewis H (1954) Deprived Children. London: Oxford University Press.

Liotti G (1999) Disorganization of attachment as a model for understanding dissociative psychopathology. In Solomon J, George C (eds) Attachment Disorganization. New York: Guilford Press, pp. 291–317.

Martorell R, Kettel Khan L, Schroeder DG (1994) Reversability of stunting: epidemiological findings in children from developing countries. European Journal of Clinical Nutrition 48: S45–S57.

Morgan P (1998) Adoption and the Care of Children: The British and American Experience. London: Institute of Economic Affairs Health and Welfare Unit.

O'Connor T, Rutter M, Beckett C, Keaveney L, Krepner J, ERA Study Team (2000) The effects of global severe privation on cognitive competence. Child Development 71: 376–90.

Pearce JW, Pezzot-Pearce TD (1994) Attachment theory and its implications for psychotherapy with maltreated children. Child Abuse and Neglect 18: 425–38.

Plomin R (1994) Genetics and Experience: The Interplay between Nature and Nurture. Newbury Park CA: Sage.

Quinton D, Rushton A, Dance C, Mayes D (1998) Joining New Families: A Study of Adoption and Fostering in Middle Childhood. Chichester: Wiley.

Rushton A, Dance C, Quinton D (2000) Findings from a UK based study of late permanent placements. Adoption Quarterly 3(3): 51–71.

Rutter M, ERA Study Team (1998) Developmental catch-up and deficit following adoption after severe global early privation. In Ceci S, Williams W (eds) The Nature–Nurture Debate. Oxford: Blackwell.

Rutter M, ERA Study Team (2000) Developmental catch-up and deficit following adoption after severe global early privation. Journal of Child Psychology and Psychiatry 39(40): 465–76.

Sadowski H, Ugarte B, Kolvin I, Kaplan C, Barnes J (1999) Early life disadvantages and major depression in adulthood. British Journal of Psychiatry. 174: 112–20.

Schaffer HR (2000) The early experience assumption: past, present and future. International Journal of Behavioral Development (March): 5–14.

Schore A (1996) The experience-dependent maturation of a regulatory system in the orbital prefrontal cortex and the origin of developmental psychopathology. Development and Psychopathology 8: 59–87.

Seglow J, Pringle M, Wedge P (1972) Growing Up Adopted. Windsor: NFER.

Smith P, Nenney S, Weinman M, Mumford D (1982) Factors affecting perception of pregnancy risk in the adolescent. Journal of Youth and Adolescence. 11: 207–17.

Solomon J, George C (eds) (1999) Attachment Disorganization. New York: Guilford Press.

Stovall KC, Dozier M (1998) Infants in foster care: an attachment theory perspective. Adoption Quarterly 2(1): 55–88.

Thoburn J (1991) Evaluating placements: survey findings and conclusions. In Fratter J, Rowe J, Thoburn J (eds) Permanent Family Placement. London: BAAF, pp. 34–57.

Thoburn J (2001) The effects on child mental health of adoption and foster care. In Gelder M, Lopez J, Andreason N (eds) New Oxford Dictionary of Psychiatry. Oxford: Oxford University Press, pp. 1841–8.

Thoburn J, Norford L, Rashid S (2000) Permanent Family Placement for Children of Minority. London: Jessica Kingsley.

Tienari P, Lahti I, Sorri A, Naarala M, Moring J, Kaleva M, Wahlberg K, Wynne L (1990) Adopted-away offspring of schizophrenics and controls. In Robins L, Rutter M (eds) Straight and Devious Pathways from Childhood to Adulthood. New York: Cambridge University Press.

Tizard B (1977) Adoption: A Second Chance. London: Open Books.

Verhulst F (2000) Internationally adopted children: a Dutch longitudinal adoption study. Adoption Quarterly 4(1): 27–43.

Versluis-den Bieman, Verhulst F (1995) Self-report and parent reported problems in adolescent and international adoptees. Journal of Child Psychology and Psychiatry 36: 1411–28.

Zeanah C (1996) Beyond insecurity: a reconceptualization of attachment disorders of infancy. Journal of Consulting Clinical Psychology 64(1): 45–52.

CHAPTER 5

Deliberate self-harm in children and adolescents

CLAIRE DORER

Self-harming behaviours are often met with strong feelings, both from professionals and those close to the self-harmer. These feelings can include revulsion, pity, bewilderment and anger. The last two are particularly likely to be evoked if the self-harmer is a child or young person. Here, the perceived waste of youthful potential or the belief that childhood provides the happiest days of one's life (and therefore no cause for such behaviours) can lead to a particular lack of comprehension of, and hostility towards, the young self-harmer. And yet, self-harm in young people is not a new or uncommon phenomenon; evidence suggests that it is an increasing problem (Hawton et al., 1997). In this chapter I will review key literature from the early 1990s to build up a more vivid picture of the characteristics and experiences of young people who self-harm. From this position, the role of professionals in supporting these young people becomes clearer and the implications for practice will be discussed.

Defining deliberate self-harm

This task is not as simple as it may first appear. Initially, we may think of a range of behaviours that we might wish to include under this definition: self-cutting, overdoses of medication, self-strangulation, gassing. We also have a bewildering array of terms for such behaviours – self-harm, self-injury, self-destructive behaviour, parasuicide and self-inflicted violence. Once we attempt to think about the purpose of the act, it becomes rather more complicated. Historically, a link has been made between self-harming behaviours and suicidal intent, with non-fatal behaviours being viewed as focal, partial or 'failed' suicide attempts (for example, Menninger, 1938). It is from such views that we get terms such as

103

'parasuicide', where the perceived intention of the behaviour is implicit in the word itself. Such views remain pervasive today – as professionals we routinely ask questions about suicidal intent, even when the self-injury is relatively minor in medical terms. This approach is not inherently unhelpful (and, indeed, is a vital part of a full psychosocial assessment), however, it does lead to gaps in our understanding of what such behaviours actually mean to the person engaging in them. If we always assume that every act of self-harm represents a suicidal wish we are unlikely to ask the questions that will help us understand the individual's experience.

Several authors (for example, Babiker and Arnold, 1997; Harrison, 1995) make the point that rather than being concerned with ending life, many self-harming behaviours are actually aimed at preserving life. Acts such as self-cutting and self-burning are often performed as a response to unbearable negative feelings, which threaten to overwhelm the person. The act of self-injury is viewed as a coping mechanism, which allows for the expression of these feelings and hence averts either literal suicide or the sense of an annihilation of self. Once we can conceive of self-harming behaviours as being a potential coping function we are put in the position of having to compare them to other coping mechanisms. Certainly, we can see links between overtly self-harming behaviours such as self-cutting and other self-destructive behaviours such as the bingeing and purging seen in anorexia – a link that many authors have noted (e.g., Miller, 1994; Levenkron, 1998). However, some authors (e.g., Harrison, 1995) have suggested that self-harming behaviours could be seen as one point on a continuum of coping behaviours, ranging from neglectful eating habits and over-work at one end, through smoking and alcohol use and abuse to deliberate self-injury at the other. Such an approach has benefits, most notably that it helps reduce the stigma faced by young people who engage in self-harming behaviours by making their acts more comprehensible. If we can understand the reasons why we might reach for an alcoholic drink at the end of a particularly bad day we are more likely to understand why a young person might take a razor blade to her arms in response to an argument with her parents. Of course, this is a simplified example – the search for the reasons for self-harm needs to go beyond an examination of the precipitating factor. The possible disadvantage of a continuum view of self-harm is that in 'normalizing' such behaviours we may become oblivious to the distress behind them. Whilst it is crucial that we understand why a young person self-harms it is also vital that we take all acts of self-harm seriously.

Within this chapter I shall examine a range of behaviours under the banner of deliberate self-harm (DSH). Given the range of functions such behaviours may provide, I have deliberately resisted giving an all-encompassing definition. However, for the purposes of this chapter deliberate self-harm will refer to any behaviour engaged in with the intent to cause physical harm or tissue damage. This may or may not refer to the ending of life. However, it will not include behaviours such as recreational drug or alcohol use where, even though there may be short or long-term risk to health, this was not the conscious intent when engaging in the behaviour.

Incidence

General

Deliberate self-harm in young people is quite common. Since the late 1960s it has greatly increased and, despite a brief period in the late 1970s and early 1980s when the rate slowed, continues to increase (Hawton and Fagg, 1992). It is relatively easy to find figures for more medically significant forms of self-harm such as overdosing and self-strangulation because medical attention is both more likely to be needed and to be sought. Other forms of self-harming behaviours, particularly superficial or 'delicate' cutting, are less likely to result in a visit to medical services and are less likely to be recorded. This is partially because there is not always a clear medical need (cuts often do not require any stitching) but also, possibly, due to the increased stigma attached to such behaviours when compared with other forms of self-harm.

It is estimated that in England and Wales 19,000 young people aged between 10–19 present at hospital each year following an act of deliberate self-harm (Burgess et al., 1998). Young people in the 15-to-19-year-old age group make up the biggest proportion of this group. In one study, the incidence of DSH was estimated to be as high as 8.3% of the general population (Shaffer and Piacentini, 1994). Looking at community-based, rather than hospital-based, samples a study of adolescents' self-report of deliberate self-harm over a 12-month period in an Australian secondary school revealed an estimated prevalence of 5.1% (Patton et al., 1997). Lifetime estimates of suicidal behaviour range from 1.3% to 3.8% among males and 1.5% to 10.1% of females (Brent, 1997).

Methods of deliberate self-harm

Research indicates that the chosen form of DSH varies greatly, depending on where the study was carried out. The relative ease of access to firearms in America is clearly reflected in studies of chosen methods of suicide (Brent et al., 1998b). However, in general, this is a method that is more likely to be chosen by males than females. In Europe, self-poisoning by overdose is the most commonly reported method of DSH in both males and females, accounting for 90% of episodes of DSH in one study

(Hawton et al., 2000). For young women, self-poisoning represents the commonest cause for medical admission to hospital (Hawton and Fagg, 1992). In recent years there has been a major increase in the use of para-cetamol in overdoses; it is now used in approximately two-thirds of all overdoses (Dorer et al., 1999; Hawton et al., 2000).

Other forms of DSH, such as self-cutting, tend to be reported far less frequently in hospital-based studies. However, in community surveys they are more common, accounting for approximately one-third of all reported acts of DSH (Patton et al., 1997). There are suggestions that those adolescents who engage in relatively less lethal methods of self-harm are at a lower risk of eventual suicide. However, this is a generalization and it is not easy to predict future self-harm by current method alone. Some adolescents who engage in an act of high potential lethality will never self-harm again; others who appear to engage in relatively superficial acts of self-harm, such as self-cutting, will go on to commit suicide (American Academy of Child and Adolescent Psychiatry, 2001). This, as with so many factors, points towards the need for a full assessment of each adolescent who self-harms, rather than assumptions that may or may not have validity.

Age

As previously noted, the majority of young self-harmers are aged between 15 and 19 years old and older age in adolescence is considered a risk factor (Brent et al., 1998b). However, younger children do harm themselves and the numbers are increasing. It is generally thought that younger children who engage in acts of self-harm are less likely to show suicidal intent than older children (Brent et al., 1998b). This, however, is a generalization. I myself have worked with an 8-year-old who had twice engaged in acts of deliberate self-harm, both with a high and apparently intentional risk of suicide. Parents, carers and some professionals may find it difficult to believe that a child so young could entertain serious thoughts of ending his or her life and often there is a particular reluctance on the part of parents to accept that the act was anything more than an accident. Whilst it might be easier for a parent to believe that their child has swallowed a bottle of tablets, believing them to be sweets, the clinician must be careful to undertake a full assessment to determine the child's mental health and the intention of the act.

Gender

There are a number of differences between boys and girls in the patterns of self-harming behaviours. Approximately six times more young men than women succeed in killing themselves (Brent et al., 1998b; Langhinrichsen-Rohling et al., 1998). This has been linked to the higher prevalence of substance abuse and disruptive disorders in males (Shaffer et al., 1996). Links have also been made to gender-role socialization theory, suggesting that young males are socialized to engage in potentially high-risk and self-destructive activities during adolescence as 'proof' of their masculinity (Clark et al., 1990). In contrast, young females learn that they are expected to internalize their distress and anger (Nolen-Hoeksema, 1994).

Unsurprisingly, young females who engage in acts of deliberate self-harm have a higher incidence of depression than young males (Langhinrichsen-Rohling et al., 1998). Whilst young women commit suicide less frequently than young men they engage in suicidal thoughts and acts of DSH more frequently (Andrews and Lewinsohn, 1992). Young women are less likely to be intoxicated at the time of their self-harm, but when substance abuse is present it is equally as strong a risk factor as for young men (Brent et al., 1998).

Ethnicity

Possible links between ethnicity and self-harming behaviours have received relatively little attention in research. However, studies have suggested that both the suicide rates and the rate of self-poisoning in adolescent Asian girls are higher than in other ethnic groups (Maniam, 1988; Merril and Owens, 1986). Research has also suggested that whilst Asian girls may have a higher rate of deliberate self-harm than their Caucasian peers, their suicidal intent is generally lower. However, their rates of social isolation, depression and hopelessness tend to be higher and their acts of self-harm premeditated for a longer time (Kingsbury, 1994). Goddard and colleagues (1996) found fewer differences in terms of referral rate, psychiatric symptoms and circumstances of DSH between black (African-Caribbean and Asian) and Caucasian adolescents. However, black adolescents reported higher levels of social stress, particularly in the form of persecution or discrimination. In considering these findings one needs to bear in mind that there is generally a low rate of service utilization in adolescents from ethnic minorities (Barker and Adelman, 1994) and, therefore, this picture may be somewhat incomplete.

Sexuality

Sexuality is another area that has tended to be overlooked in research. However, the development of a sexual identity and the establishment of sexual preferences are key tasks of adolescence and frequently a source of tension and difficulties for young people. These are compounded if one's sexual preferences are seen as being different from the 'norm' such as attraction to members of the same sex or attraction to members of both sexes. Research suggests that young lesbian, gay and bisexual youths are

two to three times as likely to engage in acts of self-harm as those identified as heterosexual (Gibson, 1989). However, most research has taken its
samples from gay, lesbian and bisexual support groups. Lock and Steiner
(1999) hypothesize that the stress of 'coming out' into a homophobic
society may contribute to the high rates of self-harm in this group and an
increase in the risk of other health problems such as substance abuse.
This homophobia can be internalized, leading to lower self-esteem in
some of this group (Rotheram-Borus et al., 1995). However, there are
many adolescents who have confusion or struggle with their sexuality but
who do not consciously identify themselves as gay, lesbian or bisexual.
Additionally, adolescents who are suspected of being gay or lesbian by
their peer group may face prejudice and increased social stress, regardless
of their actual sexual preferences.

Repetition and the link between DSH and suicide

Between 14% and 50% of self-harming children and adolescents are
repeaters (Beratis, 1990; Hawton et al., 1982), with 10% to 15% carrying
out a further act of self-harm within 12 months of the initial episode
(Hawton and Fagg, 1992). The variability in these figures might, in part,
be accounted for by the way in which repetition is recorded within studies. Studies relying on hospital records of previous admissions tend to
report lower figures than those whose information comes from adolescent self-reports. In my own study, hospital records suggested a repetition
rate of approximately 12%. Interviews with adolescents in their own
homes revealed a repetition rate of 40% (Dorer et al., 1998). It appeared
that the adolescents were wary of receiving a negative reaction to a disclosure of previous self-harm and a good working relationship is
necessary for a clinician to elicit this information. It is extremely important that this information is accessed because approximately 4% of
adolescent self-harmers go on to commit suicide within 10 to 15 years
(Otto, 1972; Kotila and Lonnqvist, 1987).

Understanding deliberate self-harm

Having looked at who self-harms, it is now useful to think about the
meaning behind self-harming behaviours. For parents or carers, professionals and even young people themselves the 'why' question is
frequently asked directly. Unfortunately, the answers, if they are given at
all, rarely give a full picture of the experience of the young self-harmer.
Many young people find it hard to give a concrete reason why they have
harmed themselves or are only able to give the final contributing factor,
which precipitates the act (Dorer et al., 1999). This section will consider

precipitating factors but it will also try to address the wider range of meanings and circumstances around DSH in children and adolescents, such as family and psychiatric factors.

Precipitating factors

Asking young people why they took an overdose or cut themselves is likely to lead to a response that reflects a final event within a context of other difficulties. To try to understand the meaning of the act from such information is similar to trying to understand the plot of a film by looking at a still photograph. In looking at the reasons adolescents give for their self-harming behaviours, particularly overdoses, a number of core factors emerge. Conflict with parents is the single biggest precipitating factor in child and adolescent self-harm (Dorer et al., 1999; McLaughlin et al., 1996). Many adolescents report having taken overdoses after arguments with their parents. School problems are also a major precipitating factor. Such problems would include bullying but also difficulties relating to work pressures or impending exams. Conflict with partners is also common, although perhaps not as common as 'conventional wisdom' on why young people self-harm would suggest. Whilst examining precipitating factors to self-harm is important, it is essential that an assessment of the act move beyond this. Focusing exclusively on these factors may trivialize the behaviour and has led to the development of 'urban myths' such as all adolescent self-harmers are 'hysterical' teenage girls who have had a row with their boyfriend. Self-harm can also be viewed as a conscious attempt on behalf of the young person to manipulate people around them or to test out the quality of the relationship. However, young people rarely characterize their own self-harm in such terms (Michel et al., 1994; Boergers et al., 1998). Such approaches may lead to clinicians failing to recognize the very real difficulties faced by such adolescents. These difficulties will now be considered in more detail.

Escape from pain and the wish to die

As mentioned earlier, it is sometimes assumed that all acts of DSH represent a wish to die. For many young people, although death may be a potential result of their self-harm (particularly when more lethal methods of self-harm are chosen) the main aim of the behaviour is to escape an unbearable situation or to stop feeling emotional pain (Kienhorst et al., 1995). In Boergers and colleagues' study (1998), over 50% of young self-harmers indicated that they had attempted suicide in order to die, obtain relief or escape from difficult intrapersonal situations. The wish to die is associated both with increased levels of hopelessness and depression.

However, of the two, depression is the greater predictor of the wish to die (Boergers et al., 1998; Lewinsohn et al., 1993).

Most of the studies mentioned above focus on adolescents whose self-harm has resulted in contact with medical services. The majority of these young people have taken overdoses. It is possible that the functions of other forms of self-harm are slightly different. As discussed earlier in this chapter, some authors have described self-injury as life-preserving, rather than life-threatening. Young people who harm themselves through methods such as self-cutting, hitting or burning often see the behaviour as something that releases unbearable tension or emotional pain. In this way, the act is believed to prevent a more conscious suicide attempt (Smith et al., 1998). For others, self-injury is seen as a self-soothing behaviour or a method of 'returning' from dissociative states (Babiker and Arnold, 1997). Viewing these behaviours as signalling an intent to die is likely to lead to a lack of understanding of the young person's experience and of their self-harming behaviours. This clearly has implications for the success and nature of any therapeutic intervention.

Family background and relationships

A range of difficulties within the family has been identified as contributing towards DSH in children and adolescents. Of these, perhaps the most overt is child abuse. In particular, young people who have been sexually abused are at an increased risk of deliberate self-harm in adolescence (Renvoize, 1993). Brown and colleagues (1999) carried out a 17-year study of a randomly selected group of children. Their findings indicated that the risk of repeated suicide attempts was eight times higher for adolescents with a history of sexual abuse. This may be both due to risks caused by the direct impact of the abuse and other less direct risks such as increased interpersonal sensitivity and impulsive aggression (Gladstone et al., 1999). There is also a strong link between childhood sexual abuse and self-injury (Babiker and Arnold, 1997). Self-injurious behaviours can be viewed as trauma repetition, a means of expressing anger or a form of self-punishment (Miller, 1994). Although not all sexual abuse takes place within the immediate family, it has been suggested that the majority of survivors knew their abuser (Courtois, 1996). Other forms of abuse and neglect also increase the risk of deliberate self-harm. Adolescents with a history of childhood maltreatment are three times more likely to become depressed or suicidal than those without such a childhood history (Brown et al., 1999). In looking at neglect, it appears that many of the observed negative effects can be linked to contextual factors such as family environment and relationships (Belsky, 1993).

Family problems need not be as overt as abuse to have a major impact on young people. Many young self-harmers have experienced communication difficulties within their families, particularly in relation to their parents. The structure of families appears to be of less importance than the quality of relationships within the family. Research suggests that there is no significant difference between young people who live in two parent families and those living in single parent families with regards to self-harming behaviour (McKeown et al., 1998). However, children who have spent time in foster or institutional care are at an increased risk of repeat self-harm (Stewart et al., 2001). Impaired communication between adolescents and their parents, and in particular the absence of a family confidant, may be important in the origins of DSH (Tulloch et al., 1997). Suicidal adolescents perceive their parents to be significantly more critical, less caring and more overprotective than their non-suicidal peers (Allison et al., 1996). Conversely, perceived family cohesiveness has been shown to be a protective factor against DSH (Wagman-Borowsky et al., 2001). Myths concerning suicide, particularly that talking about it is likely to make it happen, can also leave young people without an opportunity to share their distress with those close to them (Hill, 1995). Many young people who self-injure report having grown up in 'invalidating environments' where feelings were not approved of or spoken about, or where children were told what they were feeling by their parents (Linehan, 1993). Families of adolescent self-harmers often have high levels of conflict (Asarnow, 1992). It has been theorized that adolescent suicide attempts may function to produce an effect on a parent or caregiver to whom they are insecurely attached (Bowlby, 1980). This might either be to punish the caregiver, perhaps to push them into being more attentive, or to express distress as a means of signalling a need for attention and care. As discussed earlier, young people themselves give this as an explanation for their self-harm relatively rarely. However, research from Wagner and colleagues (2000) suggests that in the time immediately after the discovery of the episode, mothers are likely to increase their feelings of caring for their child. Feelings of hostility may also be present. However, mothers are less likely to verbalize these than they are to verbalize support.

Parental illness may also be a factor in adolescent DSH (Armistead et al., 1995). In one study, over 40% of young people interviewed after an episode of self-harm had a parent with a significant physical or mental illness (Dorer et al., 1998). Some young people within the study reported that their self-harm had been prompted by a fear that their parent would die, whereas others felt burdened by the task of caring for their parent. Parental illness may interfere with treatment efficacy and it has been suggested that assessment and treatment of parental psychopathology should be part of the overall treatment plan in working with children and adolescents who self-harm (Brent et al., 1998a). In considering this range of family problems, it is important to note that often several problems occur at once and that this may present a cumulative risk to adolescents.

Mood disorders and other psychiatric conditions

Mood disorders (specifically depression) are a well-documented risk factor in child and adolescent self-harm (Kandel et al., 1991; Brent et al., 1993). It has been suggested that the increase in deliberate self-harm in recent decades may be accounted for by an increase in mood disorders (Diekstra et al., 1995). Research suggests that the association between mood disorders and self-harm is present in completed suicide, non-fatal suicide attempts and suicidal ideation (Flisher, 1999). However, although many young people who harm themselves are depressed, not all young people who are depressed harm themselves. Characteristics that distinguish between the two include life stressors (as discussed above), hopelessness and cognitive distortion (Kovacs et al., 1993; Brent et al., 1990). Depression seems to be a specific feature in young people with repeat episodes of DSH, particularly when it is associated with high levels of aggression (Stein et al., 1998; Hawton et al., 1999). Depressive disorders tend to persist in a significant number of adolescents who have taken overdoses, 2 to 3 months after the attempt (Kerfoot et al., 1996). Given the prevalence and significance of depression, it is essential that all clinicians who work with adolescents who self-harm take steps to assess and treat it effectively. It has been suggested that low self-esteem might underlie depression and could be the focus of interventions (Overholser et al., 1995).

Depression may be implicated in repetitive self-injury, but it is often thought of as a less important factor than in overdoses or overt suicide attempts. This does not appear to be because young people who self-injure do not report feelings of low mood. However, the pattern of such feelings tends not to correspond to a pattern of major clinical depression. For example, periods of intense negative affect often appear to arrive and depart quickly, rather than following a more chronic pattern. This rapid fluctuation in mood, coupled with apparently impulsive acts of self-injury, is more likely to result in a diagnosis of personality disorder (most likely borderline personality disorder) rather than affective disorder (Smith et al., 1998). A number of authors have noted that this is an unhelpful starting place for working with people who self-injure (Herman, 1992). Borderline personality disorder is a psychiatric label with considerable stigma attached to it. There is an expectation from professionals that people with the diagnosis will be difficult to work with and often this can prevent a more thorough exploration and understanding of the meaning behind self-harming behaviours.

There have been clear links established between psychosis and both self-harm and future risk of suicide (Royal College of Psychiatrists, 1998). This can be linked both to 'positive' symptoms, such as self-harm under the influence of hallucinations or delusions, and 'negative' symptoms such as self-harm during periods of depression.

Conduct/oppositional disorder

Research suggests that conduct disorder is a particular suicide risk in adolescents, particularly in older adolescent males (Shaffer et al., 1996). This risk is increased if it coexists with substance misuse and mood disorders. There is also evidence for a link between conduct disorder and suicide in females (Shaffer et al., 1996). Flannery and colleagues (2001) suggest that violent females are more likely to be depressed and to have significantly higher suicidal potential than both control group females and violent males. In my own research, I encountered a number of teenage girls who were the lead figures in their 'gang' of friends and who had been the perpetrators of violence, generally towards other girls. One described the pressure of maintaining her position as 'top dog' within her peer group and her belief that she could never openly show her distress for fear of it being considered a weakness. Her only way of managing her feelings was to attempt suicide (Dorer et al., 1998).

The link between non-fatal DSH and conduct disorder is less clear. A variety of behaviours relating to conduct disorder, such as aggressive or criminal behaviour and running away have been identified as risk factors in suicide attempts (for example, Groholt et al., 2000; Garnefski et al., 1992). However, most studies have focused on comorbidity with mood disorders, rather than look at the independent effects of conduct disorders (Gould et al., 1998). In one study, aggressive/criminal behaviour was a co-occurring problem category in 87% of male and 49% of female suicide attempters (Garnefski and Diekstra, 1995). Gould and colleagues suggested that, when findings are adjusted for psychiatric disorders, disruptive disorders have an insignificant association with suicide attempts. However, those adolescents who have run away from home are nearly three times more likely to have engaged in suicidal ideation or self-harm, even after adjustment for psychiatric disorders. In examining the role of aggression in DSH it has been suggested that the mediating factor between adolescents who direct aggression and anger at themselves and those who direct it at others might be the level of trait anxiety (Apter et al., 1991). Whilst conduct disorders clearly play a role in some cases of DSH it is important, as with other factors, that full attention is given to the range of problems experienced by the young person in association with his or her aggressive or disruptive behaviours.

Cognitive factors and problem-solving skills

Most adolescents experience some life problems and stress and yet, although many adolescents do respond to this with self-harming behaviour, the majority do not. Whilst each group of sub-factors in DSH appears to have important mediating factors, cognitive style and problem-solving ability may have an overarching influence in determining which adolescents are more or less likely to engage in acts of self-harm.

Several studies have suggested that adolescents who self-harm have poorer problem-solving skills than their non-harming peers (for example, Sadowski and Kelly, 1993; Reder et al., 1991). McLaughlin and colleagues (1996) note that adolescents in general might be expected to have fewer problem-solving resources than adults because they have fewer life experiences to draw from. However, Kingsbury and colleagues' study (1999) indicated that self-harming adolescents had poorer problem-solving abilities than both a non-harming peer control group and a group of adolescents with psychiatric diagnoses. Adolescents who have self-harmed tend to give more passive solutions in assessments of problem-solving skills and to generate fewer solutions to problems (Kingsbury et al., 1999). Additionally, adolescents who self-harm demonstrate higher levels of wishful thinking and a greater focus on problems, rather than solutions (Rotheram-Borus and Trautman, 1990). However, it has been suggested that in 'one off' episodes of self-harm many of these deficiencies are transitory and that performance on social skills assessments in young self-harmers can be linked to their depression scores (Spirito et al., 1990). Links have been made between repetitive self-injury and problem-solving deficiencies (Linehan, 1993).

Hopelessness is also linked to depression but also may exist as a permanent cognitive deficiency (McLaughlin et al., 1996). Hopelessness is one possible end result of a difficulty in problem-solving, when no solution to the problem is apparent. At this point, self-harm may be viewed as an attempt to generate a solution to the problem, even though this might be considered maladaptive. This is supported by an examination of what young people thought their self-harm would achieve. The majority of adolescents expect their self-harm to influence their problems – by their removal through death, a partial escape or a communication to those around them of their distress and need for help (McLaughlin et al., 1996; Dorer et al., 1998). McLaughlin and colleagues (1996) report that hopelessness is an important variable in adolescent DSH over and above the influence of depression. This has important implications for treatment, which will be discussed later.

Linked to hopelessness is locus of control. Adolescents who have self-harmed are more likely than non self-harmers to have an external, rather than an internal, locus of control (Pearce and Martin, 1993). At times of stress, we are more likely to cope if we believe that we have some power to influence the outcome of our situations. Young people who are under stress but believe that they have no power to change their situation are more likely first to become hopeless and then self-harm.

Managing DSH in children and adolescents

Having explored the meanings of self-harming behaviours I now wish to turn to the clinical implications of these. First I wish to consider good practice and guidelines for working with those who have presented to medical services after an episode of self-harm and, in particular, first contact in accident and emergency departments. As I will indicate, engaging a young person at this first point of contact is crucial for future treatment adherence and success. I then wish to explore a range of possible treatment options for working with adolescents who have self-harmed. Throughout these sections I wish to draw particular attention to the features that young people themselves find helpful, since these are not always routinely reported in studies of self-harm management strategies. Finally I want to explore the '$64,000 dollar question' – how do we prevent young people from engaging in acts of DSH? Lest I raise expectations falsely at this point, I have to admit that I am unable to claim the full cash prize with respect to this question! However, there are strategies that may be adopted that could have an impact on improving adolescent mental health and, consequently, reducing self-harm.

Presentation at accident and emergency departments

The accident and emergency department is often the first port of call for children and adolescents presenting with deliberate self-harm. Consequently, staff in these departments carry a considerable responsibility for beginning the process of engaging the young person in treatment. This is not an easy task. The majority of young people who have self-harmed, present at accident and emergency without having first made contact with their general practitioner or family doctor. This can make the collection and dissemination of essential third-party information extremely difficult (Nadkarni et al., 2000). Often they present alone or with non-parental family members, making it difficult to obtain consent for treatment and information for a full psychosocial assessment (Nadkarni et al., 2000). Staff within accident and emergency have not always received full training in recognizing and assessing self-harming behaviours and specialist staff are not always immediately available

(Horowitz et al., 2001). Recently, a brief screening tool to detect suicide risk has been developed for use in emergency room settings (Horowitz et al., 2001). The brief questionnaire contains questions on suicide risk, such as use of drugs and alcohol, and suicidal ideation. Early results are encouraging, however, further research is needed.

Young people themselves are often extremely fearful at the time of presentation. In one study, an adolescent reported feeling extremely anxious when faced with a wait for treatment in accident and emergency. She had taken an overdose, which was rated as having low potential lethality by staff, resulting in a brief waiting time before a full assessment took place. However, she was convinced that her life was at risk after the overdose and believed that the wait was likely to increase this risk (Dorer et al., 1998). Clear explanations of the reasons for actions, or lack of them, would have helped in this situation. Research also suggests that young people expect to receive harsh treatment from staff in accident and emergency and to be 'told off' for their behaviour. Receiving a non-judgemental response from staff has been rated as a particularly strong factor in young people's satisfaction with the service they receive (Burgess et al., 1998; Dorer et al., 1999). Young people who self-harm by cutting themselves report that they are less likely to receive such a response. This is possibly linked to staff's perceptions of the meaning of the behaviour. Superficial self-cutting is not generally seen as an attempt to end one's life and often the behaviour will be interpreted instead as 'attention seeking' (Smith et al., 1998). Adults who cut themselves report receiving harsh treatment in accident and emergency, sometimes even having wounds stitched without anaesthetic (Babiker and Arnold, 1997). As noted, research indicates that the problems of young people who injure themselves are broadly similar to those who take overdoses, and that self-injury is generally a sign of emotional distress. Therefore, staff in accident and emergency departments need to treat all adolescents who present with any form of DSH with compassion and sensitivity.

Hospital admission

It is essential that all children and adolescents who present to accident and emergency after an episode of DSH receive a full psychosocial assessment. However, there is some debate over where this assessment should take place. With appropriate training and support, accident and emergency staff can, and do, carry out assessments after self-harm. In the UK, the Royal College of Psychiatrists (RCP) has issued guidelines that recommend admission to hospital in all cases of DSH, regardless of physical medical need (RCP, 1998). This is for a number of reasons. Self-harm is often the route by which problems, particularly those within the family such as sexual abuse, first come to light. Admission gives young people 'time-out' from the stressful situation and may provide the space and security for them to discus their difficulties. Admission also gives the message that the self-harming behaviour has been taken seriously by health professionals. Finally, admission can allow more time for a full assessment to take place and for the involvement of Child and Adolescent Mental Health Services (CAMHS). In the UK, admission is not routine in all cases of DSH. A recent survey of DSH policies in one geographical region suggested that only 36% of policies made reference to automatic admission (Dorer, 1998). In the majority of cases, admission relates primarily to medical need. Consequently, those who have taken overdoses are more likely to be admitted to hospital than those who have self-injured through relatively superficial self-cutting.

The value of admission has been questioned in a number of studies. For those admitted, there is no conclusive evidence that hospital admission significantly reduces suicide risk (Greenhill and Waslick, 1997). Young people's experience of admission tends to be mixed. Whilst some report appreciating their removal from stressful situations, many report feeling bored whilst in hospital and older adolescents often find it difficult to be surrounded by much younger children when placed on general paediatric wards (Dorer et al., 1998). At present, there is little in the way of research into the specific characteristics of the children and adolescents who would benefit most from admission. However, admission should always be considered for those young people presenting with a persistent wish to die and those whose families are either unable or unwilling to provide close supervision and support (American Academy of Child and Adolescent Psychiatry, 2001).

Inpatient admission can be problematic due to the risk of contagion. An episode of self-harm in one young person often triggers further episodes in other young people. Psychiatric inpatients appear to be at particular risk from self-harm contagion, both with lethal and non-lethal intent (Taiminen et al., 1992). Self-harm through self-cutting appears to have a particular influence on young people, specifically young women, hospitalized with personality disorders (Taiminen et al., 1998). Taiminen and colleagues (1998) have recommended that the concentration of young women with personality disorders within an inpatient unit should be kept as low as possible or that admission should be kept to less than two weeks to reduce the sense of a 'self-harm subculture'. Research also suggests that open communication about self-cutting, in a neutral manner reduces the number of incidents of the behaviour (Ross and McKay, 1979).

Therapeutic interventions

Improving treatment adherence

Young people who self-harm are a difficult group to engage in treatment. Adherence to outpatient treatment is poor and up to 48% of adolescents have dropped out of treatment by their third appointment (Trautman et al., 1993). Those who are non-compliant with treatment are at risk of repeat episodes of self-harm, so it is important that non-compliance is not taken to mean a lack of need for treatment (Stewart et al., 2001). This is one possible reason for locating assessment, and even some forms of intervention, in accident and emergency departments (Rotheram-Borus et al., 1996). Rotheram-Borus and colleagues suggest that a specialized emergency room programme, involving staff training, a video modifying families' expectations of treatment and an on-call family therapist improves treatment adherence in adolescents. However, mothers were less likely to complete the treatment programme and the programme was most effective for families with more cohesive relations (Rotheram-Borus et al., 1996).

Ideally, all adolescents who have engaged in an episode of self-harm should be offered an early follow-up appointment after discharge from hospital or emergency room. However, resource limitations sometimes make this impossible and adolescents can be particularly vulnerable during the intervening time. One option to reduce this vulnerability is to give young self-harmers open access to support via an emergency telephone number. Morgan et al. (1993) gave adult suicidal patients a card containing emergency contact details, which led to a reduced rate in repeated self-harm. Studies of similar approaches with adolescents have been less conclusive. Cotgrove and colleagues (1995) found that issuing a card with emergency contact details, and the right to automatic readmission to hospital on demand, led to a substantial, but not significant, reduction in the rate of repeat self-harm over a 12-month period. Dorer et al. (1998) found that the majority of cards given out to adolescents were lost or forgotten about. However, the few young people who made use of the card did not engage in any further acts of self-harm over a 6-month period.

'No harm' contracts

The establishment of 'no-harm' or 'no-suicide contract' is often a key feature of treatment programmes with young self-harmers. There are advantages and disadvantages to using such contracts. On the plus side, the clinician is able to give a strong message about wanting to keep the young person safe and alive. The young person is also given the message that they, and their family, must take some responsibility for maintaining their safety. In establishing a contract, the clinician also has some professional protection should further episodes of self-harm occur. However, it is important that this is not seen as a substitute for professional treatment. A no-harm contract will only be useful if the young person or family can make contact with services immediately if they experience suicidal ideation or the wish to self-harm (Brent, 1997). Possible disadvantages of contracts are that they may encourage clinicians and family members to relax their vigilance. Also, the young person may not be in a mental state to fully understand or agree with a contract (AACAP, 2001).

The use of no-harm contracts is particularly contentious in working with young people who self-injure. Some authors maintain that no-harm contracts are a necessary condition for an effective therapeutic alliance. Conterio et al. (1999), who run the Self-Abuse Finally Ends (SAFE) inpatient programme in America, insist that all clients refrain from self-harm whilst on the programme. They view self-injury as a maladaptive coping resource and believe that self-harmers must learn to resist the compulsion to hurt themselves. Consequently, no level of self-harm is seen as being acceptable, including coping strategies such as holding ice or drawing red marks on the body, which mimic self-injury. Other authors (for example, Babiker and Arnold, 1997; Harrison, 1995) view no-harm contracts as problematic. Self-injury is often used as means of controlling and coping with an aspect of the young person's life, particularly strong emotions that might be perceived as overwhelming. Denying access to this coping mechanism may leave the young person extremely vulnerable. Also, young people who have self-injured have reported finding covert ways to hurt themselves whilst apparently contained by no-harm contracts. For example, an adolescent who has previously injured herself by cutting her arms may chose to cut more easily hidden parts of her body such as her breasts or stomach, or choose less visible forms of self-injury such as head banging. Clearly, when a contract that has been established to form a therapeutic alliance actually leads to the very behaviour being treated simply being driven out of sight, but maintained, the value must be questioned. It may be possible that some compromise can be reached through the formation of safety-planning agreements (for example, Alderman 1997). Here, the expectation can be created that the clinician expects the young person to refrain from self-harm and either seek support from another person or use an alternative strategy, should they experience the urge to hurt themselves. However, the agreement also recognizes that further episodes of self-harm may occur and seeks to minimize harm in such situations, for example by asking the young person only to use clean cutting implements or to only make a single cut.

Pharmacological treatments

The use of pharmacological treatments for adolescents who have self-harmed has received mixed support. Since depression is such an important risk factor for repeated self-harm, anti-depressants may be considered as a treatment option. However, the use of tricyclic anti-depressants is generally not recommended for adolescents because of relative lack of effectiveness, side-effects and the risk of lethality in overdose (Hazell et al., 1995). However, anti-depressants that are less toxic in overdose, such as the SSRIs, may have a role to play in treating depression in adolescents who self-harm, in conjunction with other approaches (Ambrosini et al., 1995). Depot flupenthixol has been found to have some effectiveness for adults who engage in repetitive self-injury (Montgomery et al., 1979). However, it is unlikely that this would prove to be a popular choice of treatment for children and adolescents.

Psychotherapeutic interventions

A range of psychotherapeutic interventions has been used in working with self-harming children and adolescents. Unfortunately, to date, there have been insufficient large-scale studies to conduct a full comparison of approaches, or recommend which might be the most effective (Hawton et al., 1998). However, a number of approaches have been identified that appear to have strengths in working with this clinical population. Cognitive behavioural therapies (CBT) have been found to be particularly useful with children and adolescents who self-harm. In a number of studies (for example, Brent et al., 1998a) CBT has been found to be more effective than non-directive supportive therapy. Cognitive behavioural therapy addresses key risk factors such as depression whilst modifying high-risk cognitions, such as hopelessness and perfectionism, and addressing deficits such as problem-solving and affect-regulation skills (Brent, 1997). Marsha Linehan's dialectical behaviour therapy (1993), which contains many elements of CBT, has also been shown to be effective with young harmers, specifically those who have repeatedly self-injured.

Given the difficulties in engaging this client group, Kerfoot and colleagues (1995) have pioneered a home-based programme for young self-harmers. This programme involves working with the whole family to address issues such as family communication and problem-solving skills. However, a recent evaluation did not indicate that this approach was any more effective than the range of treatments received by the control group, including outpatient appointments with psychiatrists and psychiatric nurses (Harrington et al., 1998). The programme did have the benefits of high compliance and high parent satisfaction at the 2-month assessment point. Wagner and colleagues (2000) suggest that, in working with families of self-harmers, it may be helpful to discuss common family reactions. This may help to 'normalize' parents' experiences and allow them to process feelings that they may have found unacceptable, such as anger towards their child. Other family-based interventions such as systemic family therapy have been suggested to be less effective than CBT (Brent et al., 1998a) in treating depression in young people. Controlled studies of family therapy, which relate specifically to self-harm, are difficult to find. However, the American Academy of Child and Adolescent Psychiatry do suggest that family therapy could be considered as a treatment option. Psychodynamic psychotherapy receives a similar endorsement, however, again, controlled studies are thin on the ground.

Helpful responses to self-harm – using the views of young people who self-harm

Young people consistently report the value of being listened to when talking about stress or difficulties in their lives (Hill, 1995). However, they do not always find it easy, either to initiate discussions on these topics or even to find the language to express their distress. Clinicians need to find ways of facilitating discussion and of indicating a willingness to listen and tolerate the adolescent's distress. As mentioned earlier, young people expect to be judged harshly for their self-harm and this can result in them attempting to minimize their distress or suggest that causal problems have been resolved. It may be difficult for adolescents to discuss their difficulties but it can also be a relief when someone is able to see beyond the self-harming behaviour to think about them as people and their current experiences and problems. This is particularly true when working with young people who self-injure. Often work becomes entirely focused on the self-harming behaviour itself when in fact it is just an expression of other difficulties. A reduction in self-harming behaviour is desirable but it should be achieved as an effect of addressing other difficulties, with a focus on the person, rather than the behaviour.

Preventing self-harm and suicide

It is encouraging that there is now a range of treatments to support children and adolescents who have harmed themselves. However, it would be even more encouraging if we could find a way of preventing them from doing it in the first place! Unfortunately, this challenge has yet to be met fully, despite a range of programmes designed to prevent self-harm. Telephone hotlines, either aimed specifically at children (such as Childline) or at the general population (such as The Samaritans) clearly have a role to play in supporting suicidal young people. However, early evaluation studies had a number of methodological problems and failed to show that hotlines reduce the incidence of self-harming behaviours (AACAP, 2001). Anecdotal evidence suggests that such services can play a very important role in supporting individual adolescents, but their widespread effectiveness as a general preventative tool remains untested to date.

There have been a number of school-based programmes introduced with the aim of encouraging suicide awareness and self or third-party disclosure of self-harming behaviours. Klingman and Hochdorf (1993) designed a school-based, cognitive behavioural programme to improve students' ability to cope with distress and to encourage them to act as 'gatekeepers' for each other with regard to self-harming behaviours. The programme appeared to have a positive effect on attitudes, knowledge and awareness of coping skills. However, there is no longer term information about how participation in this programme contributed to a reduction in self-harming behaviours among the student group. This has tended to be a problem in evaluating similar programmes and, to date, there is little evidence to support the efficacy of school-based suicide education programmes (Burns and Patton, 2000). It has been suggested that programmes that focus on improving the general mental health of adolescents and, in particular, addressing depression, might have a bigger impact on self-harming behaviour than addressing the topic directly, in isolation of other factors (AACAP, 2001).

The 'broad brush' approach to self-harm prevention does not appear to be highly effective, so it has been suggested that interventions should focus on identifying young people who are particularly at risk of self-harm (Burns and Patton, 2000). Thompson and Eggert (1999) have recently developed the Suicide Risk Screen. This aims to identify young people at risk of suicide amongst the already high-risk group of school dropouts. Other similar scales have been developed (for example, Lewinsohn et al., 1996; Larzelere et al., 1996), however, they have proved to be relatively inaccurate at detecting youths who later attempted suicide and there has been a high rate of 'false positives'. The Suicide Risk Screen has shown encouraging early findings, identifying young people by risk factors rather than only past episodes of self-harm. However, the rate of false positives was again high, suggesting that this may be something that must be tolerated when introducing screening programmes.

Conclusion

Self-harm is a growing problem amongst children and adolescents. As health and social care professionals we must always take acts of self-harm seriously and as an indication of difficulties and distress within the young person's life. We can now identify a number of factors that put young people at an increased risk of repeated self-harm and suggest a range of treatments that are effective in reducing the depression and cognitive distortions that lead to self-harming behaviours. Our ability to prevent self-harm remains somewhat limited. However, it is now possible to identify, with some confidence, risk factors that make young people particularly vulnerable. With sensitive, responsive treatment the difficulties that lead young people to self-harm can be effectively addressed. However, this is an area of work where the clinician must remain particularly vigilant and ongoing research is essential, particularly in the areas of preventative strategies and effective treatment programmes.

References

Alderman T (1997) The Scarred Soul: Understanding and Ending Self-inflicted Violence. New York: New Harbinger Publishers.

Allison S, Pearce C, Martin C, Miller K, Long R (1996) Parental influence, pessimism and adolescent suicidality. Archives of Suicide Research 1: 229–42.

Ambrosini PJ, Emslie GJ, Greenhill LL, Kutcher S (1995) Selecting a sequence of antidepressants for treatment of depression in youth. Journal of Child and Adolescent Psychopharmacology 5: 233–40.

American Academy of Child and Adolescent Psychiatry (2001) Summary of the practice parameters for the assessment and treatment of children and adolescents with suicidal behaviour. J Am Acad Child and Adolescent Psychiatry 40: 495–9.

Andrews JA, Lewinsohn PM (1992) Suicide attempts among older adolescents: prevalence and co-occurrence with psychiatric disorders. J Am Acad Child and Adolescent Psychiatry 31: 655–62.

Apter A, Kotler M, Sevy S, Plutchick R, Brown S, Foster H, Hillbrand M, Korn ML, van Praag HM (1991) Correlates of risk of suicide in violent and non-violent psychiatric patients. American Journal of Psychiatry 148(7): 883–7.

Armistead L, Klein K, Forehand R (1995) Parental physical illness and child functioning. Clinical Psychology Review 15: 409–22.

Asarnow JR (1992) Suicidal ideation and attempts during middle childhood: associations with perceived family stress and depression among child psychiatric inpatients. Journal of Clinical Child Psychiatry 21: 35–40.

Babiker G, Arnold L (1997) The Language of Injury – Comprehending Self-Mutilation. Leicester: BPS Books.

Barker LA, Adelman H (1994) Mental health and help-seeking among ethnic minority adolescents. Journal of Adolescence 17: 251–63.

Belsky J (1993) Etiology of child mistreatment: a developmental-ecological analysis. Psychological Bulletin 111: 413–34.

Beratis S (1990) Factors associated with adolescent suicide attempts in Greece. Psychopathology 23: 161–8.

Boergers J, Spirito A, Donaldson D (1998) Reasons for adolescent suicide attempts: associations with psychological functioning. J Am Acad of Child and Adolescent Psychiatry 37: 1287–93.

Bowlby J (1980) Attachment and Loss. Vol. III: Loss. New York: Basic Books.

Brent DA (1997) Practitioner review: the aftercare of adolescents with deliberate self-harm. J Child Psychology and Psychiatry 38: 277–86.

Brent DA, Kolko DJ, Allan MJ, Brown RV (1990) Suicidality in affectively disordered adolescent inpatients. J Am Acad Child and Adolescent Psychiatry 29: 589–93.

Brent DA, Johnson B, Bartle S, Bridge J, Rather C, Matta J, Connolly J, Constantine D (1993) Personality disorder, tendency to impulsive violence and suicidal behaviour in adolescents. J Am Acad Child and Adolescent Psychiatry 32: 69–75.

Brent DA, Kolko D, Birmaher B, Baugher M, Bridge J, Roth C, Holder D (1998a) Predictors of treatment efficacy in a clinical trial of three psychosocial treatments for adolescent depression. J Am Acad Child and Adolescent Psychiatry 37: 906–14.

Brent DA, Baugher M, Bridge J, Chen T, Chiapetta L (1998b) Age and sex-related risk factors for adolescent suicide. J Am Acad Child and Adolescent Psychiatry 98: 1497–505.

Brown J, Cohen P, Johnson JG, Smailes EM (1999) Childhood abuse and neglect: specificity of effects on adolescent and young adult depression and suicidality. J Am Acad Child and Adolescent Psychiatry 38: 1490–6.

Burgess S, Hawton K, Loveday G (1998) Adolescents who take overdoses: outcome in terms of changes in psychopathology and the adolescents' attitudes to care and to their overdose. Journal of Adolescence 21: 209–18.

Burns JM, Patton GC (2000) Preventative interventions for youth suicide: a risk factor-based approach. Australian and New Zealand Journal of Psychiatry 34: 388–407.

Clark DC, Sommerfeld L, Schwartz M, Hedeker D, Watel L (1990) Physical recklessness in adolescence. Trait or byproduct of depressive/suicidal states? Journal of Nervous and Mental Disease 178: 423–33.

Conterio K, Lader W, Kingson Bloom J (1999) Bodily Harm: The Breakthrough Healing Programme for Self-injurers. New York: Hyperion Books.

Cotgrove A, Zirinsky L, Black D, Weston D (1995) Secondary prevention of attempted suicide in adolescence. Journal of Adolescence 18: 569–77.

Courtois C (1996) Healing the Incest Wound. New York: WW Norton Company.

Diekstra RFW, Kienhorst CWM, De Wilde EJ (1995) Suicide and suicidal behaviour among adolescents. In Rutter M, Smith DJ (eds) Psychosocial Disorders in Young People Time Trends and their Causes. Chichester: Wiley, pp. 686–761.

Dorer C (1998) An evaluation of protocols for child and adolescent deliberate self-harm. Child Psychology and Psychiatry Review 3: 156–60.

Dorer C, Vostanis P, Feehan C, Winkley L (1998) Self-harming Behaviours in Young People. Unpublished report for Birmingham Children's Hospital.

Dorer C, Feehan C, Vostanis P, Winkley L (1999) The overdose process – adolescents' experience of taking an overdose and their contact with services. Journal of Adolescence 22: 413–17.

Flannery DJ, Singer MI, Webster K (2001) Violence exposure, psychological trauma and suicide risk in a community sample of dangerously violent adolescents. J Am Acad Child and Adolescent Psychiatry 40: 435–42.

Flisher AJ (1999) Mood disorder in suicidal children and adolescents: recent developments. Journal of Child Psychology and Psychiatry 40: 315–24.

Garnefski N, Diekstra R (1995) Suicidal behaviour and the co-occurrence of behavioural, emotional and cognitive problems among adolescents. Archives of Suicide Research 1: 243–60.

Garnefski N, Diekstra RFW, De Heus P (1992) A population-based survey of the characteristics of high school students with and without a history of suicidal behaviour. Acta Psychiatrica Scandinavica 86: 189–96.

Gibson P (1989) Gay male and lesbian youth suicide. In Report of the Secretary's Task Force on Youth Suicide. Washington DC: US Government Printing Office, pp. 110–42.

Gladstone G, Parker G, Wilhelm K, Mitchell P, Austin M (1999) Characteristics of depressed patients who report childhood sexual abuse. Am J Psych 156: 431–7.

Goddard N, Subotsky F, Fombonne E (1996) Ethnicity and adolescent deliberate self-harm. Journal of Adolescence 19: 513–21.

Gould MS, King R, Greenwald S, Fisher P, Schwab-Stone M, Kramer R, Flisher A, Goodman S, Canino G, Shaffer D (1998) Psychopathology associated with suicidal ideation and attempts among children and adolescents. J Am Acad Child and Adolescent Psychiatry 37: 915–23.

Greenhill LL, Waslick B (1997) Management of suicidal behaviour in children and adolescents. Psychiatr Clin North Am 37: 915–23.

Groholt B, Ekeberg O, Wichstrom L, Rouleau M, Wagner KD (2000) Young suicide attempters: a comparison between a clinical and an epidemiological sample. J Am Acad Child and Adolescent Psychiatry 39: 876–80.

Harrington R, Kerfoot M, Dyer E, McNiven F, Gill J, Harrington V, Woodham A, Byford S (1998) Randomised trial of a home-based family intervention for children who have deliberately poisoned themselves. J Am Acad Child and Adolescent Psychiatry, 37: 512–18.

Harrison D (1995) Vicious Circles. London: GPMH.

Hawton K, Fagg J (1992) Deliberate self-poisoning and self-injury in adolescents: a study of characteristics and trends in Oxford 1976–1989. B J Psych 161: 816–23.

Hawton K, Osborn M, O'Grady J, Cole D (1982) Classification of adolescents who take overdoses. B J Psych 140: 124–31.

Hawton K, Fagg J, Simkin S, Bale E, Bond A (1997) Trends in deliberate self-harm in Oxford, 1985–1995. B J Psych 171: 556–60.

Hawton K, Arensman E, Townsend E, Bremner S, Feldman E, Goldney R, Hazell R, Van Heeringen K, House A, Owens D, Sakinofsky I, Traksman-Bendz L (1998) Deliberate self-harm: systematic review of efficacy of psychosocial and pharmacological treatments in preventing repetition. British Medical Journal 317: 441–7.

Hawton K, Kingsbury S, Steinhardt K, James A, Fagg J (1999) Repetition of deliberate self-harm by adolescents: the role of psychological factors. Journal of Adolescence 22: 369–78.

Hawton K, Fagg J, Simkin S, Bale E, Bond A (2000) Deliberate self-harm in adolescents in Oxford, 1985–1995. Journal of Adolescence 23: 47–55.

Hazell P, O'Connell O, Heathcote D, Robertson J, Henry D (1995) Efficacy of tricyclic drugs in treating child and adolescent depression: a meta-analysis. British Medical Journal 310: 897–901.

Herman J (1992) Trauma and Recovery. London: HarperCollins.

Hill K (1995) The Long Sleep. Young People and Suicide. London: Virago.

Horowitz LM, Wang PS, Koocher GP, Burr BH, Fallon Smith M, Klavon S, Cleary PD (2001) Detecting suicide risk in a paediatric emergency department: development of a brief screening tool. Paediatrics 107: 1133–7.

Kandel DB, Ravies VH, Davies M (1991) Suicidal ideation in adolescence: depression, substance use and other risk factors. Journal of Youth and Adolescence 20: 289–309.

Kerfoot M, Harrington RC, Dyer E (1995) Brief home-based intervention with young suicide attempters and their families. Journal of Adolescence 18: 557–68.

Kerfoot M, Dyer E, Harrington V, Wordham A, Harrington R (1996) Correlates and short-term course of self-poisoning in adolescents. B J Psych 168: 38–42.

Kienhorst CWM, DeWilde EJ, Diekstra RFM (1995) Adolescents' image of their suicide attempt. Journal of the American Academy of Child and Adolescent Psychiatry 34: 623–8.

Kingsbury S (1994) The psychological and social characteristics of Asian adolescent overdose. Journal of Adolescence 17: 131–5.

Kingsbury S, Hawton K, Steinhardt K, James A (1999) Do adolescents who take overdoses have specific psychological characteristics? A comparative study with psychiatric and community controls. J Am Acad Child and Adolescent Psychiatry 38: 1125–31.

Klingman A, Hochdorf Z (1993) Coping with distress and self-harm: the impact of a primary prevention program among adolescents. Journal of Adolescence 16: 121–40.

Kotila L, Lonnqvist J (1987) Adolescents who make suicide attempts repeatedly. Acta Psychiatrica Scandinavica 79: 453–9.

Kovacs M, Goldstone D, Gastonis C (1993) Suicidal behaviours and childhood-onset depressive disorder: a longitudinal investigation. J Am Acad Child and Adolescent Psychiatry 32: 8–20.

Langhinrichsen-Rohling J, Lewinsohn P, Rohde P, Seley J, Monson CM, Meyer KA, Langford R (1998) Gender differences in the suicide-related behaviours of adolescents and young adults. Sex Roles: A Journal of Research 39: 839–54.

Larzelere RE, Smith GL, Batenhorst LM, Kelly DB (1996) Predictive validity of the Suicide Probability Scale among adolescents in group home treatment. Journal of the American Academy of Child and Adolescent Psychiatry 35: 166–72.

Levenkron S (1998) Cutting – Understanding and Overcoming Self-mutilation. New York: Norton.

Lewinsohn PM, Rhode P, Seeley JR (1993) Psychosocial characteristics of adolescents with a history of suicide attempt. Journal of the American Academy of Child and Adolescent Psychiatry 32: 60–8.

Lewinsohn PM, Langhinrichsen-Rohling J, Langford R, Rhode P, Seeley JR, Chapman J (1995) The life attitudes schedule: a scale to assess adolescent life-enhancing and life-threatening behaviours. Suicide and Life-Threatening Behaviour 25: 458–74.

Linehan M (1993) Cognitive behavioural treatment of borderline personality disorder. New York: Guilford Press.

Lock J, Steiner H (1999) Gay, lesbian and bisexual youth risks for emotional, physical and social problems: results from a community-based survey. J Am Acad Child and Adolescent Psychiatry 38: 297–304.

Maniam T (1988) Suicide and parasuicide in a hill resort in Malaysia. B J Psych 153: 222–5.

McKeown R, Garrison CZ, Cuffe SP, Waller JL, Jackson KL, Addy CL (1998) Incidence and predictors of suicidal behaviours in a longitudinal sample of young adolescents. J Am Acad Child and Adolescent Psychiatry 37: 612–20.

McLaughlin J, Miller P, Warwick H (1996) Deliberate self harm in adolescents: hopelessness, depression, problems and problem-solving. Journal of Adolescence 19: 523–32.

Menninger K (1938) Man Against Himself. London: Harvest Books.

Merril J, Owens J (1986) Ethnic differences in self-poisoning: a comparison of Asian and Caucasian Groups. B J Psych 148: 708–12.

Michel K, Valach L, Waeber V (1994) Understanding deliberate self-harm: the patients' views. Crisis 15: 172–8.

Miller D (1994) Women who Hurt Themselves. New York: Basic Books.

Montgomery SA, Montgomery DB, Jayanthi-Rani S, Roy DH, Shaw PJ, McAuley R (1979) Maintenance therapy in repeat suicidal behaviour: a placebo-controlled trial. Proceedings of the 10th International Congress for Suicide Prevention and Crisis Intervention, Ottawa, pp. 227–9.

Morgan H, Jones E, Owen J (1993) Secondary prevention of non-fatal deliberate self-harm. The Green card study. B J Psych 163: 111–12.

Nadkarni A, Parkin A, Dogra N, Stretch DD, Evans PA (2000) Characteristics of children and adolescents presenting to accident and emergency departments with deliberate self-harm. Journal of Accident and Emergency Medicine 17: 98–102.

Nolen-Hoeksema S (1994) An interactive model for the emergence of gender differences in depression in adolescence. Journal of Research on Adolescence 4: 519–34.

Otto U (1972) Suicidal acts by children and adolescents (Suppl. 233) Acta Psychiatrica Scandinavica 306: 7–123.

Overholser J, Adams D, Lenhert K, Brinkman D (1995) Self-esteem deficits and suicidal tendencies among adolescents. J Am Acad Child and Adolescent Psychiatry 34: 919–28.

Patton GC, Harris R, Carlin JB, Hibbert ME, Coffey C, Schwartz M, Bowes G (1997) Adolescent suicidal behaviours: a population-based study of risk. Psychological Medicine 27: 715–24.

Pearce CM, Martin G (1993) Locus of control as an indicator of risk for suicidal behaviour among adolescents. Acta Psychiatrica Scandinavica 88: 409–14.

Reder P, Lucey C, Fredman G (1991) The challenge of deliberate self-harm by young adolescents. Journal of Adolescence 14: 135–48.

Renvoize J (1993) Innocence Destroyed. A Study of Child Sexual Abuse. London: Routledge.

Ross RR, McKay HB (1979) Self-Mutilation. Toronto: Lexington Books, DC Heath.

Rotheram-Borus MJ, Trautman PD (1990) Cognitive style and pleasant activities among adolescent female suicide attempters. Journal of Consulting and Clinical Psychology 58: 554–61.

Rotheram-Borus MJ, Rosario M, Reid H, Koopman C (1995) Predicting patterns of sexual acts among homosexual and bisexual youths. American Journal of Psychiatry 152: 588–95.

Rotheram-Borus M, Piacentini J, Rossem R, Graae F, Cantwell C, Van Castro-Blanco D, Miller S, Feldman J (1996) Enhancing treatment adherence with a specialized emergency room program for adolescent suicide attempters. J Am Acad Child and Adolescent Psychiatry 35: 654–63.

Royal College of Psychiatrists (1998) Managing deliberate self-harm in young people. Council Report CR64. RCP: London.

Sadowski C, Kelly ML (1993) Social problem solving in suicidal adolescents. Journal of Consulting and Clinical Psychology 61: 121–7.

Shaffer D, Piacentini J (1994) Suicide and attempted suicide. In Rutter M, Taylor E, Hersov L (eds) Child and Adolescent Psychiatry: Modern Approaches. 3 edn. Oxford: Blackwell, pp. 407–24.

Shaffer D, Gould MS, Fisher P, Trautman D, Moreau D, Kleitman M, Flory M (1996) Psychiatric diagnosis in child and adolescent suicide. Archives of General Psychiatry 53: 339–48.

Smith G, Cox D, Saradjian J (1998) Women and Self-harm. London: Women's Press.

Spirito A, Hart K, Overholser J, Halverson J (1990) Social skills and depression in adolescent suicide attempters. Adolescence 25: 543–52.

Stein D, Apter A, Ratzoni G, Har-Even D, Avidan G (1998) Associations between multiple suicide attempts and negative affects in adolescents. J Am Acad Child and Adolescent Psychiatry 37: 488–94.

Stewart SE, Manion IG, Davidson S, Cloutier P (2001) Suicidal children and adolescents with first emergency room presentations: predictors of six-month outcome. J Am Acad Child and Adolescent Psychiatry 40: 580–7.

Taminen TJ, Salmenpera T, Lehtinen K (1992) A suicide epidemic in a psychiatric hospital. Suicide and Life-Threatening Behaviour 22: 350–63.

Taiminen TJ, Kallio-Soukainen K, Nokso-Koivito H, Kaljonen A, Helenius H (1998) Contagion of deliberate self-harm among adolescent inpatients. J Am Acad Child and Adolescent Psychiatry 37: 211–17.

Thompson EA, Eggert LL (1999) Using the Suicide Risk Screen to identify suicidal adolescents among potential high school dropouts. J Am Acad Child and Adolescent Psychiatry 38: 1506–14.

Trautman PD, Stewart N, Morishma A (1993) Are adolescent suicide attempters noncompliant with outpatient care? J Am Acad Child and Adolescent Psychiatry 32: 89–94.

Tulloch AL, Blizzard L, Pinkus Z (1997) Adolescent-parent communication in self-harm. Journal of Adolescent Health 21: 267–75.

Wagman-Borowsky I, Ireland M, Resnick MD (2001) Adolescent suicide attempts: risks and protectors. Paediatrics 107: 485–93.

Wagner BM, Aiken C, Mullaley M, Tobin J (2000) Parents' reactions to adolescents' suicide attempts. J Am Acad Child and Adolescent Psychiatry 39: 429–36.

SECTION 2

FAMILY-RELATED ISSUES

CHAPTER 6

Gene-environment transactions and family process: implications for clinical research and practice

KIRBY DEATER-DECKARD, BERNADETTE MARIE BULLOCK

From the beginning of the evolving field of psychology there has been a strong emphasis placed on the role of the family in children's healthy and maladaptive development. From Freud (1995) to Bronfenbrenner (1986), the family context has been regarded as critical. Parents are considered by many to be the primary and most powerful socializing agents in children's lives and, as we describe in more detail later, this view is warranted. However, it is equally important to consider the 'genetic' context of the family – that is, in addition to providing environments for their children, in most families the parents are also transmitting genetic material to their offspring (Scarr, 1992). In nearly every family, the family members share genes as well as experiences. Furthermore, the 'familiality' of individual outcomes (for example, parent-child similarity in aggression or sibling similarity in cognitive performance) is thought to arise not as a result of independent genetic and environmental influences but rather from a complex interplay between genes and the environment (Plomin, 1994).

This is not a new realization. Scientists have long grappled with the roles of heredity and the environment in human development. Historically, empirical research has generally fallen into either a biological or a psychosocial/environmental rubric, with relatively few researchers attempting to address the interplay between genes and environments. More recently, quantitative and molecular genetic as well as medical and psychological researchers have come to acknowledge the dynamic interplay between genetic and environmental factors and the necessity of exploring this synergy in the study of mental health throughout the lifespan. It is our contention that research and practice is informed by an integrative approach that addresses the ways in which genetic and environmental influences work together. Thus, our goal in this chapter is to examine the operation of genes and environments within the family context with respect to individual differences in mental health outcomes. We begin with a general overview of research on family environments and genetic influences, followed by a discussion of gene-environment transactions. We then examine the implications of behavioural genetic approaches on our understanding of family process, mental health and the efficacy of interventions.

Family influences

The literature regarding the influence of the environment on mental health is vast and provides substantial support for the role of environmental factors on nearly all aspects of development. A review of the environmental literature is beyond the focus of this chapter, so the following synopsis will focus on family relationship processes and their links to mental health outcomes in offspring.

Of the many environmental influences that have been and continue to be explored, family relationships – and parent-child relationships in particular – have received the most attention, in part because of the consistent findings linking these factors to mental health outcomes. These factors can be conceptualized as direct effects, such as harsh or coercive parenting strategies and poor monitoring (Deater-Deckard and Dodge, 1997; Patterson, Reid and Dishion, 1992), indirect effects that are mediated through relationships with siblings (Bank, Patterson and Reid, 1996; Bullock and Dishion, in press), or bidirectional effects between family members (Dishion and Bullock, in press; Lollis and Kuczynski, 1997).

Parenting

A substantial literature supports the relation between parenting practices and child and adolescent behavioural adjustment. Factors such as coercive discipline (Patterson, 1982), inconsistent limit setting (Gardner, 1989), poor family management skills (Baumrind, Moselle and Martin, 1985; Block, Block and Keyes, 1988; Loeber and Dishion, 1983), ineffective parent monitoring and discipline (Conger, Patterson and Ge, 1995; Forgatch, 1991) and inadequate supervision (Wilson, 1980) have each been found to be related to the development and course of antisocial problem behaviour.

Clinical research regarding the effects of parenting on ameliorating child problem behaviour also supports the relationship between parenting practices and child outcomes. Interventions targeting family management practices have resulted in a significant decline in problem behaviour with young children (Webster-Stratton, 1990; Patterson,

1984) as well as adolescents (Dishion, Andrews, Kavanagh and Soberman, 1996; Henggeler, Schoenwald, Borduin, Rowland and Cunningham, 1998), suggesting that changes in the rearing environment can result in changes in child outcomes. Moreover, longitudinal intervention studies that focus on fostering the development of effective parenting in domains such as parent-child communication and family management skills have resulted in significantly lower rates of academic difficulty and emotional and behavioural problems in the target children and their siblings (Arnold, Levine and Patterson, 1975; Seitz and Apfel, 1994).

Internalizing problems (for example, anxiety, depression) among children and adolescents are also influenced by parent-child interaction, particularly when one or both parents are themselves depressed (Downey and Coyne, 1990). For example, studies of parental 'expressed emotion' – the extent to which the parent is critical of or overly emotionally involved with a child – suggest that there is an association between maternal expressed emotion and child internalizing problems. Some of this research has shown that high maternal expressed emotion, particularly criticism, is more common among mothers of adolescents diagnosed with depressive disorder, mania, substance abuse and conduct disorder (Schwartz, Dorer, Beardslee, Lavori and Keller, 1990), and among mothers of children with major depressive disorder or dysthymia (Asarnow, Tompson, Hamilton, Goldstein and Guthrie, 1994). In one study, high maternal expressed emotion ratings predicted one-year, postdischarge outcomes of children with major depressive or dysthymic disorder, even after statistically controlling for mediating variables such as medication and psychological intervention, age, gender, and socioeconomic status (Asarnow, Goldstein, Tompson and Guthrie, 1990). In another, higher rates of anxiety disorders in children were found for children whose parents expressed high levels of emotional overinvolvement when compared with the remainder of the sample (Stubbe, Zahner, Goldstein and Leckman, 1993).

In sum, parenting practices and the quality of parent-child relationships are important with respect to the onset and course of child and adolescent externalizing and internalizing problems. These data clearly implicate the rearing environment in youth mental health and psychosocial adjustment. We hasten to add that these findings do not necessarily imply uni-directional causal processes in the parent-child dyad, with parenting behaviour causing child maladjustment. Instead, parenting should be conceptualized as part of a dynamic and reciprocal exchange between parent and child, whereby child attributes and behaviour can also serve to elicit certain parenting behaviours and vice versa (Dishion and Bullock, in press; Deater-Deckard and O'Connor, 2000; Rothbart and Bates, 1998).

This 'bidirectional' conceptualization of the parenting environment is critical to our understanding of transactions between genes and environments, a point to which we return later.

Siblings

The contribution of parents to the mental health and wellbeing of their children is well established, but family systems theory suggests that the sibling relationship also makes an important contribution (Minuchin, 1985). Thus, the sibling relationship is another component of the family environment that should be considered. Sibling interaction has been shown to be prognostic of mental health outcomes in several domains. For example, high levels of sibling conflict are associated with each child's problems in peer relationships, academic difficulties and antisocial behaviours (Bank, Patterson and Reid, 1996; Loeber and Tengs, 1986; Patterson, 1982). Conversely, supportive sibling relationships may serve to actually protect children from other adverse circumstances (for example, parental divorce, poverty) and lead to better outcomes for some high-risk children who would otherwise show more severe signs of impairment (Brody, 1998).

Sibling relationships are important because they function as an additional and unique socialization influence within most families. Sibling interactions serve as a training ground for negotiating conflict, particularly in families that are characterized by high rates of negativity and discord. For instance, verbal and physical aggression between siblings operates as a form of escape conditioning whereby children learn to use hostile behavioural strategies to terminate conflict (Patterson, 1982; Patterson, Reid and Dishion, 1992). This approach to conflict resolution, in turn, has been shown to predict problems in peer relations, substance use, behaviour problems and emotional problems (Bank et al., 1996; Dunn, Slomkowski, Beardsall and Rende, 1994; Loeber and Tengs, 1986; Stormshak, Bellanti and Bierman, 1996). Importantly, these socializing influences are by no means limited to conflicted interactions.

Outwardly positive interactions between siblings may also contribute to the development and escalation of maladaptive behaviour. Sibling collusion, a process whereby siblings conspire to participate in problem behaviour that effectively diminishes their parents' efforts to socialize, has also been implicated. In these collusive sibling relationships, children and adolescents often encourage or reward one another for antisocial talk through the use of positive affect and subtle behavioural cues. What is remarkable about these sibling exchanges is that parents are present. Recent studies have indicated that sibling collusion is readily employed in families with an adolescent at risk for problem behaviour, yet virtually absent in families of normative controls. In addition, collusion among siblings predicts early adolescent concurrent and future problem behaviour, even after controlling for the influence of deviant peer association (Bullock and Dishion, 2000; Bullock and Dishion, in press).

Emotional negativity in the sibling relationship can also serve a maladaptive function (Brody, 1998). A recent study of young adult siblings revealed that the older sibling's negative, hostile attitudes toward a younger brother were associated with that younger brother's concomitant and future antisocial behaviour, substance use, friendship with similarly antisocial peers, higher criminality, and earlier onset of sexual activity (Bullock, Bank and Burraston, 2002). Siblings of poorly adjusted younger brothers were more likely to be critical and report negative sibling relationships than siblings of well-adjusted brothers. Moreover, negative attitudes of an older sibling predicted younger brother maladjustment 1 to 2 years later after controlling for sibling conflict and parental discipline. These findings indicate that the sibling affective relationship is also relevant to mental health outcomes.

In sum, the family environment is important to the development and maintenance of healthy and maladaptive outcomes for children and adolescents. However, the family also provides a genetic context, whereby (in nearly all families) parents and their children share genes as well as environments. We turn next to this important aspect of 'family'.

Genetic influences

A growing body of behavioural genetic research has revealed that the role of genes in the development of individual differences is practically ubiquitous. These human behavioural genetic studies have employed various family designs where the genetic similarity of siblings or parents and their offspring is considered. This information has been used to provide estimates of the relative contribution of genetic and nongenetic sources of variance in individual differences in outcomes (see Neale and Cardon, 1992, for a detailed overview of this quantitative genetic methodology). Not surprisingly, genetic influence has been found to be significant for numerous physical maladies including diabetes mellitus, a spectrum of cardiopulmonary diseases, and ulcers, to name but a few (Plomin, Rende and Rutter, 1991). Genetic influence is also implicated in a broad variety of mental health outcomes.

The research on schizophrenia represents perhaps the most widely documented relation between genetic factors and mental illness. Despite the fact that about 90% of persons who develop schizophrenia have no relatives with the illness, a number of studies using twin designs indicate that monozygotic (MZ) or identical co-twins have significantly higher concordance rates for schizophrenia compared to dizygotic (DZ) or fraternal co-twins (approximately 50% and 13% respectively – Farmer, McGuffin and Gottesman, 1987; Onstad, Skre, Torgersen and Kringlen, 1991). Likewise, the Danish Adoption Study reported high frequencies of schizophrenia among biological relatives of individuals with schizophrenia that had been placed for adoption, and these rates were comparable to those for diagnosed persons who resided with their biological families (Kendler, Gruenberg and Kinney, 1994a). Consistent with this finding, adopted individuals without schizophrenia have also been reported to have few biological relatives with the disorder (Onstad et al., 1991).

Studies of genetic transmission of personality and personality disorders have also provided evidence of heritability of certain behavioural traits. Several studies comparing twins reared together and apart provide evidence for genetic influences on individual differences in neuroticism, extraversion-introversion, openness to experience and conscientiousness (Bergeman, Chipuer, Plomin et al., 1993; Pedersen, McClearn, Plomin et al., 1991). Likewise, researchers have reported that numerous forms of personality disorder probably include genetic influences (Kendler, Heath and Martin, 1987; Kendler and Hewitt, 1992; Livesley, Jang, Jackson and Vernon, 1993; Torgersen, Skre, Onstad, Evardsen and Kringlen, 1993). These findings are not consistent across studies though, due in part to differences in methodology, measurement (for example, variations in the way in which personality variables are defined), and the heterogeneity of personality disorder classifications in the DSM criteria (Diagnostic and Statistical Manual of Mental Disorders; American Psychiatric Association, 1980). Nevertheless, these data point to a broad genetic influence in the presentation of individual differences in personality (Nigg and Goldsmith, 1994).

Evidence for genetic influences on mood disorders is more consistent, with diagnoses of major depression being observed among the biological relatives of persons diagnosed with bipolar disorder and dysthymia. Twin studies have provided evidence for a genetic association between bipolar disorder and major depression and for genetic associations among the spectrum of mood disorders (Kendler, Neale, Kessler, Heath and Eaves, 1993; Kendler, Walters, Truett et al., 1994b; Torgersen, 1986; Wender, Kety, Rosenthal et al., 1986). Genetic factors have also been implicated in the development of anxiety disorders in a number of twin studies. These data suggest that prevalence of panic disorders, anxiety disorders with panic attacks, and post-traumatic stress symptoms also may be influenced by genetic factors (Kendler et al., 1987; Torgersen, 1983; True, Rice, Eisen et al., 1993).

Substance abuse and externalizing behaviour problems (for example, conduct disorder, aggression) are also genetically variable. Twin and adoption studies of substance use suggest that genetic factors account for some of the individual differences in drug/alcohol abuse (Bohman, Sigvardsson and Cloninger, 1981; Cadoret, Yates, Troughton, Woodworth and Stewart, 1995a; Grove, Eckert, Heston, et al., 1990; Kendler, Neal, Heath, Kessler and Eaves, 1994; McGue, Pickins and Svikis, 1992). Antisocial behaviour, including conduct problems and aggression, are also genetically influenced (Miles and Carey, 1997; Reiss, Neiderhiser, Hetherington and Plomin, 2000). Farrington and others have found a compelling familial pattern in delinquency and criminal behaviour, with 50% of crimes being committed by members of only 5% of the families in their study populations (see, for example, Loeber and Dishion, 1983; West and Farrington, 1973). This presentation of antisocial behaviour within families has been documented in numerous studies that have utilized genetically informative designs, and all of which suggest genetic influence (Eaves, Silberg, Meyer et al., 1997; Eaves, Rutter, Silberg et al., 2000; Ge, Conger, Cadoret et al., 1996; Gjone and Stevenson, 1997; O'Connor, Neiderhiser, Reiss et al., 1998; and others). Recent work by Taylor, Iacono and McGue (2000) suggests that genetic liability may be greater for early onset forms of antisocial behaviour, in contrast to late-onset forms that are more likely influenced by exposure to deviant peers. This developmental finding serves as an important reminder that genetic influences are likely to be dynamic over the course of the lifespan. It is possible that different genes become involved at different stages of development, or that different genes are associated with different subtypes of a particular disorder or outcome – subtypes that differ based on their developmental trajectories (for example, age of onset).

As indicated by this brief review, there remains little doubt that genetic influence is an important part of the etiology of mental health outcomes. What is not discernible from these studies is the process by which genetic factors influence the onset, course and severity of psychological problems or the directionality of such influence. However, several mechanisms have been proposed. The most simple form of genetic influence is Mendelian inheritance, with a single gene being responsible for the presentation of a particular outcome. While this explanation is plausible, the evidence from behavioural genetic studies is that most mental health outcomes are very complex and arise as a result of the influence of multiple genes (Rutter, Dunn, Plomin et al., 1997a; Torgersen, 1997). It is likely that maladjustment is due to polygenic inheritance, in which several to many genes function independently or interactively to lead to a probabilistic risk for a particular disorder. To date, little is known about these various mechanisms and their impact on specific forms of psychopathology. However, this will change rapidly as molecular genetic studies lead to new discoveries regarding specific genes that are

associated with individual differences in mental health outcomes (Plomin
and Rutter, 1998; Rutter, Silberg, O'Connor and Simonoff, 1999).

Integration: gene-environment transactions

We have provided a brief and selective overview of the major findings
regarding genetic and family environmental factors pertaining to mental
health outcomes among children and adolescents. However, the difficult
task that lies ahead for researchers and clinicians is understanding how
genes and environments work together in development. In the following
section, we focus on two specific types of gene-environment transactions:
gene-environment correlation and gene-environment interaction.

Gene-environment correlation

Three models of gene-environment correlations have been proposed:
passive, evocative and active (Plomin, DeFries and Loehlin, 1977). Passive
gene-environment correlation refers to the process that occurs in all families that include genetically related children and parents, whereby
parents provide a family environment that is correlated with the genes of
themselves and their children. For example, parents who are musicians
may create an environment for their children that stimulates musical
development. They are likely to expose their children to many different
types of music, to teach them to play instruments and sing, and to learn
how to read music. In addition, to the extent that an aptitude for musi-
cality is genetically variable, the parents are also transmitting these genes
to their children. Thus, the musically enriched family environment is correlated with the presence of genes that influence musical abilities in both
the parents and the children. The same concept applies to other family
processes and child outcomes, including those pertaining to the mental
health of family members. These passive gene-environment effects are
believed to be most prominent during early childhood, a developmental
period when children spend a large proportion of their time in the home
(Scarr and McCartney, 1983). The main point to consider with respect to
this passive form is that what may appear to be a purely environmental
process linking parenting behaviour to children's outcomes may in fact be
a gene-environment process, whereby parents' genetically influenced
behaviours create environments that are correlated with their children's
genetically influenced behaviours.

The second type, called evocative gene-environment correlation, is said
to be present when an individual's genetically influenced behaviours
induce or evoke particular responses from the environment that in turn

further shape the experiences of that individual. This does not mean that the environment is epiphenomenal. Instead, it means that one of the ways in which the genetic influences operate on the child's behaviours is through the environments and experiences that those behaviours elicit or induce. For example, heritable components of a child's temperament and behavioural adjustment are likely to have a significant influence on the reciprocal parent-child exchanges that occur within the family. These behaviours can, but do not necessarily, elicit particular responses from parents and other family members (Deater-Deckard, 2000; Rothbart and Bates, 1998). For example, one might predict that children who tend to be consistently oppositional and defiant (behaviours that are likely to include genetic influences) would evoke greater negativity from family members, whereas pleasant, compliant children would elicit greater positivity. Importantly, these processes may differ across families and cultural groups, given that parents are likely to respond differently to different child behaviours depending on the family and broader cultural context.

Experimental designs examining parent-child interaction and child conduct problems have demonstrated such effects (Anderson, Lytton and Romney, 1986), although the experimental approach typically does not employ genetically informative samples. Thus, there also have been attempts to model these evocative gene-environment correlation processes using quasi-experimental behavioural genetic designs. For example, we have known for some time that evocative gene-environment correlation may be present and accounting for some of the covariation between parents' self-reported feelings of negativity and warmth toward their children, and those parents' perceptions of their children's behavioural and emotional problems (Plomin, 1994). At the same time, more recent studies indicate that these evocative gene-environment correlations also may be present in observed child behaviours and observed parent-child interactions (Deater-Deckard and O'Connor, 2000; Leve, Winebarger, Fagot, Reid and Goldsmith, 1998; Reiss et al., 2000).

These evocative gene-environment correlational processes are also likely to be operating in sibling relationships and interaction. As noted previously, a formulation of family dynamics should include parent-child and sibling relationships. By comparison to the genetic studies of parenting and parent-child relationships, there have been relatively few investigations of gene-environment transactions in sibling dyads. One recent example involved a large sample of young twins (Lemery and Goldsmith, in press). These researchers found that the instigation of cooperation with a sibling showed no genetic influence but considerable environmental influence, whereas the instigation of conflict with a sibling included both genetic and environmental sources of variance. Furthermore, the links between the temperament of the child and his or her relationship with the sibling were mediated by genetic influences, suggesting gene-environment correlation. Genetic studies like this one – those that examine both sibling and parent-child relationships – represent an exciting new direction in family process research, because they bring us one step closer to a complete representation of the family dynamics that are contributing to each individual's mental health outcomes.

The third type, called active gene-environment correlation or 'niche picking', operates by producing experiences through selection of environments that are most consistent with or reinforcing of the individual's genetically influenced attributes. Scarr and McCartney (1983) proposed that these effects become increasingly salient over the course of development as children gain more control over situations and experiences that are more likely to be compatible with their genetically influenced characteristics. The major developmental transitions in childhood and adolescence, such as starting school and puberty, come with new opportunities to meet and interact with other children and adults. In this regard, most of the attention in the literature has been given to children's peer relationships because these are usually relationships that involve a selection process – for better or worse, we do not get to choose our parents and siblings.

Once again, the development of conduct problems provides a good example. Longitudinal studies have demonstrated that there are links between children's behavioural and emotional problems, troubled family relationships, and problems in peer relationships and the formation of friendships with antisocial peers (Ary, Duncan, Duncan and Hops, 1999; Fergusson and Horwood, 1999; Fergusson, Woodward and Horwood, 1999). It is clear that by adolescence and probably earlier in development, friendship similarity in antisocial behaviour emerges (Haselager, Hartup, van Lieshout and Riksen-Walraven, 1998; Laird, Pettit, Dodge and Bates, 1999). Furthermore, it is this selection of similarly antisocial friends that mediates the associations between maladaptive family relationships and children's antisocial behaviours (Dishion, Bullock and Owen, 2001; Kim, Hetherington and Reiss, 1999). There is also evidence that antisocial parents are more likely to provide environments for their children that increase the likelihood that those children will be antisocial (Rowe and Farrington, 1997; Rutter, Maughn, Meyer, Pickles et al., 1997; Rutter, Giller and Hagell, 1998). Given that these antisocial behaviours include genetic influences, it is likely that the link between an antisocial family environment and children's selection of antisocial peers is genetically mediated via these active processes.

This leads us to perhaps the most important point to be raised in this chapter – that the presence of gene-environment correlation processes like those just described does not relegate the environment to a secondary role. Using the example of the selection of antisocial peers, the essential environmental factors involving peer socializing influences are seen as part of an integrated process linking children's genetically-influenced behaviours and their peer experiences. It is not surprising that parental monitoring of their children's whereabouts and friendships is critical to these children's long-term trajectories (Flannery, William and Vazsonyi, 1999; Pettit, Bates, Dodge and Meece, 1999). Parents of children with some genetic risk for antisocial behaviour who effectively minimize their at-risk children's opportunities to form friendships with deviant peers are intervening in a process that, if left unchecked, would lead to an escalation in these genetically-variable behavioural problems.

Gene-environment interaction

Another type of transaction – gene-environment interaction – is said to exist when genetic influences are conditioned upon the environments that are present, or when environmental influences are conditioned upon the genetic influences that are present (Plomin et al., 1997). A particular set of genes may have different effects depending on the presence of certain family environments. Similarly, a particular set of environmental factors may have different effects depending on the presence of certain types of genes. Plomin and Rutter (1998) provide a hypothetical example whereby the effects of dopamine receptor genes on the development of hyperactivity and inattention are amplified in those families where parenting is inconsistent and harsh, but are attenuated in those families where parenting is warm, supportive and contingent.

Some research using the adoption design does suggest that gene-environment interactions are present in the development of antisocial behaviour in adolescence and adulthood. For example, Bohman (1996) reported that, in the presence of a combined genetic and environmental risk for adult criminality, the rate of criminal outcome was three times greater than that found for individuals who had only a genetic risk, and about six times greater than the rate found for individuals who had only an environmental risk. Likewise, other studies that have assessed the intergenerational transmission of antisocial behaviour indicate that it is the interaction between a genetic liability and adverse environmental influences that account for the wide range of outcomes (Cadoret, Cain, Troughton and Heywood, 1985; Cadoret et al., 1995b; Mednick, Gabrielli and Hutchings, 1984). However, behavioural genetic designs are a fairly weak test of gene-environment interaction. Therefore, researchers are eager to apply the current molecular genetic technologies to answering questions about gene-environment transactions. Although by no means a panacea, these molecular genetic approaches will permit more precise assessment of gene-environment interaction in a much wider array of research designs (Plomin and Rutter, 1998).

In considering this brief review of gene-environment transactions, it is apparent that neither nature nor nurture explanations alone can capture the links between family processes and developmental outcomes. Both genes and environments are important sources of variability when considering family environments and mental health, and yet these conceptually distinct influences are most likely bound together in many complex gene-environment transactions. Most recently, Turkheimer (2000: 161) has provided a concise description of this gene-environment process.

> Individual genes . . . and their environments (which include other genes) interact to initiate a complex developmental process that determines adult personality. Most characteristic of this process is its interactivity: Subsequent environments to which the organism is exposed depend on earlier states, and each new environment changes the developmental trajectory, which affects future expression of genes and so forth. Everything is interactive, in the sense that [nothing] proceeds from cause to effect; any individual gene or environmental event produces an effect only by interacting with other genes and environments.

Implications for research and practice

What do clinicians and clinical scientists gain from this perspective? In what ways does consideration of these gene-environment transactions improve our understanding of the development of family dysfunction and mental illness, and in so doing, lead to more optimal prevention and intervention? Turkheimer's (2000) proposition – that it is important to consider continuous dynamic gene-environment interplay when formulating hypotheses regarding development – is central to our conceptualization of family process. Herein lie the opportunities and challenges for prevention and intervention scientists and clinicians.

It is worth emphasizing from the outset that the benefits of considering genetic factors for complex disorders are not likely to be fully realized until molecular genetic approaches yield the specific genes in question. This work is proceeding at a rapid pace, and it is worthwhile to consider now the implications of these future discoveries. Nevertheless, the current state of knowledge regarding gene-environment transactions suggests that mental illnesses and problematic behaviours that are genetically influenced can be affected by environmental interventions. By conducting research examining likely environmental influences within the context of potential genetic influences, we are more likely to identify precisely those mechanisms that will be most effectively manipulated in environmental interventions. It would be a mistake to assume that genetic influences are intractable and unchangeable, just as it would be to conclude this about environmental influences. In the final section of this chapter, we discuss some of the clinical implications of this perspective.

Before interpreting these behavioural genetic results, it is worth considering some methodological limitations. Method effects (for example, informant, procedure and setting effects) can lead to disparate findings (Turkheimer and Waldron, 2000), a concern when one considers that most of the previous studies have relied on only survey methods based on self or parents' reports (Manke, McGuire, Reiss, Hetherington and Plomin, 1995). With respect to the adoption design, adoptive families do not represent the wide range of family environments that exist in the populations to which we would like to generalize findings, because in most cases the adoptive parents are screened prior to being allowed to adopt (Stoolmiller, 1999). Twin studies can yield inflated estimates of heritability on mental health outcomes for a variety of reasons (Wachs and Plomin, 1991). Studies of full-siblings and half-siblings living in stepfamilies can be problematic in that the children have experienced multiple family transitions (for example, parental divorce, the arrival of stepparents and stepsiblings), experiences that may have profound effects on the types of processes we discover (Deater-Deckard, Dunn, O'Connor, Davies and Golding, in press). No single design is perfect. What is needed is an integration in our research whereby we use designs that use a full complement of sibling subtypes (twins, full- and half-siblings, unrelated adoptive siblings), employ multi-agent multi-method data collection strategies, and apply multivariate statistical procedures that can account for gene-environment correlations and interactions (Reiss et al., 2000).

Already, the extant family process literature has informed research and practice with respect to optimizing child and adolescent developmental outcomes. Clinical research has shown that child behaviour is directly influenced by parent actions (Baumrind et al., 1985; Mason, Cauce, Gonzales and Hiraga, 1996; and others). For example, the coercion model for the development of antisocial behaviour demonstrates that escape conditioning – a recurring pattern of using aversive behaviour to terminate disputes – can occur in the context of family conflict, and contributes to an escalation in aggressive and non-aggressive conduct problems in childhood and adolescence (Patterson, 1982; Patterson et al., 1992). Additional evidence is found in the intervention literature, based on studies in which parents were randomly assigned to treatment or control conditions (for example, families receiving no intervention). These experimental studies have shown that changes in parent behaviour directed toward their offspring can lead to changes in child behaviour (Dishion,

Patterson and Kavanagh, 1992; Forgatch and DeGarmo, 1999; Webster-Stratton, 1990). At the same time, evidence exists for genetic influence on a broad array of psychiatric illnesses and developmental outcomes more generally. These include, but are not limited to, schizophrenia (Onstad et al., 1991; Plomin et al., 1991), personality disorders (Kendler et al., 1987; Kendler and Hewitt, 1992; Livesley et al., 1993), mood disorders (Kendler et al., 1994b; Wender et al., 1986), substance use and dependency (Cadoret et al., 1995a; McGue et al., 1992), and behaviour problems (Eaves et al., 2000; Gjone and Stevenson, 1997; O'Connor et al., 1998a). More importantly, psychopathology research regarding the effects of genes on maladjustment suggests that such disorders arise as a result of the complex interplay of multiple genes and multiple environmental factors. A particular complement or configuration of genes may result in a diathesis for one or more psychological disorders, raising the likelihood of developing that disorder when the individual also experiences a rearing environment that contains risk factors.

Consistent with this view, research has shown evidence for bidirectionality in parent-child relations, with characteristics of both the child and the parent contributing to the emergent attributes of that dyadic relationship and the child's social-emotional adjustment (Lollis and Kuczynski, 1997). For instance, negative emotionality and irritability in young children have been found to elicit greater negativity and avoidance from caregivers (Rutter and Quinton, 1984), and conduct-disordered boys' noxious behaviours have been shown to evoke more negative reactions from adults (Anderson, Lytton and Romney, 1986). It is likely that this process is mediated genetically. In a study of adoptees, children who had a genetic liability for behavioural problems tended to evoke greater parental negativity from their adoptive parents than did children who did not have this genetic risk (O'Connor et al., 1998a). Together, these findings suggest that parental behaviour mediates some of the genetic effects found on child maladjustment, highlighting the importance of parenting quality and the significance of rearing environments in the socialization of children.

Studies of human and non-human primates point to a link between parenting behaviour and child adjustment, and suggest that the environments that parents provide may directly influence the observable (phenotypic) expression of underlying genetic vulnerabilities in their children. There are data suggesting that it is the combination of certain aspects of temperament and parenting environments such as the child's resistance to parental control and harsh discipline practices that in combination predict individual differences in behavioural problems in early and middle childhood (Bates, Pettit, Dodge and Ridge, 1998). Research with non-human primates complements these findings (Suomi, 1997).

Cross-fostering studies of non-human primates, in which surrogate mothers raise infants, demonstrate these gene-environment interaction effects. For example, when monkeys that had a powerful genetic risk for extreme emotional reactivity were reared with calm surrogate mothers during the first 6 months of their lives, the infants displayed an ability to cope with stressors and typical development of social competence. However, there was also a main effect of parenting – infant monkeys that were not genetically at risk for emotional reactivity but were reared by highly reactive surrogate mothers were easily perturbed by interpersonal or environmental stressors and were not socially competent. In nature, these combinations of calm mothers and reactive infants or reactive mothers and calm infants would be relatively rare because the mothers and infants would share many of the genetic factors that contribute to this emotional reactivity. The presence of these sorts of gene-environment interactions suggests that the family environment moderates genetic effects on child outcomes.

Consideration of these gene-environment correlation and interaction processes may lead to greater precision in diagnoses when problems arise. Current approaches typically result in the identification of heterogeneous groups of children who are showing evidence of multiple problems in development. The simultaneous consideration of genetic and environmental factors may lead to further improvements in diagnostic procedures that solve some of these problems surrounding the heterogeneity and comorbidity of disorders. Knowing which genes are associated with particular behavioural or emotional problems will be only part of the process of diagnosis and intervention, because these genetic influences will need to be considered in light of the environmental contexts in which they are operating.

An emphasis on understanding gene-environment interaction may be particularly useful when considering the implementation of preventative measures. Currently, prevention science focuses on using early behavioural or environmental indicators of risk for subsequent disorder for determining the population that should be targeted. Knowledge about the underlying genetic architecture of a particular outcome, when coupled with information regarding the ways in which those genetic influences operate in transaction with specified environmental factors, has the potential to improve prevention effectiveness by allowing clinicians to match the preventative measure to the particular complement of gene-environment risks for any given individual child and family. Accordingly, some children with genetic risk factors for a particular disorder may not yet be exhibiting symptoms of the disorder only due to the absence of environmental risk factors – a result of gene-environment interaction. For these children, the goal will be to provide preventative measures that mitigate the onset of environmental risk, or offer treatment when environmental risks become ev'dent.

Consideration of gene-environment correlation processes is also informative. Even if a particular set of environmental risk factors have been eliminated for a child who has a known genetic risk for a particular disorder, those genetic risk factors may still operate in such a way as to elicit or select risk-inducing experiences in settings that are not so easily controlled through intervention (for example, idiosyncratic events). Consider the genetic risk factors for conduct problems in childhood. These are likely to be influencing the child's abilities to self-regulate emotions, attention and thoughts, and desire for novelty and arousal. When coupled with exposure to a harsh parenting environment, it is likely that these children will show increases in behavioural problems at home and at school. However, even if one intervenes by improving the parenting environment, the child may still elicit or select experiences in environments where the parents or interventionist have little control (for example, unsupervised peer interaction). The most successful prevention and intervention efforts will require comprehensive knowledge of the multitude of gene-environment correlational processes underlying any particular disorder, ranging from those that are easily identified and controlled to those that are not easily identified and manipulated.

Given the theoretical and clinical relevance of these and other integrative approaches, it is not surprising that 'socialization' researchers are collaborating more frequently with 'biological' researchers. Nonetheless, much remains to be done. In particular, we need more studies that examine family processes and developmental outcomes using genetically informative designs such as twin and adoption studies. Ideally, these new studies will be parts of programmes of research that test for replication in processes across alternative designs (Reiss et al., 2000), but there are practical concerns to consider. Rather than focusing on the additive genetic and environmental variance in separate developmental outcomes – the traditional behavioural genetic approach – these designs must also incorporate state-of-the-art measures of environmental factors and family relationship processes. Without this component, gene-environment correlation and interaction processes cannot be tested and elucidated. In addition, behavioural genetic findings are sometimes interpreted to suggest that 'heritability is destiny' – that a genetically variable outcome is somehow fixed or impervious to change. Such reasoning is flawed because these genetic influences operate in transactions with environments and are probabilistic in their prediction of outcomes (Collins et al., 2000; Plomin and Rutter, 1998; Scarr, Webber, Weinberg and Wittig, 1981). The inclusion of family environment measures in behavioural genetic studies – using both participants' and observers' reports – will continue to move us toward more effective interventions.

In conclusion, this review of the findings regarding families and mental health indicated that the existence of pathology in one or more biological parents or siblings poses an elevated genetic liability for other immediate family members. Moreover, environments characterized by risk factors including parental mental illness and substance use, harsh or ineffective parenting and family management, and high degrees of internal and external stressors may also increase the likelihood of child maladjustment. Children of parents who themselves suffer from behavioural or emotional disturbances possess the 'double' risk of being exposed to suboptimal rearing environments in addition to inheriting genetic risk (O'Connor, Deater-Deckard and Plomin, 1998b). In this sense, the 'family' is a genetic and environmental context for the emergence of psychopathology and the consideration of both types of influences and the transactions between genes and environments is critical. Preventative programmes that target parenting behaviour and family management skills may serve to mitigate the environmental risk and, possibly, attenuate or even eliminate the phenotypic expression of child behavioural and emotional problems.

Acknowledgement

We wish to thank Gretchen Lussier and Kathryn Becker for their helpful comments on an earlier version of this chapter. During the writing of this chapter, the first author was supported by research funds from the National Science Foundation, and the second author was supported on a predoctoral fellowship on a National Institute of Mental Health training grant (Tom Dishion, University of Oregon). Address correspondence to Kirby Deater-Deckard, Department of Psychology, 1227 University of Oregon, Eugene, OR, 97403-1227, USA; Email: kirbydd@darkwing.uoregon.edu.

References

American Psychiatric Association (1980) Diagnostic and Statistical Manual of Mental Disorders. 3 edn. Washington DC: American Psychiatric Association.

Anderson K, Lytton H, Romney DM(1986) Mothers' interaction with normal and conduct-disordered boys: who affects whom? Developmental Psychology 22: 604–9.

Arnold JE, Levine AG, Patterson GR (1975) Changes in sibling behaviour following family intervention. Journal of Consulting and Clinical Psychology 43: 683–8.

Ary DV, Duncan TE, Duncan SC, Hops H (1999) Adolescent problem behaviour: the influence of parents and peers. Behaviour Research and Therapy 37: 217–30.

Asarnow JR, Goldstein MJ, Tompson M, Guthrie D (1990) One–year outcomes of depressive disorders in child psychiatric inpatients: evaluation of the prognostic power of a brief measure of expressed emotion. Journal of Child Psychology and Psychiatry 34: 129–37.

Asarnow JR, Tompson M, Hamilton EB, Goldstein MJ, Guthrie D (1994) Family-expressed emotion, childhood-onset depression, and childhood-onset schizophrenia spectrum disorders: is expressed emotion a nonspecific correlate of child psychopathology or a specific risk factor for depression? Journal of Abnormal Child Psychology 22: 129–46.

Bank L, Patterson GR, Reid JB (1996) Negative sibling interaction patterns as predictors of later adjustment problems in adolescent and young adult males. In Brody GH (ed.) Sibling Relationships: Their Causes and Consequences Advances in Applied Developmental Psychology. Norwood NJ: Ablex, pp. 197–229.

Bates JE, Pettit GS, Dodge KA, Ridge B (1998) Interaction of temperamental resistance to control and restrictive parenting in the development of externalizing behaviour. Developmental Psychology 34: 982–95.

Baumrind D, Moselle K, Martin JA (1985) Adolescent drug abuse research: a critical examination from a developmental perspective. Advances in Alcohol and Substance Abuse 4: 41–67.

Bergeman CS, Chipuer HM, Plomin R, Pedersen NL, McClearn GE, Nesselroade JR, Costa PT Jr, McCrae RR (1993) Genetic and environmental effects on openness to experience, agreeableness, and conscientiousness: an adoption/twin study. Journal of Personality 61: 159–78.

Block J, Block JH, Keyes S (1988) Longitudinally fortelling drug usage in adolescence: early childhood personality and environmental precursors. Child Development 59: 336–55.

Bohman M (1996) Predisposition to criminality: Swedish adoption studies in retrospect. In Bock GR, Goode JA (eds) Genetics of Criminal and Antisocial Behaviour (Ciba Foundation Symposium 194). Chichester: Wiley, pp. 94–114.

Bohman M, Sigvardsson S, Cloninger CR (1981) Maternal inheritance of alcohol abuse: cross–fostering analysis of adopted women. Archives of General Psychiatry 38: 965–9.

Brody G (1998) Sibling relationship quality: its causes and consequences. Annual Review of Psychology 49: 1–24.

Bronfenbrenner U (1986) Ecology of the family as a context for human development: research perspectives. Developmental Psychology 22: 723–42.

Bullock BM, Bank L, Burraston B (2002) Adult sibling expressed emotion and fellow sibling deviance: a new piece of the family process puzzle. Journal of Family Psychology 16(3): 307–17.

Bullock BM, Dishion TJ (in press) Sibling collusion and problem behaviour in early adolescence: toward a process model for family mutuality. Journal of Abnormal Child Psychology.

Bullock BM, Dishion TJ (2000) Sibling collusion as a predictor of concurrent and one-year outcomes in early adolescents: toward a process model for family mutuality. In Dishion TJ, Bullock BM (chairs) Advances in family process research on the development of antisocial behaviour: implications for an evolving behaviour therapy paradigm. Paper presented at the annual meeting of the Association for Advancement of Behaviour Therapy, New Orleans.

Cadoret RJ, Cain CA, Troughton E, Heywood E (1985) Alcoholism and antisocial personality: interrelationships, genetic and environmental factors. Archives of General Psychiatry 42: 161–7.

Cadoret RJ, Yates WR, Troughton E, Woodworth G, Stewart MA (1995a) Adoption study demonstrating two genetic pathways to drug abuse. Archives of General Psychiatry 52: 42–52.

Cadoret RJ, Yates WR, Troughton E, Woodworth G, Stewart MA (1995b) Genetic–environmental interaction in the genesis of aggressivity and conduct disorders. Archives of General Psychiatry 52: 916–24.

Collins WA, Maccoby EE, Steinberg L, Hetherington EM, Bornstein MH (2000) Contemporary research on parenting: the case for nature and nurture. American Psychologist 55(2): 218–32.

Conger RD, Patterson GR, Ge X (1995) A mediational model for the impact of parents' stress on adolescent adjustment. Child Development 66: 80–97.

Deater-Deckard K (2000) Parenting and child behavioural adjustment in early childhood: a quantitative genetic approach to studying family process. Child Development 72(2): 468–84.

Deater-Deckard K, Dodge KA (1997) Externalizing behaviour problems and discipline revisited: nonlinear effects and variation by culture, context, and gender. Psychological Inquiry 8: 161–75.

Deater-Deckard K, O'Connor TG (2000) Parent-child mutuality in early childhood: two behavioural genetic studies. Developmental Psychology 36: 561–70.

Deater-Deckard K, Dunn J, O'Connor TG, Davies L, Golding J (in press) Using the step–family genetic design to examine gene-environment processes in family functioning. Marriage and Family Review.

Dishion TJ, Andrews DW, Kavanagh K, Soberman LH (1996) Preventive interventions for high-risk youth: the adolescent transitions program. In Peters RD, McMahon RJ (eds) Preventing Childhood Disorders, Substance Abuse, and Delinquency. Thousand Oaks CA: Sage Publications.

Dishion TJ, Bullock BM (in press) Parenting and adolescent problem behaviour: an ecological analysis of the nurturance hypothesis. In Borkowski JG (ed.) Parenting and Your Child's World. Hillsdale NJ: Erlbaum.

Dishion TJ, Bullock BM, Owen LD (2001) Deviant Norms in Families: Constructing a Process Bridge to Peer Culture. Manuscript in preparation.

Dishion TJ, Patterson GR, Kavanagh K (1992) An experimental test of the coercion model: linking theory, measurement, and intervention. In McCord J, Trembley R (eds) The Interaction of Theory and Practice: Experimental Studies of Interventions. New York: Guilford Press, pp. 253–82.

Downey G, Coyne JC (1990) Children of depressed parents: an integrative review. Psychological Bulletin 108: 50–76.

Dunn J, Slomkowski C, Beardsall L, Rende R (1994) Adjustment in middle child-hood and early adolescence: links with earlier and contemporary sibling relationships. Journal of Child Psychology and Psychiatry 35: 491–504.

Eaves L, Rutter M, Silberg J, Shillady L, Maes H, Pickles A (2000) Genetic and environmental causes of covariation in interview assessments of disruptive behaviour in child and adolescent twins. Behaviour Genetics 30(4): 321–34.

Eaves L, Silberg JL, Meyer JM, Maes HH, Simonoff E, Pickles A, Rutter M, Neale MC, Reynolds CA, Erikson MT, Heath AC, Loeber T, Truett TR, Hewitt JK (1997) Genetics and developmental psychopathology: 2 The main effects of genes and environment on behavioural problems in the Virginia Twin Study of Adolescent Behavioural Development. Journal of Child Psychology and Psychiatry 38: 965–80.

Farmer AE, McGuffin P, Gottesman II (1987) Twin concordance for DSM–III schizophrenia: scrutinizing the validity of the definition. Archives of General Psychiatry 44: 634–41.

Farrington DP, Barnes GC, Lambert S (1996) The concentration of offending families. Legal and Criminological Psychology 1: 47–63.

Fergusson DM, Horwood LJ (1999) Prospective childhood predictors of deviant peer affiliations in adolescence. Journal of Child Psychology and Psychiatry 40: 581–92.

Fergusson DM, Woodward LJ, Horwood LJ (1999) Childhood peer relationship problems and young people's involvement with deviant peers in adolescence. Journal of Abnormal Child Psychology 27: 357–69.

Flannery DJ, Williams LL, Vazsonyi AT (1999) Who are they with and what are they doing? Delinquent behaviour, substance use, and early adolescents' after–school time. American Journal of Orthopsychiatry 69: 247–53.

Forgatch MS (1991) The clinical science vortex: developing a theory for antisocial behaviour. In Peppler DJ, Rubin KH (eds) The Development and Treatment of Childhood Aggression. Hillsdale NJ: Erlbaum, pp. 219–315.

Forgatch MS, DeGarmo D (1999) Parenting through change: an effective prevention program for single mothers. Journal of Consulting and Clinical Psychology 67(5): 711–24.

Freud S (1995) The Basic Writings of Sigmund Freud. New York: The Modern Library.

Gardner FEM (1989) Inconsistent parenting: is there evidence for a link with children's conduct problems? Journal of Abnormal Child Psychology 71: 223–33.

Ge X, Conger RD, Cadoret RJ, Neiderhiser JM, Yates W, Troughton E, Stewart MA (1996) The developmental interface between nature and nurture: a mutual influence model of child antisocial behaviour and parenting. Developmental Psychology 32: 574–89.

Gjone H, Stevenson J (1997) The association between internalizing and externalizing behaviour in childhood and early adolescence: genetic and environmental common influences. Journal of Abnormal Child Psychology 25: 277–86.

Gottesman II, Carey G, Hanson DR (1983) Pearls and perils in epigenic psychopathology. In Guze SB, Earls ED, Barrett JE (eds) Childhood Psychopathology and Development. New York: Raven Press, pp. 287–300.

Grove WM, Eckert ED, Heston L, Bouchard TJ Jr, Segal N, Lykken DT (1990) Heritability of substance abuse and antisocial behaviour: a study of monozygotic twins reared apart. Biological Psychiatry 27: 1293–304.

Haselager GJT, Hartup WW, Van Lieshout CFM, Riksen–Walraven JMA (1998) Similarities between friends and nonfriends in middle childhood. Child Development 69: 1198–208.

Henggeler SW, Schoenwald SK, Borduin CM, Rowland MD, Cunningham PB (1998) Multisystemic treatment of antisocial behaviour in children and adolescents. New York: Guilford Press.

Jary ML, Stewart MA (1985) Psychiatric disorder in the parents of adopted children with aggressive conduct disorder. Neuropsychobiology 13: 7–11.

Kendler HS, Hewitt JK (1992) The structure of self–report schizotypi in twins. Journal of Personality Disorders 6: 1–17.

Kendler HS, Heath A, Martin ND (1987) A genetic epidemiologic study of self–report suspiciousness. Comprehensive Psychiatry 28: 187–96.

Kendler KS, Neale MC, Kessler RC, Heath AD, Eaves LJ (1992) Major depression and generalized anxiety disorder: same genes, (partly) different environments? Archives of General Psychiatry 49: 716–22.

Kendler HS, Gruenberg AD, Kinney DK (1994a) Independent diagnoses of adoptees and relatives as defined by DSM–III in the provincial and national samples of the Danish Adoption Study of Schizophrenia. Archives of General Psychiatry 51: 456–68.

Kendler HS, Neale MC, Kessler RL, Heath AC, Eaves LJ (1993) The lifetime history of major depression in women: reliability of diagnosis and heritability. Archives of General Psychiatry 50: 863–70.

Kendler HS, Walters EF, Truett KR, Heath AC, Neale MC, Martin NG, Eaves LJ (1994b) Sources of individual differences in depression symptoms: analysis of two samples of twins and their families. Archives of General Psychiatry 151: 1605–14.

Kim JE, Hetherington EM, Reiss D (1999) Associations among family relationships, antisocial peers, and adolescents' externalizing behaviours: gender and family type differences. Child Development 70: 1209–30.

Laird RD, Pettit GS, Dodge KA, Bates JE (1999) Best friendships, group relationships, and antisocial behaviour in early adolescence. Journal of Early Adolescence 19: 413–37.

Lemery KS, Goldsmith HH (in press) Genetic and environmental influences on preschool sibling cooperation and conflict: associations with difficult temperament and parenting style. Marriage and Family Review.

Leve LD, Winebarger AA, Fagot BI, Reid JB, Goldsmith HH (1998) Environmental and genetic variance in children's observed and reported maladaptive behaviour. Child Development 69(5): 1286–98.

Livesley WJ, Jang KL, Jackson DN, Vernon PQ (1993) Genetic and environmental contributions to dimensions of personality disorder. American Journal of Psychiatry 150: 1826–31.

Loeber R, Dishion TJ (1983) Early predictors of male delinquency: a review. Psychological Bulletin 94: 68–99.

Loeber R, Tengs T (1986) The analysis of coercive chains between children, mothers and siblings. Journal of Family Violence 1: 51–70.

Lollis S, Kuczynski L (1997) Beyond one hand clapping: seeing bidirectionality in parent – child relations. Journal of Social and Personal Relationships 14: 441–61.

Manke B, McGuire S, Reiss D, Hetherington EM, Plomin R (1995) Genetic contributions to adolescents' extrafamilial social interactions: teachers, best friends and peers. Social Development 4(3): 238–56.

Mason CA, Cauce AM, Gonzales N, Hiraga Y (1996) Neither too sweet nor too sour: problem peers, maternal control, and problem behaviour in African American adolescents. Child Development 67: 2115–30.

McGue M, Pickens RW, Svikis DS (1992) Sex and age effects on the inheritance of alcohol problems: a twin study. Journal of Abnormal Psychology 101(1): 3–17.

Miles DR, Carey G (1997) Genetic and environmental architecture of human aggression. Journal of Personality and Social Psychology 72: 207–17.

Minuchin P (1985) Families and individual development: provocations from the field of family therapy. Child Development 56: 289–302.

Neale MC, Cardon LR (1992) Methodology of Genetic Studies of Twins and Families. Dordrecht: Kluwer.

Nigg JT, Goldsmith HH (1994) Genetics of personality disorders: perspectives from personality and psychopathology research. Psychological Bulletin 115: 346–80.

O'Connor TG, Deater-Deckard K, Fulker D, Rutter ML, Plomin R (1998a) Genotype-environment correlations in late childhood and early adolescence: antisocial behaviour problems and coercive parenting. Developmental Psychology 34: 970–81.

O'Connor TG, Deater-Deckard K, Plomin R (1998b) Contributions of behavioural genetics research to clinical psychology. In E Walker (ed.) Comprehensive Clinical Psychology. Volume 1 – Foundations. Oxford: Elsevier Science, pp. 88–114.

O'Connor TG, Neiderhiser JM, Reiss D, Hetherington EM, Plomin R (1998c) Genetic contributions to continuity, change and co–occurrence of antisocial and depressive symptoms in adolescence. Journal of Child Psychology and Psychiatry 39: 332–6.

Onstad S, Skre I, Torgensen S, Kringlen E (1991) Twin concordance for DSM–III–R schizophrenia. Acta Psychiatrica Scandanavica 83: 463–7.

Patterson GR (1982) A Social Learning Approach: III. Coercive Family Process. Eugene OR: Castalia.

Patterson GR (1984) Siblings: fellow travelers in a coercive system. In Blanchard RJ, Blanchard DC (eds) Advances in the Study of Aggression. Vol. 1. New York: Academic, pp. 173–215.

Patterson GR, Reid J, Dishion TJ (1992) A Social Interactional Approach. IV: Antisocial Boys. Eugene OR: Castalia.

Pedersen NL, McClearn GE, Plomin R, Nesselroade JR, Berg S, De Faire U (1991) The Swedish adoption/twin study of aging: an update. Acta Geneticae Medicae et Gemellologiae 33: 243–50.

Pettit GS, Bates JE, Dodge KA, Meece DW (1999) The impact of after-school peer contact on early adolescent externalizing problems is moderated by parental monitoring, perceived neighborhood safety, and prior adjustment. Child Development 70: 768–78.

Plomin R (1994) Genetics and Experience: The Interplay between Nature and Nurture. Thousand Oaks: Sage Publications.

Plomin R, DeFries JC, Loehlin JC (1977) Genotype–environment interaction and correlation in the analysis of human behaviour. Psychological Bulletin 84: 309–32.

Plomin R, Rende R, Rutter M (1991) Quantitative Genetics and Developmental Psychopathology. In Cicchetti D, Toth SL (eds) Internalizing and Externalizing Expressions of Dysfunction: Rochester Symposium on Developmental Psychopathology. Vol. 2. Hillsdale NJ: Erlbaum, pp. 155–202.

Plomin R, Rutter M (1998) Child development and molecular genetics: what to do with genes once they are found. Child Development 69(4): 1223–42.

Reiss D, Neiderhiser J, Hetherington EM, Plomin R (2000) The Relationship Code: Deciphering Genetic and Social Influences on Adolescent Development. Cambridge MA: Harvard University Press.

Rothbart MK, Bates JE (1998) Temperament. In Eisenberg N (ed.) Handbook of Child Psychology. Vol. 3. Social, Emotional and Personality Development. 5 edn. New York: Wiley.

Rowe DC, Farrington DP (1997) The familial transmission of criminal convictions. Criminology 35: 177–201.

Rutter M, Quinton D (1984) Parental psychiatric disorder: effects on children. Psychological Medicine 14: 853–80.

Rutter M, Dunn J, Plomin R, Simonoff E, Pickles A, Maughan B, Ormel J, Meyer J, Eaves L (1997a) Integrating nature and nurture: implications of person-environment correlations and interactions for developmental psychology. Developmental and Psychopathology 9: 335–64.

Rutter M, Maughan B, Meyer J, Pickles A, Silberg J, Simonoff E, Taylor E (1997b) Heterogeneity of antisocial behaviour: causes, continuities, and consequences. In Dienstbier RD, Osgood DW (eds) Nebraska Symposium on Motivation. Vol. 44. Motivation and Delinquency. Lincoln NE: University of Nebraska Press, pp. 44–118.

Rutter M, Giller J, Hagell A (1998) Antisocial Behaviour by Young People. Cambridge: Cambridge University Press.

Rutter M, Silberg J, O'Connor T, Simonoff E (1999) Genetics and child psychiatry: I Advances in quantitative and molecular genetics. Journal of Child Psychology and Psychiatry 40: 3–18.

Scarr S (1992) Developmental theories for the 1990s: development and individual differences. Child Development 63: 1–19.

Scarr S, McCartney K (1983) How people make their own environments: a theory of genotype–environment effects. Child Development 54: 424–35.

Scarr S, Webber PL, Weinberg RA, Wittig MA (1981) Personality resemblance among adolescents and their parents in biologically related and adoptive families. Journal of Personality and Social Psychology 40(5): 885–98.

Schwartz CE, Dorer EJ, Beardslee WR, Lavori PW, Keller MB (1990) Maternal expressed emotion and parental affective disorder: risk for childhood depressive disorder, substance abuse, or conduct disorder. Journal of Psychiatric Research 24: 231–50.

Seitz V, Apfel NH (1994) Parent-focused intervention: diffusion effects on siblings. Child Development 65: 677–83.

Stoolmiller M (1999) Implications of the restricted range of family environments for estimates of heritability and nonshared environment in behaviour – genetic adoption studies. Psychological Bulletin 125: 302–409.

Stormshak EA, Bellanti CJ, Bierman KL (1996) The quality of sibling relationships and the development of social competence and behavioural control in aggressive children. Developmental Psychology 32: 79–89.

Stubbe DE, Zahner GEP, Goldstein MJ, Leckman JF (1993) Diagnostic specificity of a brief measure of expressed emotion: a community study of children. Journal of Child Psychology and Psychiatry 34: 139–54.

Suomi SJ (1997) Long-term effects of different early rearing experiences on social, emotional and physiological development in nonhuman primates. In Kesheven MS, Murra RM (eds) Neurodevelopmental Models of Adult Psychopathology. Cambridge: Cambridge University Press, pp. 104–16.

Taylor J, Iacono WG, McGue M (2000) Evidence for a genetic etiology of early-onset delinquency. Journal of Abnormal Psychology 109(4): 634–43.

Torgersen S (1983) Genetic factors in anxiety disorders. Archives of General Psychiatry 40: 1085–9.

Torgersen S (1986) Genetic factors in moderately severe and mild affective disorders. Archives of General Psychiatry 43: 222–6.

Torgersen S (1997) Genetic basis and psychopathology. In Turner SM, Hersen M (eds) Adult Psychopathology and Diagnosis. 3 edn. New York NY: John Wiley & Sons, pp. 58–85.

Torgersen S, Skre I, Onstad S, Evardsen Il, Fringlen E (1993) The psychometric-genetic structure of DSM-III-R personality disorder criteria. Journal of Personality Disorders 7: 196–213.

True WR, Rice J, Eisen SA, Heath AC, Goldberg J, Lyons MJ, Nowack J (1993) A twin study of genetic and environmental contributions to liability for post-traumatic stress symptoms. Archives of General Psychiatry 50: 257–64.

Turkheimer E (2000) Three laws of behaviour genetics and what they mean. Current Directions in Psychological Science 9(5): 160–4.

Turkheimer E, Waldron M (2000) Nonshared environment: a theoretical, methodological, and quantitative review. Psychological Bulletin 126(1): 78–108.

Wachs TD, Plomin R (1991) Conceptualization and Measurement of Organism-Environment Interaction. Washington DC: American Psychological Association.

Webster-Stratton C (1990) Long-term follow-up of families with young conduct problem children: from preschool to grade school. Journal of Clinical Child Psychology 19: 144–9.

Wender PH, Kety SS, Rosenthal D, Schulsinger F, Ortmann J, Lunde I (1986) Psychiatric disorders in the biological and adoptive families of adopted individuals with affective disorders. Archives of General Psychiatry 43(10): 923–9.

West DJ, Farrington DP (1973) Who Becomes Delinquent? London: Heinemann Educational Books.

Wilson H (1980) Parental supervision: a neglected aspect of delinquency. The British Journal of Criminology 20: 203–35.

CHAPTER 7

An intergenerational perspective on parent-child relationships: the reciprocal effects of tri-generational grandparent-parent-child relationships

CATHERINE A LAVERS-PRESTON, EDMUND J SONUGA-BARKE

Recent changes in family constitution and the role of grandparents

Until recently nuclear families were the norm in western society and the mother was considered the key socialization agent for her child. There are now, however, an increasing number of lone parents for whom maternal grandparents are a primary source of support (Chase-Lansdale et al., 1994), reconstituted families and greater employment opportunities for women in the workplace. The importance of the contemporary grandparent role in supporting single mothers, cannot be underestimated in light of the association between the absence of a father and negative behavioural functioning in children (Herrenkohl et al., 1995). Marital satisfaction has also been consistently associated with child behaviour problems (Shaw et al., 1994). The children of single or divorcing mothers are therefore at an increased risk of developing conduct problems. Thus the buffering role grandparents can play in protecting children and mothers from the negative effects of stress in such situations, may prove invaluable to the psychosocial functioning of their grandchildren. This is especially true in the case of teenage mothers whose numbers have escalated (Thomas et al., 1990) now making up nearly one quarter of first births in America (Mott Foundation, 1991). These young mothers tend to remain in the family home, and are profoundly reliant upon maternal grandmother support and involvement in the care of their infants (Davis et al., 1997; Taylor et al., 1993). Thus the important role played by grandmothers may explain the particular research interest that has been paid to teenage mother-grandmother relations when considering the role of intergenerational support in child rearing.

Traditional role differences have been identified between motherhood and grandmotherhood. These differences tend to be characterized by a grandmother's role shift from that of a parent, who is responsible for all child rearing issues including limit setting and discipline, to that of a less responsible playmate and confidant (Neugarten and Weinstein, 1964; Tinsley and Parke, 1984). However this clear and simple delineation between grandparenting and parenting quite obviously does not represent the reality or complexity of intergenerational role differences within many families. For example the shift towards mothers now remaining in full or part-time employment whilst their children are of preschool age, may have an effect on parents' and grandparents' perceptions of ideal grandparental roles and levels of involvement. It is now relatively common for grandparents to take on a routine childcare role thereby circumventing the requirement for paid childminding. Intergenerational attitude differences may, however, be a source of friction in this area, with grandparents feeling that their daughters should be at home with their children. There is also the potential for grandparental resentment at having to remain at home with small children at a time in their lives when they expected to be enjoying freedom from such responsibilities (Hansen and Jacob, 1992). In this way intergenerational attitude differences towards the respective roles of parents and grandparents have the potential to cause discrepancies in parent/grandparent perceptions of appropriate grandparenting involvement.

Much of the research exploring teenage mother-grandmother relationships indicates that grandmothers take an equal parenting role to that of their daughters, with no significant differences between mothers' and grandmothers' parenting practices being identified (Chase-Lansdale et al., 1994). The findings from a significant number of studies exploring the role of grandmother support within African American communities, have identified grandmothers as holding authoritative or influential grandparenting styles, which involve high levels of support and/or parentlike influence (Cherlin and Furstenberg, 1985; Burton, 1990; Hogan et al., 1990; Kivett, 1993; Pearson et al., 1990; Wilson, 1984; Wilson et al., 1990).

Intergenerational links and role transitions

The literature regarding transitions to both parenthood and grandparenthood is central in understanding the complex processes by which intergenerational relationships are renegotiated in order to meet the changing needs of family members. An awareness of the issues relating to the demands and potential stresses associated with family role transitions is of importance in aiding clinical understanding of individual and family difficulties during such times. Within this section the importance of inter-generational links and role transitions in relation to risk and protective factors for mental health will be discussed, alongside an overview of the literature within this field.

The significance of intergenerational links is characterized by the say-ing, 'you can choose your friends, but you can't choose your family'; for better or for worse an individual's parents, grandparents, siblings and eventually their own children, play an influential role in their lives. Intergenerational links when viewed from a life-course perspective are an integral aspect of human development. An individual's identity is often couched in terms of family relationships, as a son, a mother, a husband, a grandmother, with at times more than one role being applicable. These roles serve as an indication of an individual's place in society, shaping the way in which people are viewed by others and in many regards how indi-viduals view themselves. Individuals should not therefore, be viewed as solitary units – they are inextricably enmeshed within a network of family members who to some extent dictate their identity. This shaping of iden-tity as a function of placement within a family should be considered when exploring an individual's notion of self-esteem, worth and concept. The manner in which roles are culturally valued, or de-valued, has been found to be related to maternal mental wellbeing (Stern and Krukman, 1983). As such an understanding of how a grandparent or new parent views their role and position within the family, and more widely within their cultural group, is important in understanding their current functioning.

The transition into motherhood/grandmotherhood has been associat-ed with mothers and daughters becoming increasingly involved with each other's lives. Roles are re-evaluated and patterns of contact and support need to be renegotiated (Fischer, 1981). One influential factor in the renegotiation of interaction patterns is the need for grandmothers to establish levels of involvement which are supportive but do not encroach upon maternal desires for independence (Hansen and Jacob, 1992). Hansen and Jacob (1992) in their discussion of role transitions highlight the importance of independence versus dependence in understanding the behaviours of both parents and grandparents. The transition into parent-hood provides mothers with the opportunity to rework earlier developmental issues, for example avoiding the mistakes made by parents, perhaps by attempting to provide their children with the perfect love denied to them. This may result in an initial rejection of grandparental input, which may or may not be later accepted when the challenges of par-enthood become apparent. Thus the transition to parenthood has been identified as a time of confusion for parents, with their behaviour undu-lating between demands for support and rejection over perceived interference.

The often contradictory demands of new parents are exemplified by Hansen and Jacob's (1992) findings, that in contrast to parents' *pre-partum* express wishes to be left alone after the birth, almost two-thirds of maternal grandmothers were asked at short notice for assistance after the babies' delivery. Thus it can be seen that the demands on grandmothers in terms of their understanding and practical assistance are great. Grandparents who are emotionally mature, having a clear memory of their own early parenthood, are often understanding. Responding sensitively to their offspring's alternating demands for support and rejection. These emotionally mature grandparents experience parental swings as stressful yet manageable, often growing in their own self-esteem as they help the new parents in their transition to parenthood (Hansen and Jacob, 1992). Yet it can be envisaged that the transition to grandmotherhood poses risks to individuals' mental wellbeing on a number of levels. This contention is supported by the findings of Troll (1985), which suggest that, when the grandparenting role is not realized as expected, grandparents may feel disappointed, deprived and distressed.

Evidence from Kornhaber and Woodward's (1981) and Cherlin and Furstenberg's (1986) studies suggests that the majority of mothers decide the levels of grandparent contact their children may experience. Kornhaber and Woodward's (1981) findings also indicate such decisions are often based on what the mother considers to be best for her own needs to the exclusion of either the grandparent's or grandchild's best interests. Kornhaber (1985) argues that parental gatekeeping, as to the extent grandparents should nurture their grandchildren, has resulted in a new trend in dysfunctional grandparent-grandchild relationships. It is argued that these 'dysfunctional relationships' feature a lack of vital cross-generational connectedness associated with the move away from the 'natural family arrangement', in which children were reared within a three-generational system enjoying long-lasting emotional attachments across all generations. Kornhaber argues that this lack of connectedness leads to detrimental effects on both grandparents and grandchildren.

It may be argued that current social trends valuing individual independence over the need for cohesive family relationships result in grandparents needing to be especially sensitive in negotiating their active role within the extended family. Hagestad (1985) reports that in an effort to minimize intergenerational conflict many grandparents avoid contentious topics via the employment of 'demilitarized zones'. This tendency for grandparents to seek intergenerational harmony may be driven by the fact mothers mediate the level of contact between grandchildren and grandparents (Cherlin and Furstenberg, 1986). The possibility of limited contact with grandchildren, or at worst estrangement, may be of significance to grandparents on two levels. Firstly on a conscious level, women are likely to desire interactions with their grand-babies (Sticker, 1991) wanting to experience the joys of grandparenthood alongside their contemporaries (Burton, 1996). Secondly, there may be a subconscious need for an intergenerational continuity of the family line, from both a biological perspective and a psychological need to pass on experiences to a third generation in order to feel secure with the prospect of mortality (Neugarten and Weinstein, 1964; Leek and Smith, 1991).

One finding that is not as compatible with grandparents' desires for continuity, is that grandmothers have also reported tensions between dependence and independence. Some grandmothers express a feeling of conflict, between wanting to be needed and anxiety about being bur-dened or even exploited by new parents (Hansen and Jacob, 1992). This may be explained by the young age of a proportion of Hansen and Jacob's sample, some of whom were still in their forties. A proportion of these grandmothers may have regarded the role transition as being early and, as such, were not welcoming of the demands associated with their new role. This demonstrates the importance of the timing of role transitions when considering intergenerational links.

The timing of role transitions

The life-course approach to developmental psychology identifies the tim-ing of role transitions as a potential cause of conflict and mental health problems for new mothers and grandmothers. This approach has been operationalized in two main ways: from a sociological perspective (for example, Hagestad and Burton, 1986) and from a humanistic viewpoint (Erikson, 1950).

The sociological perspective on role transitions

The sociological approach is primarily concerned with the impact of cul-turally prescribed timings which determine when individuals are expected to take on new roles, and the effects of off-time role transitions on an individual's wellbeing.[1] This approach is of particular interest in the case of grandparenthood, as this is a hinged role transition, with an individual's entrance into grandparenthood being facilitated by his or her offspring's entrance into parenthood. The timing of such counter-transitions present a source of potential friction between generations. For example if the role transition is deemed 'too early' or 'too late' it may lead the grandparent to put pressure on their offspring, either to begin a fam-ily or because they consider their off-spring too young for parenthood.

Hagestad and Burton (1986) propose a number of ways in which 'off-time' role transitions may be problematic for grandmothers:

- early transitions do not allow individuals time to re-orientate their expectations and other role investments in preparation for the transition to grandparenthood;
- mothers entering grandparenthood at a non-prescribed time may also encounter problems due to societal assumptions about their maturity and physical role investments;
- 'off-time' grandparents may experience a lack of empathy and support from friends not entering grandparenthood themselves, possibly resulting in feelings of isolation and deviance.

Any of the above situations may negatively affect the mental wellbeing of grandmothers and lead to intergenerational tension, thus presenting a source of stress to the dyad and inhibiting the grandmother from fulfilling a supportive role. It can be hypothesized that intergenerational discord may pose a risk to maternal mental wellbeing and ability to cope with the new demands of parenthood. As the literature clearly identifies maternal depression as a risk factor in relation to infant outcomes (Puckering, 1989) discord in relation to the timing of role transitions may have a tri-generational impact. Off-time role transitions may also be seen to have a secondary detrimental impact upon mother-infant dyads via the absence of grandparental support.

How an individual conceptualizes and deals with the transition to grandparenthood may be significant in understanding their interactions with family members. The transition to grandmotherhood, and other role transitions that may occur around this time, for example retiring from the work place, may represent a time of significant emotional stress for older women (Hansen and Jacob, 1992). For example it might be the case, in view of the media-promoted youth ideal, that the entrance into grandmotherhood marks a time of identity crisis for women (Euler and Weitzel, 1996). In contrast to this negative reaction that may occur in some cases, the majority of women entering grandmotherhood receive their first grandchild with a sense of pride and joy rather than loss (Fischer, 1981). The view of entrance into grandparenthood as a positive transition is supported by the findings of Neugarten and Weinstein (1964) who report that the majority of grandparents judge their lives to have changed for the better. Having a new focus and something to look forward to were commonly mentioned themes, indicating that grandparenthood normatively represents a positive role change. Thus, although we would like to highlight the importance of exploring issues related to role transitions during assessment and formulations with this client group of grandparents, it is important to note that in most cases this role shift does not represent a risk factor for mental health problems.

The humanistic view of role transitions

The humanistic view adopted by Erikson (1950) regards off-time role transitions as problematic, not because they clash with culturally pre-scribed timetables but because they are incompatible with an individual's developmental stage and their associated level of maturity (Burton et al., 1995; McLaughlin and Micklin, 1983). Role transitions that occur at a time incompatible with the need to complete a developmental task are thought to disrupt development and lead to maladjustment (Erikson et al., 1986). This is exemplified by the premature transition to motherhood of teenage girls, where an early off-time transition to parenthood whilst still a teen-ager may hinder the acquisition of identity. Some research has even suggested that adolescent motherhood may delay, or even preclude, the development of a stable maternal identity and family unit (Elder and Rockwell, 1976). The problems associated with teenage mothering may therefore arise due to the apparently direct opposition between the nor-mative characteristics of adolescence, such as identity fluctuation, dependence on parents and age-appropriate role experimentation, with the desirable qualities of parenting which centre around stability, assertiveness and established relationships (Schellenbach et al., 1992).

The importance of considering the timing of role transitions, with regard to clashes in developmental tasks, is therefore of particular impor-tance in understanding the problems associated with adolescent pregnancy and motherhood.

Cultural differences in grandparent-parent relationships

The increased awareness of cultural differences in child-rearing practices has been of influence in shaping the current understanding of tri-generational relationships and their impact upon mental health and parenting practices. It was therefore felt to be of importance to explore some of these findings within the current chapter.

Cross-cultural studies indicate that differences in the grandparent-parent relationship arise largely as a function of the ideologies, beliefs, traditions, and values, prescribed by the dyad's cultural group. For exam-ple Burton et al. (1995) suggest that the traditional cultural background of African-American families results in grandparents more frequently assuming parenting responsibilities than their white-American counter-parts, whilst white families are more likely than black families to provide financial support for extended family members (Hofferth, 1984). Whereas some cultures, such as Hispanic, value kinship interdependence, result-ing in the implementation of child-rearing practices that place emphasis on compliance, co-operation and obligation (MacPhee et al., 1996). The

closeness of kinship networks in interdependent cultures, places grandmothers in a highly influential position.

The importance of accounting for socioeconomic factors, alongside
cultural differences, should also be noted at this juncture. For example,
research carried out by Kivett (1993) suggests that when the economic
and living circumstance of white and African-American families are comparable, the degree of racial differences in co-residence rates and levels of
grandmother involvement are reduced. This may, however, be a function
of the common values held by the southern rural families that made up
Kivett's (1993) sample. This illustrates the importance of recognising the
differences found between the values held by families regardless of their
racial background: in the case of southern American rural families strong
intergenerational ties and financial strains are themes common to both
black and white families. The importance of racial differences should not,
however, be overlooked. For example a comparison of working class
grandparents from the Washington DC metropolitan area showed that
African-American grandparents perceive themselves to be more actively
involved with their grandchildren than are white-American grandparents
(Watson and Koblinsky, 1997). Thus, the above research demonstrates
that both ethnic and socioeconomic factors may be influential in shaping
grandparenting behaviours.

Cultural variations in family life have also been explored in the context
of grandmother-mother relationships, with research suggesting that family structure may have an impact upon mothers', grandmothers' and
children's mental health and adjustment (Chase-Lansdale et al., 1994;
Shah and Sonuga-Barke, 1994; Taylor et al., 1993a; Unger and Cooley,
1992). The contrasting results provided by these studies may in some
cases be explained as a function of their cultural settings, suggesting that
the rearing of children within a three generational setting may have either
a positive or a negative impact, depending upon the family's culture. For
example Shah and Sonuga-Barke's (1994) study indicated that, within the
Pakistani Muslim immigrant community of Britain, first generation mothers living in extended families were more anxious and depressed than
mothers living outside the extended family.

Conflict between mothers and grandmothers over issues of cultural significance is one likely cause of stress amongst immigrant families,
potentially being of detriment to a mother's mental health (Hansen and
Jacob, 1992). For example first generation mothers born and raised in the
country of their residence, are likely to hold differing beliefs and values to
those of the grandmother who spent her formative years in their country
of origin (Frankel and Roer-Bornstein, 1982). The degree of similarity in
parent-grandparent attitudes is likely to vary as a function of their assimi-
lation of the host country's values. When the parent is more acculturated

(i.e. socialized into an alternative set of cultural roles, values and beliefs) than the grandparent, for example in situations where the grandparent has not learned the language of their host country, differences within the dyad have the capacity to be marked, particularly if offspring have entered into cross-cultural relationships. This potential for increased grandparent-daughter conflict and disagreement amongst immigrant families when the daughter becomes a mother herself has been suggested as a possible cause of the high levels of maternal depression apparent within British Muslim families (Sonuga-Barke et al., 1998). This contention is supported by research carried out with Puerto Rican adolescent mothers, which suggests that the effects of high levels of grandmother involvement in childcare is moderated by the daughter's level of acculturation. The daughter's adjustment did benefit from high levels of grandmother involvement and support when acculturation scores were low, but led to more parenting stress and symptomatology when scores were high (Contreras et al., 1999).

This theory relating to acculturation levels is supported by Sonuga-Barke et al.'s (1998) finding that first generation immigrant grandmothers displayed markedly different parenting strategies to those employed by their daughters. The grandmothers were far more authority orientated and traditional than mothers, who held more liberal child-rearing beliefs and were generally more child centred. It was found that differences in child-rearing beliefs between the mother and the grandmother, predicted mother's depression and anxiety levels independently of other factors such as social class (Sonuga-Barke et al., 1998).

Thus it can be seen that cultural differences are integral in shaping the nature of grandparent-parent relationships, particularly in relation to the level of conflict experienced within dyads. Factors associated with elevated levels of grandmother-mother discord may be of particular significance, when considering the importance of grandmother-mother relationships, due to the multidimensional routes through which they may effect the maternal and infant wellbeing.

The impact of intergenerational relationships on mother-infant wellbeing: discrepancies in the grandparenting literature

In order to fully appreciate the complexity of factors that shape the outcomes associated with intergenerational relationships, it is helpful to review briefly the grandparenting literature. This fragmented body of literature demonstrates the potential for extended family support in some instances to be protective of mother-infant relations and wellbeing, whilst in other cases being detrimental. One of the aims of this chapter is to explore the possible root causes of such discrepancies and suggest the complex combination of factors that should be borne in mind when considering the quality of intergenerational relationships.

The positive effects of grandparent involvement

Grandparents' support has been identified as a significant influence in the life satisfaction of mothers. Wan et al. (1996) found that mothers who experienced poor relationships with grandparents received lower levels of support from them, which in turn led to decreased life satisfaction and support seeking by the mother. Hence, the grandmother's key role within the mother's support network renders her effectual in reducing the incidence of maternal depression and anxiety (Davis et al., 1997).

The findings of Stevens (1984) suggest that African-American teenage mothers from low-income backgrounds turn to maternal grandmothers for their primary source of support and childcare advice. African-American maternal grandmothers have also been identified as fostering sensitive parenting behaviour in their daughters by providing a positive role model, a source of parenting information and support (Colletta, 1981; MacLoyd, 1990). The extent of family support has been positively related to teenage mothers' nurturance and negatively related to restrictiveness (Thomas et al., 1990). The positive impact of such extended family support on the subsequent adjustment of mother and child has also been demonstrated, with the quality of childcare; the mother's reported self reliance and the level of child behaviour problems being associated with levels of kinship support (Taylor et al., 1993). Thus the role of maternal grandmothers in shaping teenage daughters' parenting behaviours has been established.

In situations where the mother is at risk from a number of psychosocial stressors grandmothers have an important role to play in protecting mothers' and infants' wellbeing. High levels of contact with grandmothers who provide positive stimulation has beneficial effects on the social, cognitive and motor development of teenage mothers' infants (Cooley and Unger, 1991; Tinsley and Parke, 1987). The infants of teenage mothers co-habiting with the grandmother, have also been found to be more securely attached when grandmothers take increased responsibility for childcare and are highly supportive (Frodi et al., 1984). Mother and infant co-residence with the grandmother was also associated with increased infant persistence on tasks, indicating that for this sample of mothers living with the grandmother was of benefit to their infants' future cognitive · and psychosocial wellbeing (Frodi et al., 1984). Grandmother-teenage

mother co-habitation may affect better child outcomes due to the beneficial effect it has on mother-infant interaction style, being associated with
less restrictive, punitive parenting practices (King and Fullard, 1982).
Oyserman et al. (1993) also found that where grandmothers took responsibility for childcare teenage mothers perceived there to be lower levels of
family conflict, suggesting one possible route through which high levels
of grandmother childcare may lead to positive mother-infant outcomes.

However, Frodi et al.'s (1984) findings also indicated that high levels of
grandmother support for her daughter and active involvement in the care
of her grandchild, were associated with more secure mother-infant attachment bonds when they 'lived independently'. It may, therefore, be seen
that co-habitation is not necessarily a prerequisite for grandmother
involvement to result in improved mother-infant interaction patterns.

The role played by grandfathers in the rearing and wellbeing of their
grandchildren has also been the subject of research studies. Findings suggest that grandfathers may have a particularly important role to play in the
lives of grandchildren reared within 'single mother' headed family units, as
in such cases grandfathers may act as a paternal substitute (Oyserman et
al., 1993; Crnic et al., 1983). Oyserman et al. (1993) assessed the direct
influence of grandfather involvement upon the babies of their teenage
daughters, as these infants do not normally have contact with their fathers.
It was found that grandfather nurturance was positively related to more
child compliance with maternal requests, and that grandfather involvement in childcare was positively associated with less child-exhibited
negative affect. As well as affecting child outcomes through direct grandfa-
ther-grandchild interactions, it is seems likely that grandfathers also play an
important role in shaping the parenting strategies employed by their
daughters. Oyserman et al. (1993) present evidence that suggests that
teenage mothers who feel more supported, employ parenting techniques
that are more responsive and affectionate. Thus it might be argued that
grandfathers who are supportive of their adolescent daughters indirectly
encourage more sensitive mothering behaviour. Research carried out by
Crnic et al. (1983) proposes that social behaviour modelling (Bandura,
1977) may provide an alternative route through which grandfathers might
impact upon the mothering received by their grandchildren, as mothers
may model their parenting upon grandparent-infant interactions.

Research has shown that teenage mothers who receive high levels of
support (including guidance, social reinforcement, emotional support,
practical assistance, and social stimulation from their parental families)
experience reduced emotional distress and greater wellbeing than less
supported mothers (Cooley and Unger, 1991). Cooley and Unger (1991)
also found that direct childcare by the grandmother had the secondary
effect of allowing their daughter to complete her education, leading to a

richer environment for her infant. This can be partly accounted for through the increased incidence of stable marital relationships with a father who interacts positively with their child, as the completion of a full-time education is also associated with relationship longevity. Having the opportunity to complete her education may also allow the mother to avoid some of the stressors associated with mental ill health, such as unemployment and poverty, thereby reducing their risk of experiencing a depressive episode. The above research demonstrates the multiple routes grandmother involvement may take in influencing the wellbeing of mothers and infants.

Neutral or negative effects of grandmother involvement

Despite this evidence for the benefits of grandmother involvement, several studies have found either no effects or have actually discovered negative effects of grandmother involvement on mothers and their infants. For example, although teenagers' own mothers provide the richest source of support to them, demonstrating a wider variety of positive support more often even than partners, this does not necessarily result in the employment of more positive parenting practices (Nitz et al., 1995; Voight et al., 1996). Grandmothers are also a source of conflict; with findings somewhat counterintuitively showing that the greater the range of support provided by the grandmother, the more negative the daughter's experience of parenting (Voight et al., 1996). This suggests that although grandmother involvement may improve their daughter's parenting technique, the daughter may not enjoy this process.

Neither do all studies confirm the positive effects of grandmother support on the mother's parenting practices and child outcomes (Gordon, 1999). Unlike most studies exploring the impact of grandmother support for young mothers, Oyserman et al. (1993) did not find any positive effects associated with emotional support from the parents of teenage mothers. This finding was mirrored by Frodi et al.'s (1984) study, which found that infant competence and affect were not related to grandmother involvement. An important distinction that should be highlighted when discussing teenage mothers' parenting abilities and adjustment is between adolescents who have made a life choice to become parents and those whose parenting is associated with problem adolescent behaviours (Wakschlag and Hans, 2000). The failure of studies to make this distinction may go some way in explaining the diversity of findings regarding the mothering behaviours of adolescents, however, an alternative factor that must be considered is the impact of grandmother-mother co-residence.

The effects of family structure and living arrangements have been brought into question by a number of studies. Burchinal et al. (1996) found no significant effects of family structure on the quality of maternal caregiving in their sample of young disadvantaged African-American mothers. Black and Nitz's (1996) study also found co-residence was not associated with teenage mothers' warmth towards their infants. In fact, some studies have found that grandmother-mother co-residence causes infant care to deteriorate, thus indicating that some types and levels of grandmother involvement may be detrimental to infants (Chase-Lansdale et al., 1994). Spieker and Bensley (1994) found that grandmother support had no beneficial effects on infant attachment when the mother and grandmother lived together. Unger and Cooley (1992) found that for white adolescent mothers, increased grandmother contact (including childcare) was related to more child behaviour problems; whereas for black American adolescent mothers the length of time residing in the grandmother's home was associated with lower maternal responsiveness.

In an earlier study Cooley and Unger (1991) found that if the mother remained in their parental home for too long, the positive effects of grandmother support for her were reversed. Maternal responsiveness and stimulation were found to reduce, thus jeopardizing infant outcomes, despite the mother's increased ability to complete her education and enjoy its associated benefits. This is supported by the findings of Unger and Wandersman (1985) who found that high family support predicts low levels of parenting anxiety at 1 month but not at 8 months. The findings of Crockenberg (1987) also suggest that more frequent grandmother help at 2 years is unrelated to mothering, but is associated with higher levels of angry non-compliant infant behaviour at 2 years. This deterioration in the quality of mother-infant relations could, however, be a function of poor teenage parenting, which has resulted in the grandmother attempting to alleviate the situation by being highly supportive.

Factors contributing to the quality of intergenerational relationships

In order to address why there is discrepancy in relation to child and mother outcome variables within the grandparenting literature, it is necessary to consider the nature of grandparent-parent relationships and the routes via which intergenerational influences may be affected.

There are two primary ways in which relatives can exert their influence over an individual's developmental life course, immediately through their *direct* actions and *indirectly*. This indirect route may take a number of concurrent forms, for example via the *historic* influence this relationship has on the individual's psyche, or *currently* through an intermediary family member.

These dimensions of *current-historic* and *direct-indirect* provide a useful means of conceptualizing the routes via which intergenerational influences may be mediated. They enable thinking, in terms of transgenerational relationships, to be carried out on more than one level, thereby facilitating a broader understanding of extended family process and context. For example, rather than limiting exploration of those factors determining the usefulness of intergenerational input to *current* present-day circumstances, these dimensions encourage the consideration of *historic* relationship history and thereby pose questions regarding the appropriateness of grandparental input. It would seem that in families where there has been a history of problematic grandparent-parent relations, the grandparent might not be the most suitable supportive agent. This may seem to be an obvious point, however it has often been overlooked within the grandparenting literature.

Influences of grandparents on their grandchildren: current-direct

This route of influence describes the role of grandparenting in its most obvious form; the immediate relationships between a grandchild and their grandparent. In its traditional form, as outlined above, this is likely to include spoiling of grandchildren and a more lax approach to discipline than might be employed by a parent. The grandparent-grandchild relationship is often a unique and special one, in which children experience an unconditional provision of love and security, with very few demands being placed on them with regards to responsibility and reciprocal behaviours. However, as has already been outlined, grandparents are increasingly being asked to play an active childcare role in the care of their grandchildren, for example in the case of infants born to teenage and or working mothers (Lavers and Sonuga-Barke, 1997; Taylor et al., 1993a; Taylor and Roberts, 1995). Thus it can be seen that grandparents are often in a powerful position to directly influence the wellbeing of infants.

Influences of grandparents on the care received by their grandchildren: current-indirect

The majority of *current-indirect* routes through which grandmothers may affect the care their grandchildren receive may be roughly broken down into those that are advice based and those that are support based. The quality of current grandparent-parent relationships and the level of grandparenting involvement in childcare during their off-spring's transition into parenthood may also provide another opportunity for the modelling of parenting strategies on those of the grandparents.

Childcare advice

There has been a limited amount of research focusing specifically on the advisory role of maternal grandmothers in influencing the type of parenting practices employed by new mothers. Findings indicate that in some instances high levels of childcare help and advice are associated with the provision of more age-appropriate stimulation by the mothers of preschoolers (Cotterell, 1986). Although highly directive grandmothering is associated with more secure teenage mother-infant attachments in the short term, in the long term this level of involvement appears to be associated with less competent mothering (Cooley and Unger, 1991). It is, therefore, conceivable that high levels of inappropriate or unwanted childcare advice are detrimental to mothering, with the stress and conflict associated with intergenerational interference providing one possible mechanism through which this effect may be mediated.

Grandparental support

Grandparents are an obvious source of support for families, and the support provided by grandmothers is of more benefit and wider in scope than partner support (Spieker and Bensley, 1994; Voight et al., 1996; Dalla and Gamble, 1999). Research has highlighted the importance of social support in buffering the effects of parenting stress on parenting behaviours (Burchinal et al., 1996; Herrenkohl et al., 1995; Macphee et al., 1996; Rogers, 1998; Webster-Stratton, 1990), thereby demonstrating the significant role intergenerational support plays in directly modifying the care experienced by children.

Environmental stressors have long been recognized as a major risk factor for mental ill health (Brown and Harris, 1978). Social support can, therefore, be identified as an influential factor in shaping mothers' parenting behaviour and efficacy indirectly, through the role it plays in moderating the effects of stress on maternal functioning and mental wellbeing. Thus, through her supportive role the grandmother can positively or negatively influence the mother's parenting behaviour directly, as well as influencing the mother's parenting through the promotion of maternal mental wellbeing.

Studies have revealed that parenting self-esteem (comprised of parenting efficacy and parenting satisfaction) plays an important role in the transmission of psychosocial functioning and adjustment between mothers and their infants (Bornstein, 1995a; Bugental, 1987; Cutrona and Troutman, 1986; Johnston and Mash, 1989). Grandparent support may also be important in shaping mothers' parenting efficacy and satisfaction (Abernathy, 1973, cited by Hagestad, 1985 and Voight et al., 1996), making parenting self-esteem a potentially important route through which grandmother involvement may impact upon the wellbeing of her daughter and grandchild.

Current grandparent-parent relationships: the importance of context

When exploring the role of grandparenting within the setting of contemporary family life, and in relation to parent and child functioning and outcomes, it is vital to consider the context within which families are functioning. By context we are referring to a number of situational and relational variables that are likely to affect the need for intergenerational involvement.

Situational factors

These would include the following factors:

- Economic variables: housing; childcare needs and financial independence.
- Social resources: the availability of alternative support networks.
- Personal resources: for example cognitive maturity and depression are both important factors relating to parenting ability, being influential in shaping infant adjustment and development (Van IJzendoorn et al., 1992). Low socioeconomic status is also a major risk factor to mothers' and infants' psychosocial functioning and the mothers' parenting behaviour (Brown and Harris, 1978; Herrenkohl et al., 1995; Hops, 1995).
- Finally child-related variables: physical, cognitive or temperament related difficulties (Bornstein, 1995b; Hubert et al., 1982).

The quality of current grandmother-mother relations

The current quality of the grandmother-mother relationship has the propensity to shape appropriate levels of grandmaternal involvement in childcare in a number of ways, with intergenerational similarities and differences in childcare attitudes being an integral factor. The potential for intergenerational differences in child rearing attitudes to affect the receipt of grandmaternal support negatively as well as positively have been illustrated by cross-cultural studies (Contreras et al., 1999; Frankel and Roer-Bornstein, 1982; Sonuga-Barke et al., 1998).

Bearing the complexity of the factors influencing appropriate levels of grandmother involvement in mind, attempting to produce an exhaustive list of the innumerable factors potentially affecting mother-grandmother relationships would not be advantageous at this juncture. Rather it is important to summarize that both situational and personal factors undoubtedly shape the ways in which individual grandmother-mother dyads interact and to highlight the multifaceted factors that constitute the risk and protective factors impacting upon parent-infant wellbeing.

Grandmother-mother relationship history

The importance of the *historic* route of influence, with regard to mothering behaviour, is restricted to maternal grandparents: in the case of fathering paternal grandparents assume this position.[2] This leads to a division between maternal and paternal grandparents due to the *historical* context underpinning mother-maternal grandparents' relations, extending their influence over mothers' parenting from their *current* involvement to factors that have shaped parents across their developmental lifespan. Despite the potentially significant role paternal grandmothers play in advising and supporting many mothers, the absence of an *historic* context through which the mother views parenting advice and support may mean that even *current* paternal grandmother involvement carries differing significance to that of maternal grandmother support.

The history between a mother and maternal grandmother is a potentially important factor influencing the suitability of the grandmother as a provider of support. Research by Hansen and Jacob (1992) illustrates the importance of developmental history in determining current grandmother-mother relationships. They have suggested that resentment left over from feelings of rejection during childhood, revived when a woman enters motherhood and realises the strength of her maternal love, may cause her to question further her own childhood experiences (Kornharber, 1986). Alternatively, on entering motherhood a woman may realize the extent of demands and difficulties associated with the role of motherhood, leading to the development of a closer relationship with her mother and a forgiveness over the perfect parenting she previously felt denied.

The attachment history of the mother–grandmother dyad offers a number of routes through which the appropriateness of current grandmaternal involvement might be shaped. This is not least because the nature of attachment relationships during infancy have been shown to influence an individual's concept of self, personality, future functioning and later relationships, through the formation of internal working models of the attachment relationship (Bowlby, 1980; Cassidy, 1988; Hazen and Shaver, 1994).

An insecure attachment history is also indicative of the grandmother's insensitivity towards her daughter's feelings (Ainsworth, 1973), suggesting that the dyad may currently experience difficulties in the giving and receiving of support. Thus the formation of an insecure attachment relationship

during infancy may lead to difficulties with the acceptance of grandmaternal assistance in the future. Hence it is arguable that grandmother-
mother attachment history is a significant determinant of their present-day
relationship (Shaw and Vondra, 1993; Sroufe, 1983; Sroufe and Fleeson,
1986; Waters et al., 1979). The type of attachment bond formed between
the mother and grandmother can therefore be seen to have a contemporary influence on mother-infant interaction, as mediated via the reception
current grandmother involvement. Alongside this current influence of
attachment there is an historic impact via the mother's subsequent parenting ability, as shaped by her interactional style, and the development
and nature of the mother-infant attachment bond (Greenberg et al., 1993).

Mothers whose memories of childhood rejection remain repressed tend
to go on to form 'dismissive' adult attachment relationships, redirecting the
frustration they feel towards their mothers onto others (George et al.,
1985). As a result of this such individuals have difficulties forming open,
trusting, secure adult relationships (Hazen and Shaver, 1994). These mothers are therefore placed doubly at risk of experiencing parenting difficulties
due to the absence of a cohesive support network and their own inability
to form an intimate secure relationship with their baby. The presence and
involvement of the grandmother during their daughter's transition to motherhood presents an interesting scenario; will the grandmother's
participation lead the mother to deflect even more frustration onto their
infant? Or will they express their frustrations towards their mothers? It
seems plausible that new mothers may re-assess and explore their own
childhood relationships at this time of transition (Hansen and Jacob, 1992;
Benedek, 1959), a contention that is supported by Epstein's theory of personality (Bretherton, 1985). Epstein's theory postulates that changes in
mental representations are only likely to occur through a significant emotional experience. Since working models of attachment figures and self are
formed during childhood, experiences causing the reappraisal of childhood
experiences may be especially significant. Therefore grandmother–mother
interactions during the first few months of motherhood present women
with an opportunity to update the working model of their own attachment
relationships. These contentions help to illustrate the complexity of factors
influencing the reception grandparent assistance may engender and illustrate the importance of considering the historic context within which
current grandparent-parent relations are founded.

Conclusions and suggestions for future research

In this chapter we have attempted to illustrate the complexity of the
grandparental role and the numerous ways in which intergenerational

influences may be enacted. We have also proposed that in order to understand the nature and likely outcomes associated with grandparenting, it is necessary to look beyond absolute levels and types of intergenerational involvement and explore the context in which they are set. It is our contention that much of the heterogeneity in research exploring the role and impact of grandmothering is indicative of a fine line between levels of grandparent involvement that are of benefit to mothers and their infants, and levels of involvement that are unhelpful or even detrimental.

It is arguable that discrepancies in research findings examining impact of intergenerational relationships might be explained by a more in-depth view of grandmother involvement, which looks beyond the levels of grandmother support and explores how well this support matches with the needs and wishes of the mother. This contention is supported by recent shifts in the literature, which is now recognizing the importance of issues related to the quality of grandmother-mother relationships when making quantitative assessments of the impact of intergenerational involvement levels (Davis et al., 1997; Kalil et al., 1998).

Recent shifts in family constitution and the increasing number of teenage mothers have resulted in policy changes, making an understanding of grandparent-mother relationships of even more importance within clinical work and research. An example of such policy change is demonstrated by the stipulation that unmarried, minor adolescent girls must co-reside with a parent or adult guardian in order to qualify for cash support in some American states (Kalil et al., 1998). The social and political significance of research focusing on the impact of grandparent-daughter co-residence on maternal and infant wellbeing is therefore clear. In light of these implications the need for further research exploring the impact of tri-generational co-habitation is heightened: especially in view of the discrepant nature of past research findings regarding the benefit of grandparent-mother co-residence (Lavers and Sonuga-Barke, 1997).

Within clinical work with families an understanding and sensitivity towards some of the complex relationship issues raised within this chapter may be of importance in facilitating successful resolution of intergenerational tensions.

Notes

1. Off-time role transitions describe role changes, for example entering motherhood, at a time your culture views as being either unusually early or late.
2. For simplicity, this discussion will be restricted to the mother and as such the maternal grandparents hold the position of having an historical as well as current influence.

References

Abernathy V (1973) Social networks and response to the maternal role. International Journal of Sociology of the Family 3: 86–96.

Ainsworth MDS (1973) The development of infant-mother attachment. In Caldwell BM, Reiccuiti HN (eds) Review of Child Development Research. Vol 3. Chicago: UCP, pp. 1–94.

Bandura A (1977) Social Learning Theory. New York: Prentice-Hall.

Benedek T (1959) Parenthood as a developmental phase: a contribution to the libido theory. Journal of the American Psychoanalytic Association 7: 389–417.

Black MM, Nitz K (1996) Grandmother co-residence, parenting, and child development among low income, urban teen mothers. Journal of Adolescent Health 18: 218–26.

Bornstein MH (1995a) Between caretakers and their young: two modes of interaction and their consequences for cognitive growth. In Bornstein MH, Bruner JS (eds) Interaction in Human Development. Hillsdale NJ: Erlbaum, pp. 197–214.

Bornstein MH (1995b) Parenting infants. In Bornstein MH (ed.) Handbook of Parenting. Volume one: Children and Parenting. New Jersey: Erlbaum.

Bowlby J (1980) Attachment and Loss. Volume 3. Loss: Sadness and Depression. London: Hogarth Press and the Institute of Psychoanalysis.

Bretherton I (1985) Attachment theory: retrospect and prospect. In Bretherton I, Waters E (eds) Growing Points of Attachment Theory and Research. Monographs of the Society for Research in Child Development 209: nos1–2.

Brown GW, Harris T (1978) The Social Origins of Depression: A Study of Psychiatric Disorders in Women. New York: Free Press.

Bugental DB (1987) Caregiver attributions as moderators of child effects. Paper presented at the meeting of the Society for Research in Child Development, Baltimore. Cited by Johnston C, Mash EJ (1989) A measure of parenting satisfaction and efficacy. Journal of Clinical Child Psychology 18: 167–75.

Burchinal MR, Follmer A, Bryant DM (1996) The relations of maternal social support and family structures with maternal responsiveness and child outcomes among African American families. Developmental Psychology 32: 1073–83.

Burton LM (1990) Teenage childbearing as an alternative life-course strategy in multigeneration black families. Human Nature 1: 123–43.

Burton LM (1996) Age norms, the timing of family role transitions, and intergenerational caregiving among aging African American women. Gerontologist 36(2): 199–208.

Burton LM, Dilworth-Anderson P, Merriweather-deVries C (1995) Context and surrogate parenting among contemporary grandparents. Marriage and Family Review 20: 349–66.

Cassidy J (1988) Child-mother attachment and the self in six year olds. Child Developments 59: 121–34.

Chase-Lansdale PL, Brooks-Gunn J (1994) Correlates of adolescent parenting and parenthood. In Fisher CB, Lerner RM (eds) Applied Developmental Psychology. Cambridge MA: McGraw-Hill.

Chase-Lansdale PL, Brooks-Gunn J, Zamsky ES (1994) Young African-American multigenerational families in poverty: quality of mothering and grandmothering. Child Development 65: 373–93.

Cherlin AJ, Furstenberg FF (1985) Styles and strategies of grandparenting. In Bengston VL, Robertson JF (eds) Grandparenthood. London: Sage, pp. 96–116.

Cherlin AJ, Furstenberg FF (1986) The New American Grandparent: A Place in the Family, a Life Apart. New York: Basic Books.

Colletta ND (1981) Social support and the risk of maternal rejection by adolescent mothers. Journal of Psychology 109: 191–7.

Contreras JM, Lopez IR, Rivera-Mosquera ET, Raymond-Smith L, Rothstein K (1999) Social support and adjustment among Puerton Rican mothers: the moderating effect of acculturation. Journal of Family Psychology 13: 228–43.

Cooley ML, Unger DG (1991) The role of family support in determining developmental outcomes in children of teen mothers. Child Psychiatry and Human Development 21: 217–34.

Cotterell JL (1986) Work and community influences on the quality of child rearing. Child Development 57: 362–74.

Crnic KA, Greenberg MT, Ragozin AS, Robinson NM, Basham RD (1983) Effects of stress and social support on mothers and premature and full term infants. Child Development 54: 209–17.

Crockenberg SB (1987) Predictors and correlates of anger toward and punitive control for toddlers by adolescent mothers. Child Development 58: 969–75.

Cutrona CE, Troutman BR (1986) Social support, infant temperament, and parenting self-efficacy: a mediational model of post-partum depression. Child Development 57: 1507–18.

Dalla RL, Gamble WC (1999) Weaving a tapestry of relational assistance: a qualitative investigation of interpersonal support among reservation-residing Navajo teenage mothers. Personal Relationships 6: 251–67.

Davis AA, Rhodes JE, Hamilton-Leaks J (1997) When parents may be a source of support and problems: an analysis of pregnant and parenting female African American adolescents' relationships with their mothers and fathers. Journal of Research into Adolescence 7(3): 331–48.

Elder GH, Rockwell RC (1976) Marital timing in women's life patterns. Journal of Family History 1(1): 34–53.

Erikson EH (1950) Childhood and Society. New York: Norton.

Erikson EH, Erikson JM, Kivinick HQ (1986). Vital Involvement in Old Age: The Experience of Old Age in Our Time. New York: Norton.

Euler HA, Weitzel B (1996) Discriminative grandparental solicitude as reproductive strategy. Human Nature 7(1): 39–59.

Fischer LR (1981) Transitions in the mother-daughter relationship. Journal of Marriage and the Family 43: 613–22.

Frankel DG, Roer-Bornstein D (1982) Traditional and modern contributions to changing infant rearing ideologies of two ethnic communities. Monographs of the Society for the Study of Child Development 44 (4).

Frodi AM, Murray A, Lamb ME, Steinberg J (1984) Biological and social determinants of responsiveness to infants in 10-15 year old girls. Sex Roles 10(7–8): 639–49.

George C, Kaplan N, Main M (1985) The Berkeley Adult Attachment Interview. Unpublished protocol. Berkeley CA: Department of Psychology, University of California.

Gordon RA (1999) Multigenerational coresidence and welfare policy. Journal of Community Psychology 27: 525–49.

Greenberg MT, Speltz ML, DeKlyen M (1993) The role of attachment in the early development of disruptive behaviour problems. Development and Psychopathology 5(12): 191–213.

Hagestad GO (1985) Continuity and connectedness. In Bengston VL, Robertson JF (eds) Grandparenthood. Beverly Hills, CA: Sage.

Hagestad GO, Burton LM (1986) Grandparenthood, life context, and family development. American Behavioral Science 29(4): 471–84.

Hansen LB, Jacob E (1992) Inter-generational support during the transition to parenthood: issues for new parents and grandparents. Families in Society: The Journal of Contemporary Human Services 73: 471–9.

Hazen C, Shaver PR (1994) Attachment as an organisational framework for research on close relationships. Psychological Enquiry 5: 1–22.

Herrenkohl EC, Herrenkohl RC, Rupert LJ, Egolf BP, Lutz JG (1995) Risk factors for behavioural dysfunction: the relative impact of maltreatment, SES, physical health problems, cognitive ability, and quality of parent-child interaction. Child Abuse and Neglect 19: 191–203.

Hofferth SL (1984) Kin networks, race, and family structure. Journal of Marriage and the Family 791–806.

Hogan DP, Hao LX, Parish WL (1990) Race, kin networks and assistance to mother-headed families. Social Forces 68 (3): 797–812.

Hops H (1995) Age- and gender-specific effects of parental depression: a commentary. Developmental Psychology 31: 428–31.

Hubert NC, Wachs T, Peters-Martin P, Gandour MJ (1982) The study of early temperament: measurement and conceptual issues. Child Development 53(3): 571–600.

Johnston C, Mash EJ (1989) A measure of parenting satisfaction and efficacy. Journal of Clinical Child Psychology 18: 167–75.

Kalil A, Spencer MS, Spieker SJ, Gilchrist LD (1998) Effects of grandmother coresidence and quality of family relationships on depressive symptoms in adolescent mothers. Family Relations 47: 433–41.

King T, Fullard W (1982) Teenage mothers and their infants: new findings on the home environment. Journal of Adolescence 5: 333–46.

Kivett V (1993) Racial comparisons of the grandmother role. Family Relations 42: 165–72.

Kornharber A (1985) Grandparenthood and the 'new social contract'. In Bengston VL, Robertson JF (eds) Grandparenthood. Beverly Hills, CA: Sage, pp. 159–71.

Kornharber A (1986) Grandparenting: normal and pathological: a preliminary communication from the Grandparent Study. Journal of Geriatric Psychiatry 19(1): 19–37.

Kornhaber A, Woodward K (1981) Grandparents – Grandchildren: The Vital Connection. New York: Anchor.

Lavers CA, Sonuga-Barke (1997) Annotation: on the grandmothers' role in the adjustment and maladjustment of grandchildren. Journal of Child Psychology and Psychiatry 38: 747–53.

Leek M, Smith PK (1991) Cooperation and conflict in three-generation families. In Smith PK (ed.) The Psychology of Grandparenthood: An International Perspective. London: Routledge.

MacLoyd VC (1990) The impact of economic hardship on black families and children: psychological distress, parenting, and socioemotional development. Child Development 61: 311–46.

MacPhee D, Fritz J, Miller-Heyl J (1996) Ethnic Variations in personal social networks and parenting. Child Development 67: 3278–95.

McLauglin SDE, Micklin M (1983) The timing of first birth and changes in personal efficacy. Journal of Marriage and the Family 45: 47–55.

Mott Foundation (1991) A State by State Look at Teenage Childbearing in the US. Flint MI: Charles Stewart Mott Foundation.

Neugarten BL, Weinstein KJ (1964) The changing American grandparent. Journal of Marriage and the Family 26: 197–205.

Nitz K, Ketterlinus RD, Brandt LJ (1995) The role of stress, social support, and family environment in adolescent mothers' parenting. Journal of Adolescent Research 10: 358–82.

Oyserman D, Radin N, Benn R (1993) Dynamics in a three-generational family: teens, grandparents, and babies. Developmental Psychology 29(3): 564–72.

Pearson JL, Hunter AG, Ensminger ME, Sheppard GK (1990) Black grandmothers in multigenerational households – diversity in family-structure and parenting involvement in ther woodlawn community. Child Development 61(2): 434–42.

Puckering C (1989) Annotation: maternal depression. Journal of Child Psychology and Psychiatry 30: 807–17.

Rogers AY (1998) Multiple sources of parenting stress and parenting behaviour. Children and Youth Services Review 20: 525–46.

Schellenbach CJ, Whitman TL, Borowski JG (1992) Towards an integrative model of adolescent parenting. Human Development 35: 81–99.

Shah Q, Sonuga-Barke EJS (1994) Family structure and the mental health of Pakistani Muslim mothers and their children living in Britain. British Journal of Clinical Psychology and Psychiatry 34: 79–81.

Shaw DS, Vondra JI (1993) Chronic family adversity and infant attachment security. Journal of Child Psychology and Psychiatry 34: 1205–15.

Shaw DS, Vondra JI, Hommerding DK, Keenan K, Dunn M (1994) Chronic family adversity and early child behaviour problems: a longitudinal study of low income families. Journal of Child Psychology and Psychiatry 35: 1109–22.

Sonuga-Barke EJS, Mistry M, Qureshi S (1998) The mental health of Muslim mothers in extended families living in Britain: the impact of intergenerational disagreement on anxiety and depression. British Journal of Clinical Psychology 37: 399–408.

Spieker SJ, Bensley L (1994) Roles of living arrangements and grandmothers social support in adolescent mothering and infant attachment. Developmental Psychology 30: 102–11.

Sroufe LA (1983) Infant-caregiver attachment and patterns of adaption in pre-school: the roots of maladaption and competence. In Perlmutter M (ed.) Minnesota Symposium in Child Psychology, XVI. Hillsdale NJ: Erlbaum, pp. 41–81.

Sroufe LA, Fleeson J (1986) Attachment and the construction of relationships. In Hartup W, Rubin Z (eds) Relationships and Development. Hillsdale: Erlbaum, pp. 51–71.

Stern G, Krukman L (1983) Multi-disciplinary perspectives on post-partum depression: an anthropological critique. Social Science and Medicine 17: 1027–41.

Stevens JH (1984) Black grandmothers' and black adolescent mothers' knowledge about parenting. Developmental Psychology 20: 1017–25.

Sticker EJ (1991) The importance of grandparents during the life cycle in Germany. In Smith PK (ed.) The Psychology of Grandparenthood: An International Perspective. London: Routledge.

Taylor RD, Roberts D (1995) Kinship support and maternal and adolescent well-being in economically disadvantaged African-American families. Child Development 66: 1585–97.

Taylor RD, Casten R, Flickinger M (1993a) Influence of kinship social support on the parenting experiences and psychosocial adjustment of African-American adolescents. Developmental Psychology 29: 382–8.

Taylor RT, Chatters LM, Jackson JS (1993b) A profile of familial relations among three-generation black families. Family Relations 42: 332–41.

Thomas E, Rickel AU, Butler C, Montgomary E (1990) Adolescent pregnancy and parenting. Journal of Primary Prevention 10(3): 195–206.

Tinsley BR, Parke RD (1984) Grandparents as support and socializing agents. In Lewis M (ed.) Beyond the Dyad. New York: Plenum.

Tinsley BR, Parke RD (1987) Grandparents as interactive and social support agents for families with young infants. International Journal of Aging and Human Development 25: 259–77.

Troll L (1985) The contingencies of grandparenthood. In Bengston VL, Robertson JF (eds) Grandparenthood. Beverley Hills, CA: Sage Publications.

Unger D, Cooley M (1992) Partner and grandmother contact in black and white teen parent families. Journal of Adolescent Health 13: 546–52.

Unger D, Wandersman L (1985) Social support and adolescent mothers: Action research contributions to theory and applications. Journal of Social Issues 41: 29–45.

Van IJzendoorn MH, Goldberg S, Kroonenberg PM, Frenkel M (1992) The relative effects of maternal and child problems on the quality of attachment: a meta-analysis of attachment in clinical samples. Child Development 63: 840–58.

Voight JD, Hans SL, Bernstein VJ (1996) Support networks of adolescent mothers: effects on parenting experience and behaviour. Infant Mental Health Journal 17: 58–73.

Wakschlag LS, Hans SL (2000) Early parenthood in context: implications for development and intervention. In Zeanah CH Jr (ed.) Handbook of Infant Mental Health. 2 edn. New York: Guilford Press, pp. 129–44.

Wan K, Jaccard J, Ramey SL (1996) The relationship between social support and life satisfaction as a function of family structure. Journal of Marriage and the Family 58: 502–13.

Waters E, Wippmann J, Sroufe LA (1979) Attachment, positive affect, and competence in the peer group: two studies in construct validation. Child Development 50: 821–9.

Watson JA, Koblinsky SA (1997) Strengths and needs of working-class African American and Anglo American grandparents. International Journal of Aging and Human Development 44: 149–65.

Webster-Stratton C (1990) Stress: a potential disrupter of parent perceptions and family interactions. Journal of Clinical Child Psychology 19: 302–12.

Wilson MN (1984) Mothers and grandmothers perceptions of parental behaviour in three-generational black-families. Child Development 55(4): 1333–9.

Wilson MN, Tolson TFJ, Hinton ID, Keirnan M (1990) Flexibility and sharing of child-care duties in black-families. Sex Roles 22(7-8): 409–25.

CHAPTER 8

Vulnerability and resilience in children in divorced and remarried families

THOMAS G O'CONNOR

Background and context for assessing the effects of separation/divorce and remarriage[1] on children

The rate of divorce has grown steadily in most western countries since the Second World War, with a levelling off of the prevalence of divorce in recent decades; the attendant rise in the prevalence of stepfamilies has been similarly dramatic. The most extensive findings on the more recent changes to influence family structure are based on samples in the US, where it is reported that, for example, approximately 40% of all marriages will end in divorce; most divorced men and women remarry (or repartner), but the rate of a subsequent separation is even higher than in first marriages; one-third of children will live in a stepfamily before the age of 18 years; and a growing number of children will experience multiple transitions (two or more parental separations) (Brody et al., 1988; Bumpass et al., 1990, 1991a; Clarke and Wilson, 1994; Martin and Bumpass, 1989). Data from Britain, Canada and Australia indicate that much the same kinds of changes are observed outside the US but there is some debate about whether the differences compared to those in the US are trivial or more substantial (Haskey, 1994, 1998; Pryor and Rodgers, 2001; UK Office of National Statistics, 1997).

The most dramatic recent changes affecting the structure of families in the UK is not the rate of divorce or remarriage. Instead, the biggest changes observed in recent population surveys concerns not the rate but the *reason* why children may be living in a single-mother family. From the 1990s, the most common reason why children were living in a single-parent family was not divorce (which was the most common reason in the

180

1970s and 1980s) but non-marital births (Haskey, 1998). That is, these children in single-parent families did not necessarily experience their parents' separation and the attendant loss of a parent. The second recent and major alteration in marital 'behaviour' that has had a substantial change on the structure of families concerns the rising rate of cohabitation over marriage, something that appears to be especially likely following a divorce (Cherlin and Furstenberg, 1994; Haskey, 1994). This, too, may be an important for understanding children's and adults' adjustment given that there are important differences between marital and cohabiting relationships – not least of which is a much higher likelihood of separation in the latter.

Sociodemographic data provide an essential starting point and backdrop for constructing empirical studies and interventions because they help to define the meaning of family structure and the normality of its many potential forms. There are, however, dangers in inferring causes and effects from demographic data alone. The extent to which these changes can explain behavioural/emotional problems and other outcomes is examined below.

Lessons for understanding causes and effects from sociodemographic findings

There is substantial crosscultural and subcultural variation in many family and relationship 'behaviours', including non-marital births, divorce and remarriage, and the choice to cohabit rather than marry. This variation raises a number of important questions for families and governments. So, for example, what do the lower rates of divorce in Spain and Italy, relative to Britain, say about how those societies value and support families? Furthermore, what does it mean that the rate of cohabitation in Scandinavian countries is higher than it is in Britain? To date, neither the causes nor the effects of these differences are certain, and neither is their relevance for understanding children's adjustment. What these crosscultural differences highlight is that there is potential value in adopting a crosscultural perspective on family change in order to assess the extent to which there are bidirectional links between family life and societal pressures (for example, rates and changes in unemployment), legal systems or tax structures. On the other hand, although there are obvious and important differences across cultures, it is important to consider that there is probably as much *sub*cultural variation in rates of marital/relationship and parenting behaviour within a specific culture as there is between different countries and cultures. What meaning this set of findings has for clinicians and policy makers remains to be seen. At any rate, given the current state of knowledge, it would be premature to draw firm conclusions about causes and effects of family change from (sub)cultural variation.

Summary points

- Children in the UK are more likely to be living in a single-parent family because of a non-marital birth than a divorce.
- Cohabitation is increasingly seen as an alternative to marriage, especially following a separation.
- Variation in patterns of family life may be as great within countries as between countries.

Overview of research findings

A great many studies have examined the connection between family-type membership and children's and adults' adjustment. Conclusions drawn from the meta-analysis of Amato and Keith (1991a) have been replicated in a number of more recent reviews and empirical studies (Dunn et al., 1998; Hetherington, 1999a; Pryor and Rodgers, 2001). This section sorts the key findings by several heuristic categories.

Behavioural/emotional problems

Behavioural/emotional problems are typically defined in research as depression, anxiety, withdrawal, aggression, oppositional behaviour and delinquency. It is also common in most studies to examine broadband types of problems rather than specific diagnostic clusters of symptoms. So, for example, it is common to see reports on 'internalizing' (such as depression, anxiety and withdrawal) and 'externalizing' problems (notably disruptive behaviours such as oppositional, conduct problems and hyperactivity). The reason for adapting broadband descriptive and measurement strategies is that most of the more rigorously empirical studies examine non-clinic referred samples, so the actual rate of diagnosable symptomatology is minor.

Behavioural/emotional problems in children are the most common outcome to be linked with membership in a single-parent or stepfamily and are remarkably consistent across samples, reporters, measures and settings. An overall impression is that children in divorced families show, on average, a fifth to a quarter of a standard deviation difference in behavioural/emotional problems (Amato, 2001; Amato and Keith, 1991a; Pryor and Rodgers, 2001). In statistical terms this would be considered small to moderate; in clinical terms these differences would be considered meaningful. An important lesson from compilations of the research is that, as is usually the case, studies based on clinic samples tend to show the greatest effects of divorce on children's behavioural/emotional problems, followed by convenience or volunteer samples, followed by community and samples selected at random (non-selected). Similar findings and lessons may be drawn from studies of children in stepfamilies, although the smaller number of studies means that the pattern is somewhat less robust.

The relationship between the kind of sample being studied and the magnitude of the effects of divorce or remarriage is sometimes lost in popular accounts of the research. An example of this is found in the accounts of the effects of divorce provided by both Wallerstein (1985) and Hetherington. Wallerstein's work in this area is helpful and interesting, but because it was based on clinic samples the overall message about the effects of divorce on children was somewhat overplayed. In contrast, the work of Hetherington (1999a, 2002) provides an equally accessible and clinically useful account of the research on divorce and remarriage that is not based on clinic samples; the implications drawn concerning the effects of divorce were more modest and point to considerable resilience of children to these events. Thus, although it may be tempting to link a child's disruptive behavioural problem to his or her parents' separation, it is also important to consider that the divorce may be a clinical red herring and have little directly to do with the origins and continuation of the child's adjustment difficulties.

A further finding that challenges conventional wisdom is that there is little evidence for a differential impact of divorce and remarriage on the range of behavioural/emotional problems assessed in children. That is, there is as yet no clear evidence that experiencing a parental separation or repartnering is any more likely to lead to emotional distress than to 'acting out'; nor is there clear evidence that the behavioural/emotional problems associated with marital transitions differ for boys or girls. It is worth remembering, however, that conclusions concerning differential impact on behavioural/emotional problems need to be prefaced with the usual concerns concerning the greater reliability (and perhaps validity) of assessments of externalizing than internalizing problems, especially when parents and teachers are the source of the information.

Most studies report mean level differences between groups of children in divorced and non-divorced families and stepfamilies. However, group differences may not necessarily translate into differences at the level of impairment and need for clinical treatment. Therefore, it is helpful that at least some studies also provide estimates of the rate of clinical distress in children of different family settings. A twofold or threefold increase in problems severe enough to warrant treatment is commonly found in children in single-parent and stepfamilies (for example, Hetherington, 1999b). A similar magnitude of difference is observed when the outcomes are defined in other ways with relatively immediate clinical and educational 'costs', such as suspension/expulsion from school and more serious academic failure requiring grade retention (Zill, 1994).

Furthermore, differences in the rates of problems are found across family type when the behavioural/emotional outcomes are defined as substance use or delinquency (see Pryor and Rodgers, 2001).

Achievement and social relationships

The finding that membership in a single-parent family or stepfamily is associated with poorer academic achievement is probably the next most well-documented finding in the research literature. Underachievement and poor achievement in childhood are of major interest because they have long-term direct and indirect impact on outcomes in adulthood, such as obtaining a good job and being seen as a desirable marriage partner. Here again, family-type differences are obtained across many different operationalizations of academic achievement, such as being held back a year, achievement and standardized test score results, dropping out of school, college or university attendance, and class rank (Amato, 2001; Fergusson et al., 1994; Pryor and Rodgers, 2001; Zill, 1994).

Given the well-documented findings on behavioural/emotional problems and school failure, it would be surprising if there were not also family-type differences in measures of social competence and social relationships. Several different kinds of findings are of interest in this regard. The first is that, compared to children in nuclear families, the social relationships of children in single-parent families and stepfamilies may be more impaired and conflicted and they may be more likely to be rejected by their peers (see, for example, Amato, 2001). Also, compared with children in nuclear families, children in single-parent and stepfamilies may also be more likely to associated with antisocial peers and to be more negatively influenced by an antisocial peer group (for example, Steinberg, 1987). However, this is not to say that peers are necessarily a source of risk for children in single-parent families and stepfamilies. For example, one recent report found that children were most likely to confide in friends and grandparents about their parents' separation (Dunn et al., 2001). In addition, it is likely that, regardless of family type, negative and non-supportive (versus positive) relationships with peers are more likely when parent-child relationships are conflicted (Dunn et al., 2001). This implies that problems in peer and social relationships derive, in part, from processes within the family rather than from family type per se.

Social, psychological and educational/occupational outcomes in adulthood

The impact of early experiences on later adjustment is not usually 'direct'. Instead, persistence of adjustment problems from childhood to adulthood can be explained by the tendency for high-risk environments (for example, family conflict or economic deprivation) to be stable and by a carrying forward of affective, behavioural and cognitive processes that hinder the successful resolution of developmental challenges. These explanations help to account for the growing evidence that the experience of divorce in childhood is associated with much greater risk of a range of adjustment problems in adulthood. What is emerging from a number of complementary studies is that parental divorce sets in progress a life-course pattern characterized by a relatively early age at leaving home, early sexual behaviour, teenage parenthood, decreased likelihood of meeting desirable partners, the adoption of unsuccessful patterns of marriage and parenthood, a closing off of opportunities for educational and occupational success, and mental health difficulties (Amato, 1996; Amato and Keith, 1991b; Cherlin et al., 1998; Furstenberg and Teitler, 1994; Kiernan and Hobcraft, 1997; Kiernan and Mueller, 1998; O'Connor et al., 1999b; Thornton et al., 1995; Wheaton, 1990; Zill et al., 1993).

An additional set of studies shows that experiencing one's own parents' divorce in childhood influences attitudes toward marriage, divorce and cohabitation in adulthood, which in turn may explain why children who experienced a divorce may be more likely to divorce as adults or to prefer cohabitation over marriage (Amato, 1996; Bumpass et al., 1991b; O'Connor et al., 1999a; Pope and Mueller, 1976). A probable related consequence is that children whose parents have divorced are more likely to report strained relationships with parents in adulthood, perhaps especially with the non-resident father (Aquilino, 1994; Amato, 1999; O'Connor et al., 1996).

What these findings indicate is that, for some children, there are multiple and long-term effects of divorce. Clinical attention provided in the early stages following separation and initial distress may be helpful not only in reducing distress but also pre-empting a life-course pattern of risk. What is needed is a clinical-developmental approach to understand the links in the chain leading from the experience of the divorce through to negotiating the challenges of becoming self-reliant, productive and content adults.

Physical health and wellbeing

Studies of the link between family type and physical health in children and adults are interesting and important because they help to define and extend the limits of the effects of family structure and associated risks. Such findings also provide another index for assessing the public health costs of divorce and remarriage.

Far fewer studies connect membership in a single-parent family or step-family with physical health outcomes than for behavioural/emotional outcomes, but what evidence there is suggests that there is a meaningful and significant association (Cockett and Tripp, 1994; O'Connor, Davies et al., 2000b; Wadsworth et al., 1983). The most consistent evidence is for accidents and injuries and health visits to the GP or emergency room among younger children. Interestingly, one reason why membership in a single-parent or stepfamily may increase the rate of accidents and injuries is explained by factors that predate the current family structure or even the child's birth, such as teenage pregnancy and early home leaving (O'Connor et al., 2000b). This may reflect the possibility that family type indexes characteristics of the parent that compromise children's health, such as poor monitoring and supervision.

Different, but equally strong, links between family type membership and adult health and mortality have been reported in a diverse set of studies using a range of alternative definitions of health and wellbeing. The reasons for this association can be explained in a number of ways. For example, unhealthy people may be less likely to get married and stay married; married people may be healthier simply because there are economic benefits of marriage over being single; individuals who have experienced relationship breakdown may be suffering from more severe stress that in turn compromises health; or, married individuals may be less inclined to take health risks (engage in excessive smoking or drinking; see Morgan, 1980; Umberson, 1992). These explanations are probably complementary rather than competing.

Summary

Research findings consistently show that, compared to children living in a nuclear family, those children in a single-parent family or stepfamily exhibit elevated rates of social, behavioural/emotional, cognitive, academic, and physical health problems. Two general lessons are worth keeping in mind when interpreting the findings, however. The first is that the stronger empirical studies typically report small but significant differences and considerable variability in children's adjustment between and within single-parent families and stepfamilies. The second general observation is that the effects are robust across reporter (child self-reports, parent reports, teacher reports and observer impressions) and evident in a surprisingly wide variety of outcomes. What these findings imply about the causes of these differences remains to be resolved; this is the focus of the following two sections.

What moderates the effects of divorce and remarriage?

It could hardly be expected that all children and adults would respond similarly to divorce (or other marital transition). Indeed, there are 'winners, losers, and survivors' (Hetherington, 1989) following family transitions. The extent of this variation is often not emphasized as much as the mean differences between groups but it as important for conceptual, methodological and clinical reasons. Some of the most important factors that may moderate children's adjustment to marital transitions are considered below.

Is divorce always an unhappy event for parents and children?

Separation or divorce is not an inevitable end result of an unhappy or conflicted relationship; that is, there are stable unhappy marriages. In addition, not all marriages that end in divorce were highly conflicted. Variation in circumstances in which divorce occurs has allowed researchers to examine the possibility that divorce in high-conflicted families may be a positive outcome for parents and children. The key comparison group in analyses of this kind is the group of children growing up in conflicted marriages that stay together – a group known to show elevated rates of behavioural/emotional problems. Limited evidence indicates that children do not seem to 'benefit', either in the short or long term, from the termination of a conflicted marriage (Hetherington, 1999b; Morrison and Coiro, 1999; but see Booth and Amato, 2001). Failure to find a reduction in children's disturbance when a conflicted relationship is terminated may be explained by a range of factors, including the likelihood that conflict between partners continued after the separation. To date, there are two take-home messages from the limited research on this issue. The first is that conflict between partners needs to be reduced, regardless of whether or not a divorce is impending or has already occurred. The second is that we should not expect that 'staying together for the sake of the children' carries any real benefit for children in conflicted families (although, somewhat controversially, the same lesson may not necessarily apply to non-conflicted marriages) (Hetherington, 1999b). However, for adults, there is evidence to indicate that the termination of an unhappy, conflicted or even abusive relationship may have beneficial effects (Aseltine and Kessler, 1993). Further clinical research is needed to consider why these potential positive effects may not be transferred to children.

Even fewer studies examine if the effects of a separation are different for children in nuclear families and stepfamilies. For instance, because children in stepfamilies may resent their mother's relationship to a new partner (the stepfather) it might follow that their separation might be greeted with less distress. One study, based on the National Longitudinal Study of Children and Youth (NLSCY) in Canada, did not support this possibility. That is, children who experienced the separation of their biological parents or parent and step-parent (usually a stepfather) were equally likely to show adjustment difficulties (O'Connor and Jenkins, 2000). More research of this kind is needed to understand how the conditions of the divorce may moderate children's and adults' post-divorce adjustment.

What protects children undergoing marital transitions?

A key consideration undergirding the vulnerability and resilience perspective is that there are factors that protect or buffer children from the adverse effects of risk. Studies identifying protective factors are, however, far fewer than those identifying risks. This is a curious finding given that most children adjust to the stresses associated with their parents' separation(s)/repartnering(s) without developing clinical disturbances. Of course, it could be argued that the absence of risk provides, in effect, a 'protective' environment. This is possible and may well be the case in families undergoing transitions. Nevertheless, it is important to distinguish, for conceptual and clinical reasons, between the absence of risk and the presence of a protective factor that compensates for, or reduces the effect of, risk. Identifying protective factors would, for example, be especially important for planning interventions.

One clear example of a protective factor moderating children's adjustment to separation was reported in the Canadian longitudinal study mentioned above (NLSCY). In that study, parental separation was associated with an increase in emotional problems over time, but the magnitude of the increase was significantly moderated by a positive parent–child relationship. Thus, those children who experienced a positive relationship with their mother were less likely to show the adverse effects of a separation (O'Connor and Jenkins, 2000). The finding of an interaction between parental separation and supportive parenting in a prospective study of separation strengthens and extends findings from studies on variation in children's post-divorce adjustment (Hetherington and Clingempeel, 1992). Extrafamilial support, for example, from peers may also protect children against some of the effects of parental divorce (Samera and Stolberg, 1993).

Do children's construction of the divorce explain their adjustment to it?

Research is beginning to add empirical weight to the clinical view that how children understand their parents' separation may influence their adjustment to it. One example is research conducted by Sandler and colleagues (Sandler et al., 2000). They asked children to rate how often they engaged in active coping (for example, 'you tried to figure out why things like this happen', 'you did something to make things better') and avoidant coping (for example, 'you tried to put it put of your mind'). In addition, the researchers asked children to rate coping efficacy, or the children's reports of how well they handled recent problems. Longitudinal follow-up of children in divorced families indicated that active coping efforts led to an enhanced view of coping efficacy, and that this was in turn associated with lower levels of internalizing symptoms. The pattern of findings is generally consistent with other research on children's coping and adjustment, and points out a potential cognitive intervention strategy for promoting competence in children.

What role do child age and sex play in explaining children's adjustment?

It is natural to suppose that the age at which the child experiences a separation/divorce or remarriage might influence how that event may or may not be linked with short-term and long-term adjustment. What is not clear is whether or not the 'advantage' may be for younger or older children. For example, compared with preschool and school-aged children, adolescents may adapt better to transitions because they may draw from an enhanced coping capacity and ability to make sense of their parents' separation; also, older children may be protected because they have greater autonomy and access to extrafamilial relationships that may reduce exposure to family conflict. Alternatively, adolescence may instead be seen as a time of increased vulnerability, especially as they are experiencing other normative transitions such as puberty and moving to secondary school. Furthermore, experiencing parents' separation, courtship and repartnering may be especially difficult for adolescents who are negotiating their own way into opposite-sex intimate relationships. In further support of this position, it could be argued that infants and young children may not process (for example, remember) the divorce/separation and the associated conflict, and so may not be 'affected' to a similar degree as older children who retain memories of the divorce process – so long as there is no repeat of conflict and separation.

Compounding the variability in expectations concerning age is the fact that age is used very differently across studies. For example, there is age at which the child experienced a separation and time since separation; there may even be an interaction between these two dimensions (Bray, 1999; Hetherington and Clingempeel, 1992). There is also a suggestion that certain developmental periods may 'rekindle' earlier effects (Bray,

1999; Wallerstein, 1985). Thus, for example, Bray (1999) reported that the onset of adolescence may reignite problems (or initiate problems in those without pre-existing problems) in those children in stepfamilies who were thought by the investigators to have resolved their parent's remarriage in middle childhood. Of course, many children will also experience a subsequent transition, and for them there are the additional complications of age at, and time between, these subsequent transitions. A final consideration is that, whatever the effects of age may be, it is important to recognize that age *per se* carries no particular explanatory value. What will be needed is some demonstration of what it is about being older or younger that may modify children's adjustment to their parents' marital transitions. Given the diverse manner in which age may moderate children's adjustment to parental separation it may not be a surprise to find that the findings are inconclusive.

Research findings on the connections between marital transitions and child sex are somewhat more consistent, and may be moderated by age. In her studies of children's adjustment to divorce and remarriage, Hetherington (Hetherington, 1989; Hetherington and Clingempeel, 1992) observed that boys may have greater difficulty adjusting to a single-mother family but that girls may have more trouble adjusting to a remarriage. By adolescence, however, few sex differences are found. What it is about adolescence that diminished rather than accentuated sex differences in children's adjustment requires further attention.

Does historical and cultural context modify the effects of divorce?

One of the intriguing findings from Amato and Keith's (1991a) meta-analysis is that the effects of parental divorce were somewhat greater in older studies than in more recent reports. Although this apparent time trend may be explained by improvements in the methodological rigor of studies over time, there may also be a substantive interpretation. For example, when the frequency of divorce was rare the effects might be somewhat greater, because, for example, of greater stigma and/or because society was less able to provide necessary supports to families. Whatever the 'real' effect, if any, of historical epoch, it is worth noting that even very recent studies of comparatively young samples of children have found significant and meaningful differences in children's adjustment according to family structure (Dunn et al., 1998). It is also worth noting that a more recent review did not find a simple decrease in effects of divorce on children's adjustment in research published in the 1950s through to the 1990s (Amato, 2001).

If the magnitude of the effects of divorce were moderated by the prevalence of divorce in the (sub)culture, then we might also expect to find substantial differences in the effects of divorce across countries that differ in the prevalence of divorce. Limited available evidence suggests that this is not the case. For example, compared to findings from the US, the magnitude of effect of divorce are relatively comparable in China (Liu et al., 2000) and Greece (Hatzichristou, 1993) – countries with increasing but still lower rates of separation than the US. The extent to which within-country, subcultural differences in the rates of separation and remarriage predict responses in children is an issue that also requires further research before firm conclusions can be made.

Summary

The adoption of a risk and resilience perspective, which focuses on this variability in children's adjustment to marital transitions, means that we are beginning to understand which children may be most vulnerable to the effects of a divorce or remarriage and what circumstances may increase the likelihood of disturbance. Conversely, research is also beginning to characterize the children who may be more resilient to transitions and the circumstances that may protect children from developing short- and long-term adjustment difficulties.

What is the meaning of family structure?

Research on children's adjustment in diverse family types assumes that there is something about membership in a single-parent family or stepfamily that explains the observed group differences in children's wellbeing. Recent findings raise some intriguing questions about that assumption and point to new directions for research. Three areas are highlighted: the nature of co-occurring psychosocial risks, family type as an unstable risk, and the distinction between family-wide and child-specific risk processes.

The effects of family type are mediated by co-occurring risks

Risks for children's adjustment pre-date divorce/remarriage

Children's post-divorce maladjustment may be partly attributable to long-standing, pre-divorce stresses in the family. Specifically, families who eventually divorce are distinguishable from non-divorcing families in terms of less optimal parenting, especially from fathers, and poorer marital relationships – prior to the separation (Amato and Booth, 1996; Block et al., 1986; Shaw et al., 1993). In line with these findings is evidence that there are pre-divorce elevations in adjustment problems in children, and that these pre-divorce differences may explain some, but not all, of post-divorce differences (Cherlin et al., 1991; Emery et al., 1999b; Forehand et al., 1997; Furstenberg and Teitler, 1994; O'Connor and Jenkins, 2000).

'Proximal' risks explain family-type differences in children's adjustment

More generally, it is important to consider that single-parent family and stepfamily constellations appear to be a proxy for many psychosocial risks known to be associated with children's adjustment difficulties, including parental mental health, poor parent-child relationships, socioeconomic disadvantage and many others besides (Amato and Keith, 1991a; Dunn et al., 2000; Hetherington, 1999a; O'Connor et al., 1998a). As the preceding paragraph noted, some of these risks predate the divorce or remarriage. Furthermore, when the collective set of risk factors is considered family structure is typically no longer significantly associated with child adjustment problems (O'Connor et al., 2001; Simons et al., 1999). That is, family type per se may not be an explanatory variable, at least insofar as children's adjustment is concerned. Accordingly, rather than emphasize family type it would be more profitable for theory and clinical practice to consider the 'proximal' risks indexed by family type, such as strains in the parent-child relationship.

Family type is a dynamic and unstable variable

As demonstrated above, family type is likely to change over time. More important is the observation that the likelihood of a change in family structure is greatest among those already living in higher risk settings, namely single parents and stepfamilies (Bumpass et al., 1991b; Kiernan and Mueller, 1998; O'Connor and Jenkins, 2000; O'Connor et al., 1999a). For example, in a study of a large community sample in the UK over a 2-year period (which, significantly, included the birth of a child), rates of stability were 95% in nuclear families, 62% in blended (stepfather/stepmother) families, 57% in stepmother families and 80% in stepfather families (O'Connor et al., 1999a); equally impressive was the finding that almost half of the single-parent families changed status over the same period. By comparison, in the NLSCY in Canada, over a 2-year period, the rates of stability were 96% in nuclear families, 76% in blended and stepmother families, 81% in stepfather families, and 78% in single-parent families (O'Connor and Jenkins, 2000).

These findings raise two cautions when drawing links between children's adjustment and current membership in a single-parent or stepfamily. The first is that it would be implausible to attribute the experience of divorce in early childhood to patterns of adjustment in young adulthood because, in many cases, those individuals would have experienced a further transition(s). Second, it is probable that reports of children's adjustment across different family structures over-attribute vari-ation in child wellbeing to the *current* family setting. It may be that the current family setting provides a weaker index of child adjustment than the history and number of previous transitions (Capaldi and Patterson, 1991; Dunn et al., 1998).

The 'effects' of family type may not be 'shared' by siblings

Studies that assess more than one child per family inevitably conclude that siblings show marked differences in adjustment. The implication of these sibling differences, which are found even in genetically identical sib-lings, is that simply growing up in the same family does not make siblings similar to one another (for example, Plomin, 1994). One interpretation of this finding is that there is minimal effect of a 'shared' environment and that environments that matter for children's psychological development may not be shared by siblings. Given the evidence for differential parental treatment, different extrafamilial environments of siblings, and the likeli-hood that siblings interpret and experience a 'common' event (such as their mother's depression) differently, this is an interesting, if provocative and controversial, conclusion. Questions can then be asked about whether or not parental divorce would have similar or shared effects on siblings. This is a question with potential clinical applications. For exam-ple, should families or individual children be targeted for interventions? If interventions are delivered are the beneficial effects likely to be gener-alized to all family members?

To date, only one study has investigated the extent to which the expe-rience of divorce had 'shared' effects on siblings (O'Connor and Jenkins, 2000). In that study, based on prospective longitudinal data from the NLSCY in Canada, it was found that parental divorce was associated with significant variation in children's adjustment, and that one effect attribut-able to parental divorce was to make siblings *more* different from one another over time compared with siblings who did not experience a parental separation. The finding that parental divorce increased sibling differences over time underscores the need to examine the within-family (for example, differential parental support) or extrafamilial (for example, differential peer support) processes that explain why siblings adapted to their parents' separation differently from one another. Furthermore, stud-ies conducted in Canada and the UK found that the extent to which variability in children's adjustment is attributable to family-wide or to individual child-specific factors varies significantly according to family structure (O'Connor et al., 2001; O'Connor and Jenkins, 2000).

Family systems theorists and practitioners have long argued for the need to consider differential alliance patterns and other within-family processes that might produce different outcomes for siblings (Vogel and Bell, 1960). Within-family variation has now been taken up as a focus for research in empirical studies in developmental and clinical psychology, and this has provided an additional dimension for considering risk and vulnerability. Clinical researchers are just beginning to appreciate the implications of these ideas for understanding children's adjustment to divorce, and this will constitute an important agenda in future clinical research.

Summary

If our sole goal is to explain patterns of children's adaptation across a wide range of psychological outcomes typically examined in research, then family type is 'unnecessary' so long as we assess quality of parent-child relationships, parental mental health, psychosocial stresses and family history. In other words, after we account for the above risks, the 'effect' of family structure on children's behavioural/emotional adjustment is no longer detected. Furthermore, risks explaining children's post-divorce adjustment may predate the divorce, and there is even evidence that the effects of divorce and associated risks may be partly mediated by genetic factors (O'Connor et al., 2000a). Furthermore, family type and divorce may carry a different meaning for siblings. These points are not to suggest that family structure carries no particular meaning or that it is unimportant scientifically or clinically. Instead, the above findings highlight the need for a greater appreciation – at least in the empirical literature – for what family type means to individual family members.

Implications of the research findings

Whether or not it takes place in traditional 'academic' settings, research on the effects of divorce and remarriage naturally provides some directions for clinical work and promoting children's and adult's wellbeing. This section of the chapter considers the clinical applications of the research findings, reviews lessons from intervention studies, and considers how family process differs in diverse family types.

Clinical implications: identifying needs

Perhaps the most obvious and compelling clinical implication of the research findings concerns the identification of the needs of those children and adults who are experiencing a separation/divorce or repartnering. The literature reviewed above would point to several areas in particular. Perhaps the most important is to promote positive parent-child relationships with both parents. Parents undergoing the strain of a separation may be less inclined and less able to provide encouragement and consistent support and may be more likely to respond harshly or coercively. It is also important that parents continue to monitor their children's activities and feelings and anticipate that children may be more likely to seek attention from, and yet also be more vulnerable to, influences outside the family.

Problems in parent-child relationships may not necessarily be attributed to the particular strains of pre- and post-divorce processes, but in fact may be long-standing. This distinction may be important. 'Recovery' in the parent-child (at least resident mother-child) relationship following a divorce is likely (Hetherington and Clingempeel, 1992), that is, a return to a positive relationship with modest disruption can be expected. On the other hand, it is not likely that a separation will 'improve' parent-child relationships that were strained prior to the separation, and there may be a need for ongoing therapy that is not centred on the experience of the separation per se.

The second most likely clinical concern is for parents' mental health. Rates of depression increase dramatically following a separation, in both men and women, and there may be other individual problems, such as substance use. Again, it may be useful to assess the extent to which these problems are a response to or pre-date (and may have even contributed to) the separation.

Efforts to reduce conflict during and after the separation will also be important, given the evidence that marital conflict and post-divorce conflict are comparatively common and may compromise children's and adults' adjustment. Efforts to extend social supports and activities, for both parents and children, may also help counter the loss or absence of emotional support, which in many cases may have been long-standing. Finally, two of the more common areas of post-divorce conflict, financial support and visitation (see, for example, Thompson and Amato, 1999) are also rightly seen as areas of possible clinical attention not only because they may have some direct impact on post-divorce adjustment, but also because these topics are two of the more obvious ways in which conflicted ex-partners continue to stay in conflict.

Compared with the very substantial literature and experience of working with divorced and divorcing parents, somewhat less is known about the needs of recently remarried partners and the children in these families. What is certain is that the rate of separation in second (and subsequent) relationships is greater than in first marriages, and there is a suggestion that the first 5 years of the remarriage – that is, the transition period – may be the highest risk period for the family (for example, see Hetherington et al., 1999). Interestingly, it does not follow that remarried spouses are necessarily unhappy in their relationship. For instance, several studies of non-clinic referred families found that there are no significant differences in the marital quality of first and second marriages. If there is a difference, it is in terms of conflict about child-rearing rather than about the marital relationship as such (O'Connor and Insabella, 1999; White and Booth, 1985).

Studies of clinical intervention

A number of interventions have been proposed to reduce distress associated with parental divorce. Reviews of this literature (for example, Emery et al., 1999a) emphasize that treatment studies have not generally complied with rigorous standards that make possible a careful evaluation of the efficacy and effectiveness of these interventions. Nevertheless, there are a number of interventions and intervention strategies that have been evaluated enough to merit some discussion. Four kinds of intervention studies are highlighted in this chapter: direct interventions with divorced/divorcing families, school-based projects to support children of divorce, prevention and intervention studies to improve marital quality and alternative ways of resolving post-divorce arrangements.

The first, most direct kind of intervention is designed to help children by targeting the risk factors that explain variation in children's post-divorce adjustment. Forgatch and DeGarmo's (1999) study is a good example of this sort. They found that a parenting intervention with newly divorced mothers resulted in significant increases in effective parenting and in a positive change in children's behaviour. Two features of the study deserve special attention. The first is that the intervention involved parenting. The focus on parent-child relationship quality and particular parenting skills was based on numerous studies, virtually all of which show that children's adjustment covaries with parent-child relationship quality. Accordingly, the intervention sought to decrease coercive control attempts, improve limit-setting and management of parental anger, and improve problem-solving. Second, the study took place soon after the divorce, a time when parenting stress and child behavioural/emotional problems may be at their zenith. The lesson from that study is that even (and perhaps especially) for families in a period of high stress, parenting interventions may provide one method of improving parent and child adjustment and preventing further post-divorce maladjustment.

School-based interventions have also proven successful in aiding children's adjustment to divorce (see especially the work of Pedro-Carroll and colleagues, for example Pedro-Carroll and Alpert-Ellis, 1997). The aims of these interventions are typically to promote children's coping, enhance social skills, discuss perceptions of divorce and why they occur, and identify and express feelings about the separation. That is, the intervention has much in common with other interventions, but is focused on divorce (or separation). School-based interventions have a number of interesting and important features that merit particular discussion. The first is that the intervention occurs outside the family setting. This provides a powerful test of whether or not the 'disturbance' lies in the child or in the family. Whether or not we would expect significant and lasting changes in children's behaviour to result from a school-based intervention if there are still serious conflicts in the family remains to be seen. Second, because school-based interventions are almost invariably group-based, there are additional opportunities for the clinical intervention, such as promoting peer relationships and support. School-based interventions are now applied fairly widely in the USA, but their application in the UK is just beginning. Several obstacles will need to be overcome in order for these interventions to occur, such as the modest involvement of clinical psychology in the school setting.

Interventions directed at the marital relationship have also proven to be effective, to a significant degree, and for a significant percentage of marriages/relationships. In this context, it is worth noting that longitudinal data indicate that there is a natural decline in marital satisfaction from the point of marriage through the initial years of the relationship, and that this drop in marital satisfaction is significant and large even after excluding those couples that separate (Kurdek, 1998). This is an important background finding to prevention studies that target couple communication skills prior to the marriage taking place – and apparently before problems have been identified. Thus, what seems to be prevented in these premarital interventions is, to a large extent, this normative decline in marital satisfaction. Thus, for example, in the Halhweg et al. (1998) study, couples receiving the preventive intervention experienced virtually no change in their satisfaction compared with a drop of approximately one standard deviation in the comparison group – a substantial difference. Preventive interventions that take place before marriage show not only the prevention of marital distress but also a reduction in divorces (Halhweg et al., 1998; Markman et al., 1988). These two outcomes are not synonymous, as noted.

A distinction is needed between prevention studies and intervention studies with conflicted couples who present for treatment. Intervention studies (of couples who present for treatment) show that marital conflict can be reduced and that satisfaction, communication skills and intimacy can be improved. However, what these intervention studies have not demonstrated, at least to a sizable degree, is that they prevent separation. Couples who present for marital therapy are likely to differ in some very substantial ways from couples who do not seek counselling – not least of which may be the wish to improve the relationship – so generalization across study type is problematic.

Finally, studies have been conducted to examine if mediation is a better way of resolving disputes and improving coparenting between separated spouses and, in turn, promoting post-divorce adjustment of parents and children. Several studies (see Emery et al., 1999a) suggest that mediation is effective at engaging partners, and is certainly more cost effective than the standard legal process. However, to date, it is not clear that there are lasting beneficial effects on the psychological adjustment of parents or children. Nevertheless, even if mediation is not found to improve psychological adjustment, it may have other advantages that give it an advantage of the standard adversarial legal process.

Family process considerations

Attempts to integrate clinical and family systems concepts in empirical studies have been met with mixed success. Thus, for instance, there are an increasing number of studies that assess systemic processes such as triangulation and dysfunctional alliance patterns. How effectively these constructs are operationalized, to what extent they provide a picture of family functioning, and whether or not they adequately 'explain' child or adult adjustment is a matter of ongoing research.

Attention has also turned to consider the extent to which healthy versus dysfunctional family processes are similar in nuclear, single-parent and remarried families, and what different tasks are faced by children in different family settings (Crosbie-Burnett, 1984; Weiss, 1979). For instance, many differences between nuclear and remarried families may give rise to different and differentially healthy processes. For example, remarried families will have complex histories of marital transitions; children in stepfamilies will have spent some time in a single-parent family (prior to the remarriage); children in stepfamilies will often be members of more than one household; and stepfathers are late additions to the family and may have difficulty establishing 'parental jurisdiction'. Might these differences mean that we should set a different norm for defining healthy functioning in a stepfamily?

Clinical descriptions of and research on dysfunctional nuclear families and stepfamilies (for example, Anderson and White, 1986) suggest that there are important family type differences in what can be considered healthy family process. More interesting is the suggestion that what may be considered dysfunctional in a nuclear family may not be (as) dysfunctional in a stepfamily. An example of this is the notion of crossgenerational alliances. In healthy nuclear families, we would not expect to find a parent siding with or being caught between the spouse and a child in an argument. Indeed, in nuclear families, an especially 'strong' connection between a parent and child (over a spouse) constitutes a serious disruption of boundaries between the parent and child generations and this is thought to compromise healthy adult and child development. In stepfamilies, however, there is at least a suggestion that the centrality of the marital relationship may be less 'nuclear' to family functioning. Consequently, crossgenerational alliances may be a more natural consequence of the children and mother having spent some time in a single-parent arrangement. To the extent that this is so, such relationship patterns may hold a different meaning from the interpretation customary in nuclear families.

This notion has received indirect support from a number of different sources. First, separation in stepfamilies may be more attributable to the quality of the step-relation than to the quality of the marital relationship as such (White and Booth, 1985). Other authors (for example, Crosbie-Burnett, 1984) have also suggested that the key relationship in stepfamilies may not be the health of the marital relationship but of the step-relationship. Second, several studies using rigorous methods have shown that the normally strong overlap in the association between the quality of marital and parent-child relationships is less pronounced (or even non-existent) in stepfamilies (see, for example, Hetherington and Clingempeel, 1992). Other clinical researchers have similarly drawn attention to the finding that, compared with nuclear families, stepfamilies are less 'cohesive'.

However, in contrast to these findings, a study of 'stable' stepfamilies (those that were remarried for at least 5 years) found no differences in alliance patterns or in the association between certain alliance patterns and children's wellbeing (O'Connor et al., 1998b). It may be that as families stay together they begin to resemble a nuclear family. Alternatively, it may be that those families that remain together were more like nuclear families in the initial stages. Further longitudinal studies are needed to investigate these questions. In the meantime, it remains for clinicians and researchers to examine further how family structure (nuclear versus stepfamily) shapes family process.

A final consideration is that there is strong evidence that at least some processes seem invariant across family structure. Thus, for example, authoritative parenting (warm/supportive parenting with firm and effective control) from stepfathers appears to be as important as it is from mothers in stepfamilies and mothers and fathers in nuclear families (Hetherington and Clingempeel, 1992; Hetherington et al., 1999). The issue may be not that effective step-parenting must be different from parenting from a biological parent (although it may need to be in the early stages of the remarriage) but more the case that effective parenting may be more difficult in some family settings.

Summary

Many UK-based clinically oriented books and accessible articles about divorce and remarriage are available (Gorrell-Barnes et al., 1998). To a considerable extent, the observations made in those publications add weight and depth to the research findings emerging from a remarkably large and increasingly coherent set of research papers.

Conclusion

Given the marked frequency of marital and family transitions, it is natural that policy makers, health professionals and the general public raise questions about the implications of the changing family patterns for children's and adults' wellbeing, both in the short term and longer term. There is now a wealth of information about children's adjustment in diverse family settings and we are becoming aware of the factors that explain why some children manage the transition reasonably well whereas others exhibit marked problems.

A salutary lesson from the more recent research is the increasing applicability of research to clinical practice. The translation of research findings to the clinical setting is becoming easier, aided by three important trends in how research is carried out. The first is that there is nearly complete transformation of research away from the view that family structure per se is an explanatory variable to a more dynamic, developmental model that focuses on particular risks and protective factors associated with variation in adjustment. This means that it is now easier to identify specific processes that, because of their likely causal influence on children's adjustment, should be targeted for clinical intervention.

Second, a number of studies have directed examined concepts derived from clinical and family systems writings and their applicability to diverse family structures. On one hand, these studies show that the relations among, for example, parent-child and marital relationships do differ across diverse family types. On the other hand, it has not yet been established how and if these different processes are central for understanding children's development, or if family processes that promote optimal adjustment do differ across diverse family structures. Indeed, the importance of positive parent-child relationships seems invariant across all family types. More research of this kind is needed because it addresses important clinical and conceptual issues and focuses on the family as the unit of analysis.

Third, the number of intervention studies continues to increase and provide general encouragement concerning the role of preventive and secondary interventions for preventing and reducing distress associated with family transitions. In addition, there is good reason to believe that interventions can be effective when implemented outside the traditional clinic setting, such as the school. Extending evidence-based clinical practice to a wide audience and outside the individual treatment context will be a central goal, and challenge, for future work.

Note

1. Some terminological notes are necessary. The first concerns the term to describe families in which all children are biologically related to both parents. Previous terms such as 'nuclear' and 'intact' families have fallen out of favour. Other terms previously used in research, notably, 'non-divorced' are now, in many cases, incorrect because partners may well have experienced a separation prior to forming a new relationship and having children. Other possible terms include 'non-remarried', which is cumbersome or 'biological', which may be confusing inasmuch as it may convey a lack of social bonds. The term 'nuclear' is used to refer to families headed by two married adults that includes only their biological children. Also, throughout the chapter, the terms 'divorce' and 'separation' are used. The former is the more commonly used in research because most studies assess (previously) married couples. The more general term 'separation' is used when the couple separating may have been cohabiting rather than married.

References

(References preceded by a * are especially recommended for their conceptual importance, methodological sophistication, and/or clinical relevance.)

Amato PR (1996) Explaining the intergenerational transmission of divorce. Journal of Marriage and the Family 58: 628–40.
Amato PR (1999) Children of divorced parents as young adults. In Hetherington EM (ed.) Coping with Divorce, Single-parenting, and Remarriage: A Risk and Resiliency Perspective. Mahwah NJ: Erlbaum, pp. 147–63.
Amato PR (2001) Children of divorce in the 1990s: an update of the Amato and Keith (1991) meta-analysis. Journal of Family Psychology 15: 355–70.
Amato PR, Keith B (1991a) Parental divorce and the well-being of children: a meta-analysis. Psychological Bulletin 110: 26–46.
Amato PR, Keith B (1991b) Parental divorce and adult well-being: a meta-analysis. Journal of Marriage and the Family 53: 43–58.
Amato PR, Booth A (1996) A prospective study of divorce and parent-child relationships. Journal of Marriage and the Family 58: 356–65.

Anderson J, White G (1986) Dysfunctional intact families and stepfamilies. Family
    Process 25: 407–22.
Aquilino WS (1996) The life course of children born to unmarried mothers: child-
    hood living arrangements and young adult outcomes. Journal of Marriage and
    the Family 58: 293–310.
Aquilino WS (1994) Impact of childhood family disruption on young adults' rela-
    tionships with parents. Journal of Marriage and the Family 56: 295–313.
Aseltine RH, Kessler RC (1993) Marital disruption and depression in a communi-
    ty sample. Journal of Health and Social Behavior 34: 237–51.
*Barnes GG (1999) Divorce transitions: identifying risk and promoting resilience
    for children and their parental relationships. Journal of Marital and Family
    Therapy 25: 425–41.
Block JH, Block J, Gjerde P (1986) The personality of children prior to divorce: a
    prospective study. Child Development 57: 827–40.
Booth A, Amato PR (2001) Parental predivorce relations and offspring postdivorce
    well-being. Journal of Marriage and the Family 63: 197–212.
Bray JH (1999) From marriage to remarriage and beyond. In Hetherington EM
    (ed.) Coping with Divorce, Single-parenting, and Remarriage: A Risk and
    Resiliency Perspective. Mahwah NJ: Erlbaum, pp. 253–71.
Brody G, Neubaum E, Forehand R (1988) Serial marriage: a heuristic analysis of
    an emerging family form. Psychological Bulletin 103: 211–22.
Bumpass L, Sweet JA, Martin TC (1990) Changing patterns of remarriage. Journal
    of Marriage and the Family 52: 747–56.
Bumpass LL, Sweet JA, Cherlin AJ (1991a) The role of cohabitation in declining
    rates of remarriage. Journal of Marriage and the Family 53: 913–27.
Bumpass LL, Martin TC, Sweet JA (1991b) The impact of family background and
    early marital factors on marital disruption. Journal of Family Issues 12:
    22–42.
Capaldi DM, Patterson GR (1991) Relation of parental transitions to boys' adjust-
    ment problems: 1. A linear hypothesis; 2. Mothers at risk for transitions and
    unskilled parenting. Developmental Psychology 27: 489–504.
Cherlin AJ, Furstenberg FF (1994) Stepfamilies in the United States: a reconsid-
    eration. Annual Review of Sociology 20: 359–81.
Cherlin A, Furstenberg FF, Chase-Lansdale L, Kiernan KE, Robins PK, Morrison
    DR, Teitler JO (1991) Longitudinal effects of divorce in Great Britain and the
    United States. Science 252: 1386–9.
Cherlin AJ, Chase-Lansdale PL, McRae C (1998) Effects of parental divorce on
    mental health throughout the life course. American Sociological Review 63:
    239–49.
Clarke SC, Wilson BF (1994) The relative stability of remarriages. Family Relations
    43: 305–10.
Cockett M, Tipp J (1994) The Exeter Family Study. Exeter: University of Exeter
    Press.
Crosbie-Burnett M (1984) The centrality of the step relationship: a challenge to
    family theory and practice. Family Relations 33: 459–64.
Dunn J, Deater-Deckard K, Pickering K, O'Connor TG, Golding J, ALPSAC Study
    Team (1998) Children's adjustment and prosocial behaviour in step-, single-

parent, and non-stepfamily settings: findings from a community study. Journal of Child Psychology and Psychiatry 39: 1083–95.

Dunn J, Davies L, O'Connor T, Sturgess W (2000) Parents' and partners' life course and family experiences: links with parent-child relationships in different family settings. Journal of Child Psychology and Psychiatry 41: 955–68.

Dunn J, Davies L, O'Connor T, Sturgess W (2001) Family lives and friendships: the perspectives of children in step- single-parent and nonstep families. Journal of Family Psychology 15: 272–87.

Emery RE, Kitzman KM, Waldron M (1999a) Psychological interventions for separated and divorced families. In EM Hetherington (ed.) Coping with Divorce, Single-parenting, and Remarriage: a Risk and Resiliency Perspective. Mahwah NJ: Erlbaum, pp. 323–44.

Emery R, Waldron M, Kitzman KM, Aaron J (1999b) Delinquent behavior, future divorce or nonmarital childbearing, and externalizing behavior among offspring: a 14-year prospective study. Journal of Family Psychology 13: 568–79.

Fergusson DM, Lynskey MT, Horwood LJ (1994) The effects of parental separation, the timing of separation, and gender on children's performance on cognitive tests. Journal of Child Psychology and Psychiatry 35: 1077–92.

Forehand R, Armistead L, David C (1997) Is adolescent adjustment following parental divorce a function of pre-divorce adjustment? Journal of Abnormal Child Psychology 25: 157–64.

*Forgatch M, DeGarmo DS (1999) Parenting through change: an effective prevention program for single mothers. Journal of Consulting and Clinical Psychology 67: 711–24.

Furstenberg FF, Teitler JO (1994) Reconsidering the effects of marital disruption: what happens to children of divorce in early adulthood. Journal of Family Issues 15: 173–90.

Gorell-Barnes G, Thompson P, Daniel G, Burchardt N (1998) Growing Up in Stepfamilies. Oxford: Clarendon Press.

Halhweg K, Markman HJ, Thurmaier F, Engl J, Eckert V (1998) Prevention of marital distress: results of a German prospective longitudinal study. Journal of Family Psychology 12: 543–56.

Haskey J (1994) Stepfamilies and stepchildren in Great Britain. Population Trends 17–28.

Haskey J (1998) One-parent families and their dependent children in Great Britain. Population Trends 91: 5–14.

Hatzichristou C (1993) Children's adjustment after parental separation: teacher, peer, and self-report in a Greek sample: a research note. Journal of Child Psychology and Psychiatry 34: 1469–78.

Hetherington EM (1989) Coping with family transitions: winners, losers and survivors. Child Development 60: 1–14.

*Hetherington EM (ed.) (1999a) Coping with Divorce, Single-parenting, and Remarriage: a Risk and Resiliency Perspective. Mahwah NJ: Erlbaum.

Hetherington EM (1999b) Should we stay together for the sake of the children? In Hetherington EM (ed.) Coping with Divorce, Single-parenting, and Remarriage: a Risk and Resiliency Perspective. Mahwah NJ: Erlbaum, pp. 93–116.

Hetherington EM (2002) For Better or Worse. New York: WW Norton.

*Hetherington EM, Clingempeel WG (1992) Coping with marital transitions: a family systems perspective. Monographs of the Society for Research in Child Development 57, nos 2-3, Serial No 227.

*Hetherington EM, Henderson S, Reiss D, Anderson ER, Bridges M, Chan RW, Insabella GM, Jodl KM, Kim JE, Mitchell AS, O'Connor TG, Skaggs MJ, Taylor LC (1999) Adolescent siblings in stepfamilies: family functioning and adolescent adjustment. Monographs of the Society For Research in Child Development. Serial No. 259, 64(4).

Jocklin V, McGue M, Lykken DT (1996) Personality and divorce: a genetic analysis. Journal of Personality and Social Psychology 71: 288–99.

Johnston JR, Kline M, Tschann J (1989) Ongoing postdivorce conflict in families contesting custody: effects of children of joint custody and frequent access. American Journal of Orthopsychiatry 59: 576–92.

Kiernan KE, Hobcraft J (1997) Parental divorce during childhood: age at first intercourse, partnership, and parenthood. Population Studies 51: 41–55.

Kiernan K, Mueller G (1998) The divorced and who divorces? Centre for Analysis of Social Exclusion, paper 7. London: London School of Economics.

Kurdek LA (1998) The nature and predictors of the trajectory of change in marital quality over the first four years of marriage for first-married husbands and wives. Journal of Family Psychology 12: 494–510.

Lahey BB, Hartdagen SE, Frick PJ, McBurnett K, Connor R, Hynd G (1988) Conduct disorder: parsing the confounded relation to parental divorce and antisocial personality. Journal of Abnormal Psychology 97: 334–7.

Liu X, Chuanqin G, Okawa M, Zhai J, Li Y, Uchiyama M, Neiderhiser JM, Kurita H (2000) Behavioural and emotional problems in Chinese children of divorced parents. Journal of the American Academy of Child and Adolescent Psychiatry 39: 896–903.

Markman H, Floyd F, Stanley S, Lewis H (1988) Prevention of marital distress: a longitudinal investigation. Journal of Consulting and Clinical Psychology 56: 210–17.

Martin TC, Bumpass LL (1989) Recent trends in marital disruption. Demography 26: 37–51.

Morgan M (1980) Marital status, health, illness, and service use. Social Science and Medicine 14: 633–43.

Morrison DR, Coiro MJ (1999) Parental conflict and marital disruption: do children benefit when high-conflict marriages are dissolved? Journal of Marriage and the Family 61: 626–37.

O'Connor TG, Insabella G (1999) Marital satisfaction, relationships, and roles. In Hetherington EM, Henderson S, Reiss D (eds) Adolescent siblings in stepfamilies: family functioning and adolescent adjustment. Monographs of the Society for Research in Child Development 64(4), serial 259.

O'Connor TG, Jenkins JM (2000) Marital Transitions and Children's Adjustment: Understanding Why Families Differ from One Another and Why Children in the Same Family Show Different Patterns of Adjustment, report W-01-1-3E. Ottawa: Human Resources Development Canada.

O'Connor TG, Allen JP, Bell KL, Hauser ST (1996) Adolescent-parent relationships and leaving home in young adulthood: linking developmental transitions. In

Graber JA, Dubas JS (eds) Leaving Home. New Directions in Child Development. San Francisco CA: Jossey-Bass.

O'Connor TG, Hawkins N, Dunn J, Thorpe K, Golding J, ALSPAC Study Team (1998a) Family type and maternal depression in pregnancy: factors mediating risk in a community sample. Journal of Marriage and the Family 60: 757–70.

O'Connor TG, Hetherington EM, Reiss D (1998b) Family systems and adolescent development: shared and nonshared risk and protective factors in nondivorced and remarried families. Development and Psychopathology 10: 353–75.

O'Connor TG, Pickering K, Dunn J, Golding J, ALSPAC Study Team. (1999a) Frequency and predictors of relationship dissolution in a community sample in England. Journal of Family Psychology 13: 436–49.

O'Connor TG, Thorpe K, Dunn J, Golding J, ALSPAC Study Team (1999b) Parental divorce and adjustment in adulthood: findings from a community sample. Journal of Child Psychology and Psychiatry 40: 777–90.

*O'Connor TG, Caspi A, DeFries JC, Plomin R (2000a) Are associations between parental divorce and children's adjustment genetically mediated? An adoption study. Developmental Psychology 36: 429–37.

O'Connor TG, Davies L, Dunn J, Golding J, ALSPAC Study Team (2000b) Differential distribution of children's accidents, injuries, and illnesses across family type. Pediatrics 106, e68.

O'Connor TG, Dunn J, Jenkins JM, Pickering K, Rasbash J (2001) Family settings and children's adjustment: differential adjustment within and across families. British Journal of Psychiatry 179: 110–15.

Office of National Statistics (1997) Special Focus on Families. London: The Stationery Office.

Pedro-Carroll J, Alpert-Ellis L (1997) Preventive interventions for children of divorce: a developmental model for five- and six-year-old children. Journal of Primary Prevention 18: 5–23.

Plomin R (1994) Genetics and Experience. Newbury Park, CA: Sage Publications.

Pope H, Mueller CW (1976) The intergenerational transmission of marital instability: comparisons by race and sex. Journal of Family Issues 32: 49–66.

*Pryor J, Rodgers B (2001) Children in Changing Families: Life after Separation. Oxford: Blackwell.

Samera T, Stolberg AL (1993) Peer support, divorce, and children's adjustment. Journal of Divorce and Remarriage 20: 45–64.

Sandler IN, Tein JY, Mehta P, Wolchik S, Ayers T (2000) Coping efficacy and psychological problems of children of divorce. Child Development 71: 1099–118.

Schoen R, Klugel JR (1988) The widening gap in Black and White marriage rates: the impact of population composition and differential marriage propensities. American Sociological Review 53: 895–907.

Shaw DS, Emery RE, Tuer MD (1993) Parental functioning and children's adjustment in families of divorce: a prospective study. Journal of Abnormal Child Psychology 21: 119–34.

Simons RL, Lin K-H, Gordon LC, Conger RD, Lorenz FO (1999) Explaining the higher incidence of adjustment problems among children of divorce compared with those in two-parent families. Journal of Marriage and the Family 61: 1020–33.

Steinberg L (1987) Single parents, stepparents, and the susceptibility of adolescents to antisocial peer pressure. Child Development 58: 269–75.

Thompson RA, Amato PR (eds) (1999) The Postdivorce Family: Children, Parenting and Society. Thousand Oaks CA: Sage.

Thornton A, Axinn WG, Teachman JD (1995) The influence of school enrollment and accumulation of cohabitation and marriage in early adulthood. American Sociological Review 60: 762–74.

Umberson D (1992) Gender, social status, and the social control of health behavior. Social Science and Medicine 34: 907–17.

Vogel EF, Bell NW (1960) The emotionally disturbed child as the family scapegoat. In Bell NW, Vogel EF (eds) A Modern Introduction to the Family. Glencoe IL: The Free Press, pp. 382–97.

Wadsworth J, Burnell I, Taylor B, Butler N (1983) Family type and accidents in preschool children. Journal of Epidemiology and Community Health 37: 100–4.

Wallerstein JS (1985) Children of divorce: preliminary report of a ten-year follow-up of older children and adolescents. Journal of the American Academy of Child Psychiatry 24: 545–53.

Webster PS, Orbuch TL, House JS (1995) Effects of childhood family background on adult marital quality and perceived stability. American Journal of Sociology 100: 404–32

Weiss R (1979) Growing up a little faster: the experience of growing up in a single-parent household. Journal of Social Issues 35: 97–111.

Wheaton B (1990) Life transitions, role histories, and mental health. American Sociological Review 55: 209–23.

White LK, Booth A (1985) The quality of remarriages: the role of stepchildren. American Sociological Review 50: 689–98.

Wu L (1996) Effects of family instability, income, and income instability on the risk of a premarital birth. American Sociological Review 61: 386–406.

Zill N (1994) Understanding why children in stepfamilies have more learning and behavior problems than children in nuclear families. In Booth A, Dunn J (eds) Stepfamilies: Who Benefits? Who Does Not? Hillsdale NJ: Erlbaum, pp. 97–106.

Zill N, Morrison DR, Coiro MJ (1993) Long-term effects of parental divorce on parent-child relationships, adjustment, and achievements in young adulthood. Journal of Family Psychology 7: 91–103.

CHAPTER 9

The impact of war on children: some lessons from the Afghan conflict

ZULFIQAR AHMED BHUTTA

In some ways this chapter is on Afghanistan, one of the poorest and least fortunate countries in the world. It is about its people and not the privileged politicians and warlords who claim to represent them. It is about the infirm among its populace and especially its women and children, who have borne the brunt of the smouldering conflict over the last 25 years and continue to suffer some of the highest mortality and morbidity rates in the world.

The story of Afghanistan is an epic illustration of the myriad effects of war and conflict on children, not just on their immediate health and survival but also on their long-term development and mental health. This chapter will specifically explore the impact of war and conflict on the health and development of the children of Afghanistan. As data are limited on some long-term aspects, this chapter will of necessity draw upon the emerging body of evidence from other parts of the world (Geltman and Stover, 1997; Laor et al., 1997). An attempt will be made to evaluate the potential impact of intervention strategies that may ameliorate some of the immediate and long-term effects of war and conflict on children.

The genesis and consequences of the Afghan conflict

Afghanistan is a land of spectacular natural beauty and contrasts. The rugged landscape houses 26 million people belonging to four major ethnic groups (Pashtuns 38%, Tajiks 25%, Hazara 19% and Uzbeks 6%). Almost 99% are Muslim, with the majority (84%) belonging to the Sunni sect. The average life expectancy is barely 46 years and almost 42% of the population comprises of children under 14 years of age (CIA World Fact Book, 2001).

Although the relatively recent events in Afghanistan have been the focus of world attention, it is important to understand the background and genesis of the Afghan tragedy. The history of Afghanistan (called Khorasan in medieval times) dates back over 5,000 years and is dotted with conflict, with successive invasions by Alexander the Great, the Mongols and several Afghan expeditions by the British forces.

The history of Afghanistan is one of almost continual strife, conquest and intrigue. Because of its strategic location as the gateway to India and the central Asian states, Afghanistan was the focus of great intrigues and failed incursions (Hopkirk, 1990). The period of relative tranquillity in the post-Second World War period was interspersed with intermittent strife, military coups and draconian measures for state control. The last King, Zahir Shah, ascended to the throne following the assassination of his father in 1933 and ruled over a fractious state until he was ousted in a palace coup in 1973. The tumultuous period that followed saw a rapid rise in influence of the Communist Party and a widespread rise in popular resistance. The Soviet invasion of Afghanistan in 1979 and the brutal military campaign that followed, resulted in one of the biggest humanitarian crises of the post-war era with over six million refugees fleeing to Pakistan and Iran and an additional two million displaced internally (Miller et al., 1994). The massive exodus of almost a quarter of the Afghan population, of which three-quarters were women and children, was a consequence of several factors; these included fear of the pro-Soviet regime, destruction of homes and livelihoods, fear of the Soviet occupying army and the terror of summary imprisonment and execution (Magnus and Naby, 1998).

Events in Pakistan over the last 15 years have also had a bearing on the Afghan tragedy. Most of the Afghan conflict had occurred during the military dictatorship of General Zia ul Haq, which had seen an artificial period of prosperity and economic growth, largely as a result of a massive influx of aid. Much of this was however squandered and although several civilian and elected governments followed General Zia's death in 1988, none was able to provide stable governance. With dwindling external assistance and imposition of structural adjustment programmes, there was an exponential increase in poverty over the last decade (Bhutta, 2001). This economic decline was accelerated in no small measure by the imposition of sanctions following the tit-for-tat nuclear tests in 1998 (Bhutta 1998, 2002). Admittedly the impact of these economic sanctions was compounded by lack of governance and widespread corruption, bringing social and human development to a standstill. The major victims of this economic stagnation were programmes in social development especially those related to health and education and this has resulted in growing inequity and poverty in the region (Social Policy and Development Centre (SPDC), 2002; Bengali, 2002).

With the public education system steadily falling into ruin and disarray, there was a steady growth of Madrassahs (religious schools largely run as seminaries and funded by private organizations) throughout the 1980s, largely encouraged by the Islamic revivalist government of General Zia. Although originally conceived and run as welfare projects, it is debatable if the Madrassah system has continued to function as such. The main attraction for most poor families in sending their children to Madrassahs was the benefit of free education and board for students. Other major contributory factors to this trend were the failure of the system of primary education in the public sector and the vested interest of the religious and sectarian political parties in raising their own band of followers. The curriculum in most Madrassahs still remains a blend of archaic theological teaching and intense Islamic education. In the context of the situation in Afghanistan these Madrassahs not only provided education to the local populace but also catered to refugee children, especially orphans of war. The growth of these Madrassahs has been particularly rapid in the Northwest Frontier province of Pakistan and the tribal belt bordering Afghanistan; the diaspora of these graduates now spans both sides of the Durand line. Admittedly only a minority of such Madrassahs impart militant training and preach 'Jihad' (religious war), but those that do thrive on perceptions of widespread persecution of fellow Muslims worldwide. In an ever-shrinking world with instant communication, images of civilian casualties in Palestine, Kashmir, Kosovo and Chechnya fuel a growing number of angry young men, many willing to lay down their lives for brethren in faith in distant lands (Rashid, 2002).

The Taliban (meaning 'students') movement grew out of such religious seminaries and the schools of Baluchistan and the Northwest Frontier province of Pakistan. Many were orphans of the Afghan war or children from refugee camps and were conscripted to the Taliban army. Their rapid rise to power in 1994 must be seen in the context of the chaos and civil war of Afghanistan at the time, with complete lawlessness and warlords running amok. Although the Taliban government brought some initial respite from incessant conflict, their tribal and medieval interpretation of Islam led to the imposition of draconian policies restricting the rights of women and minorities. The imposition of this extremely orthodox version of Islamic law upon the country was not only a source of great distress to development agencies but led to much disquiet throughout the Islamic world. Despite the evidence of the impact of economic sanctions on children from other parts of the world (Ali and Shah, 2000) Afghanistan was progressively sanctioned, thus making it difficult even for humanitarian agencies to operate.

War and displacement of the Afghan population

Between the years 1979 and 1992, more than a fifth of Afghanistan's population – over six million people – was driven from the country in search of safety. Most of these refugees fled to neighbouring Pakistan and Iran; according to UN figures these numbers reached a peak in 1990 with 3,272,000 Afghan refugees in Pakistan and 2,940,000 in Iran. Between the summer of 2000 and September 2001, 956,000 people had reportedly been displaced within Afghanistan (Amnesty International, 2001).

Throughout the Soviet occupation of Afghanistan between 1979 and 1989, members of the international community funnelled vast quantities of arms and ammunition to the different groups fighting for control of Afghanistan. However, following the Soviet withdrawal, international interest in the plight of Afghan refugees waned considerably. Over the period from 1990 to 2001, the United Nations Consolidated Appeal for Afghanistan, the UN inter-agency mechanism for coordinated fundraising supporting Afghan relief projects, received far less funding from donor governments than required to maintain the necessary priority assistance programmes. This had direct implications for the support of refugees, especially the most vulnerable sections among them.

Apart from the direct effect of war in terms of injury and death, the major impact of the Afghan conflict has been through widespread displacement and economic ruin of its population, principally its women and children. Prior to the US attack on Afghanistan it was estimated that most of the Afghan refugees were living in Pakistan and Iran, either in refugee camps or in squatter settlements in major cities (Miller et al., 1994; Assefa et al., 2001). Although such high rates of childhood morbidity and mortality are well recognized among refugee populations in diverse geographic locations (Bonn, 2001; Yip and Sharp, 1993; Aldis and Schouten, 2001), the effect of war on resident populations is less evident. In a 1993 survey of representative populations in Kabul (Gessner, 1994) the daily mortality rate for children under five was found to be highest among resident families (260 compared with 190 per 100,000 population among displaced families). This is plausible because although the refugees are a focus of activities of relief organizations, the resident populations are frequently left to fend for themselves.

Global evidence of the impact of war on child health and survival

Given their vulnerability, it is no surprise that around two million children are estimated to have died as a result of armed conflict in the last decade.

In Mozambique alone, between 1981 and 1988, armed conflict caused 454,000 child deaths, whereas in Somalia, according to the World Health Organization (WHO), crude mortality rates increased seven to 25 times. Some of the highest death rates occur among children in refugee camps (Machel, 2001). It is questionable whether mortality rates are the best indicators of the effects of war on children as these can be selectively affected by targeted interventions (Ugalde et al., 2000). It may be better to use multiple indicators of health and morbidity alongside them (Kinra et al., 2002). In Afghanistan alone, where a civil war of sorts has been continuing for the past 25 years, around 300,000 to 400,000 children have died out of total population of 20 million.

Many of today's armed conflicts take place in some of the world's poorest countries, where children are already vulnerable to malnutrition and disease. The onset of armed conflict increases death rates up to 24 times. Since 1990, the most commonly reported causes of death among refugees and internally displaced persons during the early influx phase have been diarrhoeal diseases, acute respiratory infections, measles and other infectious diseases such as tuberculosis (Khan et al., 2002). Even in peacetime, these are the major killers of children, accounting for some seven million child deaths each year. Their effects are heightened during conflicts, partly because malnutrition is likely to be more prevalent, thereby increasing chances of infection. These data on the deaths are corroborated by the impact of conflict on childhood malnutrition in Ethiopia (Kaluski et al., 2002), Congo (Aldis and Schouten, 2001) and even relatively well-developed parts of Eastern Europe (Hadzihalilovic and Hadziselimovic, 2001).

The data on the burden and severity of infectious diseases among displaced children and refugee populations are particularly stark. Diarrhoea is one of the most common diseases. In Somalia during 1992, 23% to 50% of deaths in Baidoa, Afgoi and Berbera were reported to be due to diarrhoea. Cholera is also a constant threat and, following armed conflicts, it has occurred in refugee camps in Bangladesh, Kenya, Malawi, Nepal, Somalia and Zaire, amongst others. Acute respiratory infections, including pneumonia, are particularly lethal in children and, according to the WHO, kill one-third of the children who died in six refugee centres in Goma, Zaire, in 1994 (Goma Epidemiology Group, 1994). Measles epidemics have been reported in recent situations of conflict or displacement in several African countries – at the height of the conflict in Somalia, more than half the deaths in some places were caused by measles. As tuberculosis re-emerges as a dangerous threat to health the world over, its effect is heightened by armed conflict and disruption. The WHO estimates that half the world's refugees may be infected with tuberculosis as the crowded conditions in refugee camps often promote the spread of tubercular

infection. These effects are especially notable as an upsurge of tuberculosis among refugees and displaced populations in Afghanistan, especially
children (Khan and Laaser, 2002). Malaria has always been a major cause
of morbidity and mortality among refugees in tropical areas, particularly
among people who come from areas of marginal transmission and who
move through or settle in endemic areas. Children, as always, are the
most vulnerable to these collective assaults on health and wellbeing at a
population level. A survey of Afghan refugee women and children in
Quetta in 1992 indicated that over 80% were unregistered and thus ineli-
gible for assistance (Miller, 1994). Of the 112 women interviewed, the
child mortality was an incredible 31% (112/366 births). In addition, of the
surviving children 67% were severely malnourished with a trend for
increasing malnutrition with age (Miller, 1994).

For children, one of the most dangerous implications of this breakdown of health services during conflict is the disruption of rural
vaccination programmes. During Bangladesh's struggle for independence
in 1971–2, childhood deaths increased 47%. Smallpox, a disease that had
virtually disappeared prior to the conflict, claimed 18,000 lives. By 1973,
in Uganda, immunization coverage had reached an all-time high of 73%.
After the fighting started in that country, coverage declined steadily until,
according to the WHO sources, by 1990, fewer than 10% of eligible children were being immunized with anti-tuberculosis vaccine (BCG), and
fewer than 5% against diphtheria, pertussis and tetanus (DPT), measles
and poliomyelitis.

Direct war-related and landmine injuries among children

It is widely recognized that children bear the major brunt of displacement
following conflict and war. It is estimated that over two million children
have been killed in conflicts all over the world since 1990, and over five
million seriously injured (Southall and Abbasi, 1998). Despite sophisti-
cated technology and claims to the contrary, children formed a
disproportionately large group among the civilian casualties following the
recent US-led military operations in Afghanistan.

Among the weapons employed in conflict, none surpasses the landmine in its ability to cause bodily harm and suffering. Landmines and
unexploded ordnance probably pose the most insidious and persistent
danger to children in conflict zones. Today, children in at least 68 countries live amid the contamination of more than 110 million landmines
(Machel, 2001). Added to this number are millions of items of unexploded ordnance, bombs, shells and grenades that failed to detonate on

impact and are frequently picked by children scavenging for scrap and a daily meal. Afghanistan, Angola and Cambodia alone are estimated to have a combined total of at least 28 million landmines, as well as 85% of the world's landmine casualties. Angola, with an estimated 10 million land-mines, has an amputee population of 70,000, of whom 8,000 are children.

Despite the public outcry and recognition of their destructive potential to civilian populations, landmines continue to be employed in most con-flicts globally. It is recognized that landmines and unexploded ordnance pose a particular danger for children (Machel, 2001). Children are also more vulnerable to the danger of landmines than adults because they may not recognize or be able to read warning signs. Children are naturally inquisitive, more likely to pick up strange objects they come across and are also less likely than adults to recognize the tell-tale signs of land mines and impending danger. In a deplorable example of targeting children, the Soviet Union littered rural Afghanistan with brightly coloured land mines shaped like toys and 'butterflies'. The risk to children is further com-pounded by the way in which mines and unexploded ordnance become a part of daily life. Children may become so familiar with mines that they forget they are lethal weapons.

Child soldiers are particularly vulnerable to landmine injuries as they are often the very personnel used to explore known minefields. In Cambodia, a survey of mine victims in military hospitals revealed that as many as 43% had been recruited as soldiers between the ages of 10 and 16. In Afghanistan it is estimated that almost a third of all landmine vic-tims were children. The victims of mines and unexploded ordnance are also far greater among the poorest sectors of society because of the risks people face in their daily life. In conflict zones, especially rural popula-tions, the tasks of civilians may consist of cultivating their fields, herding animals or searching for firewood. In many cultures, these are the very tasks carried out by children. Although anti-personnel mines are designed to maim and not to kill, they can be potentially fatal for children. While in Cambodia almost a quarter of all children injured by mines and unex-ploded ordnance died from their injuries (Stover et al., 1994), the risk of mortality associated with landmine accidents in Afghanistan was almost 55% (Andersson et al., 1995). In a comparative evaluation of landmine accidents in four areas of conflict including Afghanistan, Bosnia, Cambodia and Mozambique (Andersson et al., 1995), the highest population-based rates of landmine accidents were seen in Afghanistan.

Among those who survive landmine injuries, the consequent medical problems and rehabilitation needs are also much greater for children, as the limb of a growing child grows faster than the surrounding tissue and may require repeated surgery. As they grow, children also need expensive new prostheses and regular care. This may not only be unaffordable but is unlikely to be offered to girls in societies with deep-seated gender imbalance. Landmine injuries are a frequent direct cause of medical impoverishment with 57% to 60% of all families involved having had to sell household goods and property in order to pay for treatment. It is estimated that, despite attempts at demining, there are still around 10 million to 15 million mines in Afghanistan (UNICEF, 1994). A survey on disability indicated that 3% to 4% of the population of Afghanistan was disabled to the point of needing some from of assistance, although only 10% to 15% had any access to treatment.

Millions of children are killed by armed conflict, but three times as many are seriously injured or permanently disabled by it. According to the WHO, armed conflict and political violence are the leading causes of injury, impairment and physical disability and primarily responsible for the condition of over four million children who currently live with disabilities. In Afghanistan alone, some 100,000 children have war-related disabilities, many of them caused by landmines. The lack of basic services and the destruction of health facilities during armed conflict usually mean that children living with disabilities get little support. Only 3% in developing countries receive adequate rehabilitative care, and the provision of prosthetics to children is an area that requires increased attention and financial support. In Angola and Mozambique, less than 20% of children needing them received low-cost prosthetic devices; in Nicaragua and El Salvador, services were also available for only 20% of the children in need.

The immediate and long-term costs of landmine injuries are also compounded by the high costs of clean-up operations and land reclamation. It is recognized that clearing landmines can be both long and extremely expensive. To illustrate, clearing each landmine takes 100 times longer to remove than to deploy. Thus a weapon that costs $3 or less to manufacture may eventually cost $1,000 to remove, limiting the resources available for essential services.

War orphans and child soldiers

During the 1990s, two million children worldwide were killed as a result of war, four to five million children were disabled, 12 million were left homeless, more than one million orphaned or separated from their parents, and approximately 10 million children have been psychologically traumatized as a result of war (UNICEF, 1996). Wars have several other effects on children including loss of parents and other close relatives. Many left their education because of poverty, displacements, disabilities, destroyed infrastructure of education and so forth. Many street children have no shelter and are dependent on relatives for a place to stay and otherwise vulnerable to abuse. According to a survey conducted by the UNHCR in 1997, there were an estimated 28,000 street children in Kabul, 20% of them girls. Following an escalation of conflict and reduction of support services, the figure rose to more than 35,000.

War orphans and refugees are subjected to great abuse, none more glaring than conscription as child soldiers or being forced to undertake menial hard labour. The latter may be necessary for survival as many such children are forced to carry out the most hazardous jobs, frequently in return for meagre wages. Other adolescents and teenagers are conscripted as soldiers. The worst examples of the latter practice were seen in Africa and cases have also been reported from Sri Lanka and Afghanistan. A detailed assessment of the dimensions of child labour and the direct effect and consequences of war on child soldiers is beyond the scope of this chapter. However, a reference must be made to the relationship of the Afghan war to the growth of the Taliban and conscription of children and adolescents to *Jihadi* (holy war) organizations.

There is general consensus that the Taliban edicts restricting access to education, health care and employment for women brought considerable suffering and impoverishment to war widows and families in Afghanistan. The impact of these policies on the health and nutrition of women and adolescent girls were corroborated by several surveys indicated the disproportionate impact of food shortages and malnutrition on Afghan girl children (Rasekh et al., 1998). Less obvious were the psychological trauma and mental stress that many resident Afghan women and families endured on an almost daily basis (Iacopino, 1999). Such effects have been well described among as residents and refugee women and children in other conflict zones as well (Bryce et al., 1989; Locke et al., 1996). On a direct level despite the passage of a law in 1998 to the contrary, the continued conscription of child soldiers by the Taliban resulted in a large number of young Madrassah students and refugee children forced to fight on the front lines.

While the growth of religious extremism and fanaticism is by no means restricted to the illiterate, the most ready conscripts to the philosophy of violence are the adolescents and youngsters who are a product of conflict, and see little future and hope in the status quo. The disenchantment of a growing number of poorly educated, if not illiterate, and unemployable youth in the region is a fertile source of recruits for right-wing religious extremist groups. This phenomenon is compounded several times by the apathy of the state towards human development and promotion of equity. Writing on inequality and the growth of obscurantism and terrorism in the region, Kaiser Bengali a prominent social scientist writes (2002):

> Unequal societies are unjust societies. And unjust societies lose their moral and political legitimacy. Attention to the problem of income and regional

inequality is thus not only important but also urgent. While poverty causes hardships and deprivation for those caught in the poverty web, inequality causes a sense of grievance and injustice, promotes despondency and anger, and generates social and political instability and even violence. Terrorism is a buzzword today, but those who are concerned about terrorism should pay close attention to the problem of inequality.

This worrisome epiphenomenon is by no means restricted to the conflict zones of Afghanistan, Pakistan and Kashmir but has found its way into the streets of Palestine in a growing number of teenage suicide bombers, as well as the murderous gangs of right-wing extremist youngsters in Indian Gujarat.

The psychosocial effects of war and its relationship to the Afghan conflict

The lasting effects of war on the psychological state of women and children have been well described in Lykes (1994). These effects may consist of post-traumatic stress disorders suffered as a consequence of witnessing or experiencing parental loss in war (Macksoud and Aber, 1996), whereas in others political repression (Locke et al., 1996) and state terror (Munczek and Tuber, 1998) have been shown to result in significant psychological sequelae. More recently a study of internally displaced children from the war in Bosnia has revealed features of post-traumatic stress disorder in 94% of the cases (Goldstein et al., 1997) and it has also been demonstrated that the negative effects of war may overwhelm coping mechanisms (Allwood et al., 2002). The same phenomenon has been observed in Kuwaiti children who lived through the Gulf war (al Eissa, 1995). More worryingly some reports suggest that children and adolescents scarred by war transmit their problems into the next generation in a quasi-genetic fashion (Sack, et al. 1995).

There are few systematic studies of the effect of conflict on Afghan children, but the landmark survey by UNICEF on the effect of war on children between 8 and 18 years of age living in Kabul (Gupta, 1997) indicated that 41% had lost one or more parents due to the war and over half had directly witnessed torture or violent death. Over 90% of the children interviewed expressed the fear of dying in the conflict. A particularly gruesome practice of encouraging children to witness public amputations and executions has an enormous impact on impressionable minds. In other instances consistent exposure to gruesome violence and death at an early age can make a young mind inured to it. The average Taliban and Mujahideen soldier is a product of the same cycle of violence and social upheaval in Afghanistan, witnessed and experienced from early child-hood. Their vision of the world is largely tainted by ignorance, isolation and a daily ritual of religious dogma. This lost generation is likely to breed many more unless action is taken to bring this cycle of violence to an end.

Potential intervention strategies and what can be done?

The aforementioned sections indicate the myriad effects of war on chil-dren in conflict zones and to the nihilistic among us, an almost irretrievable situation. However, others see in these unique circumstances enormous opportunities for intervention. The developed world may not be into 'nation building' but it owes it to the women and children of Afghanistan, a country whose people served as a bulwark in the war against communism and sacrificed a full generation in its aftermath. Although greatly traumatized by two decades of war one can draw some hope and faith from the relative resilience of Afghan children (Sellick, 1998). Although the psychological trauma of war on children has been described as permanent (UNICEF, 1996), others disagree (Summerfield, 1998) and place great faith in the potential of community and social struc-tures in buffering these effects. Kinra et al. (2002) have also highlighted the ameliorating effects of good primary care systems on the children sur-viving the Bosnian conflict. Howsoever transient, others have documented the fact that children respond rapidly to the onset of peace with remarkable adaptation (Qouta et al., 1995). Although the evidence base for effective interventions ameliorating the effect of war on children is small, there is a growing body of literature on strategies that help. The important issue is that much can be done and the impact of war on a child's psyche can be ameliorated.

These intervention strategies can be largely grouped into two categories:

- Preventive strategies and upholding child and family rights during conflicts.
- Recognition of psychological stress and early intervention (individual and public health levels).

Preventive strategies and upholding child and family rights during conflicts

Provision of security and safety to children during conflict is principally an adult responsibility and all the charters of child rights must be strictly adhered to. Psychosocial readaptation and rehabilitation also presupposes a certain degree of physical security and economic stability before an adolescent is prepared, or even able, to come to terms with the experiences of armed conflict. Thus reestablishment of primary health care services and provision of basic housing and food is of key importance.

Most children who experience violence need special care and attention. The family is the basic and most important ingredient in a child's physical and psychological rehabilitation and thus every attempt must be made to keep the family unit intact in conflict zones. In most cases, such psychosocial support must be offered to the parents as well as the children if the assistance to the children is going to make a meaningful difference.

Recognition of psychological stress and early intervention (individual and public health levels)

An important part of any intervention programme is the recognition of high-risk groups and those with urgent needs. A number of strategies and screening programmes have been identified as useful in screening children suffering from post-traumatic stress disorder in diverse situations like Bosnia, Kosovo, Chechnya and Palestine (Allwood et al., 2002; Barath, 2002). The relative prevalence of post-traumatic stress disorder and depression has been recognized to be as high as 68% and 18% respectively (Allwood et al., 2002). It is important that early recognition of these problems is coupled with rehabilitation programmes and positive interventions. Although the evidence base for effective interventions is relatively small, these may be considered under the following available categories:

- Ensuring physical and economic security. There is an inevitable risk of civilian casualties especially among children in war zones. Although some so-called 'collateral damage' is inevitable, a large proportion is avoidable. Deliberate targeting of areas where women and children seek refuge must be banned. There is a plethora of resolutions and guidelines to this effect and the key issue here is one of sensitization and implementation.
- Direct psychosocial support, counselling and community-based approaches. Avoid institutionalization at all costs and even in the case of orphans, deliberate placement with families and foster parents is important. Although psychiatrists and trained psychotherapists in conflict zones may be both rare and largely available in institutional settings it is critical that children and adolescents not be placed in such institutions. As much as possible, these interventions must be

undertaken in community settings and through support groups whenever possible. National societies of health professionals and human rights groups can play a special role in this regard.

- Education and schooling strategies. Of all the possible intervention strategies, educational approaches appear to be the most promising. These presuppose the rapid introduction of regular schooling and educational activities and the special role that teachers can play in recognising psychosocial distress and stress. There is always a paucity of mental health professionals in developing countries and teachers can play a special role in the recognition and amelioration of stress. Many children suffering from PTSD will have difficulty functioning in a school setting. Teachers describe students as having short attention spans, exaggerated startle reactions and either emotional lability or lack of affect. The child's ability to concentrate and learn can be increased by incorporating classroom activities stressing relaxation, group support and problem-solving skills. The experience from Bosnia of such approaches is both heartening and instructive (Husain, 2001). Teachers from local cultural settings can be rapidly trained in basic stress recognition and counselling strategies employing culturally relevant and acceptable tools. Such graphic and painful material that traumatized children discuss or act out can also affect the teachers. Teachers and other mental health professionals working with trauma victims often develop painful images, thoughts and feelings. This is referred to as vicarious or secondary traumatization. It is especially likely to happen when dealing with serious trauma to children. It may thus be important to put mechanisms in place to provide emotional and psychological support and stress relief for teachers and other health professionals

- Promotion of healthy sports and recreational activities. These activities have a special role in stress relief and rapid restitution of normalcy. The activities should focus in particular on group activities, team play and sportsmanship. Care must be taken however, that sports in multi-ethnic environments do not become surrogates for violence and polarization of children or groups.

- Support for healing programmes rather than focusing on the negatives and psychosocial stress alone. Although the recognition of overt and subliminal problems is crucial, it is also important that professionals and community groups focus on the positive and actively promote optimism and healing, deliberately highlighting positive outcomes and promoting concrete activities such as group activities, vocational training and extra curricular activities are important. No matter how difficult or artificial, deliberate promotion of normalcy is extremely important for children and adolescents.

- Special role of parents and truth commissions. A special mention has been made of the key role that health professionals and teachers play in rehabilitating children and adolescents after war and the importance of restoring normalcy. However, in certain circumstances communal healing may be important and particularly adolescents may benefit from such a process. Truth commissions, human rights commissions and reconciliation groups can be important vehicles for community healing. To date, 16 or more countries in transition from conflict have organized truth commissions as a means of establishing moral, legal and political accountability and mechanisms for recourse. In South Africa and Guatemala, the commissions are aimed at preserving the memory of the victims, fostering the observance of human rights and strengthening the democratic process.

To summarize, no matter how disastrous the Afghan conflict, how tragic the effect on its children, there is room for optimism in the future and hope. It is important to create, strengthen and expand programmes for family support, education, improved nutrition and protection of human rights in conflict zones such as Afghanistan and northern Pakistan. These programmes must be based on solid foundations of political stability, forgiveness and human development. The smiling faces of numerous Afghan girls attending schools are a testament to the fact that humanity can triumph when given a chance. However, the lessons of the Afghan conflict must lead to strategies that protect children in the event of such conflicts (Southall and Carballo, 1996). The ground-breaking report by the UN commission headed by Graca Machel (2001) laid the foundations for protective mechanisms to prevent and ameliorate the effects of war on children and adolescents. It is now up to the global community to ensure their implementation.

References

al Eissa YA (1995) The impact of the Gulf armed conflict on the health and behaviour of Kuwaiti children. Soc Sci Med 41:1033–7.

Aldis W, Schouten E (2001) War and public health in Democratic Republic of Congo. Lancet 358: 2088.

Ali MM, Shah IH (2000) Sanctions and childhood mortality in Iraq. Lancet 355: 1851–7.

Allwood MA, Bell-Dolan D, Husain SA (2002) Children's trauma and adjustment reactions to violent and nonviolent war experiences. J Am Acad Child Adolesc Psychiatry 41: 450–7.

Amnesty International (2001) Protect Afghan Civilians and Refugees. London: Amnesty International.

Andersson N, Da Sousa SP, Paredes S (1995) Social cost of land mines in four countries: Afghanistan, Bosnia, Cambodia and Mozambique. Br Med J 311: 718–21.

Assefa F, Jabarkhil MZ, Salama P, Spiegel P (2001) Malnutrition and mortality in Kohistan District, Afghanistan, April 2001. JAMA 286: 2723–8.

Barath A (2002) Psychological status of Sarajevo children after war: 1999-2000 survey. Croat Med J 43: 213–20.

Bengali K (2002) Creating an unequal society. Daily Dawn 10 August, p. 7.

Bhutta ZA (1998) Staring into the abyss: walking the nuclear tightrope in South Asia. Br Med J 317: 363–4.

Bhutta ZA (2001) Structural adjustments and impact on health and society: a perspective from Pakistan. Int J Epidemiol 30: 712–16.

Bhutta ZA, Nundy S (2002) Thinking the unthinkable. Br Med J 324: 1405–6.

Bonn D (2001) Infectious diseases threaten refugees entering Pakistan. Lancet Infect Dis 1: 214.

Bryce JW, Walker N, Ghorayeb F, Kanj M (1989) Life experiences, response styles and mental health among mothers and children in Beirut, Lebanon. Soc Sci Med 28: 685–95.

CIA. World Fact Book – Afghanistan (2001) http://www.cia.org/Afghanistan

Geltman P, Stover E (1997) Genocide and the plight of children in Rwanda. JAMA 277: 289–92.

Gessner BD (1994) Mortality rates, causes of death, and health status among displaced and resident populations of Kabul, Afghanistan. JAMA 272: 382–5.

Goldstein RD, Wampler NS, Wise PH (1997) War experiences and distress symptoms of Bosnian children. Pediatrics 100: 873–8.

Goma Epidemiology Group (1994) Public health impact of Rwandan refugee crisis: what happened in Goma, Zaire, in July, 1994? Lancet 345: 339–44.

Gupta L (1997) Survey on Afghan Children. New York: UNICEF.

Hadzihalilovic J, Hadziselimovic R (2001) Growth and development of male children and youth in Tuzla's region after the war in Bosnia and Herzegovina. Coll Antropol 25: 41–58.

Hopkirk P (1990) The Great Game: On Secret Service in High Asia. Oxford: Oxford University Press.

Husain SA (2001) Hope for Children: Lessons from Bosnia. Tuzla: Harfo-Graf.

Iacopino V (1999) Mental health of women in Afghanistan (reply). JAMA 281: 231.

International Crisis Group (2002) Pakistan: Madrasa, Extremism and the Military. Brussels: International Crisis Group Report.

Kaluski DN, Kaluski DN, Ophir E, Amede T (2002) Food security and nutrition – the Ethiopian case for action. Public Health Nutr 5: 373–82.

Khan IM, Laaser U (2002) Burden of tuberculosis in Afghanistan: update on a war-stricken country. Croat Med J 43: 245–7.

Kinra S, Black ME, Sanja Mandic S, Selimovic N (2002) Impact of the Bosnian conflict on the health of women and children. Bulletin of the World Health Organization 80: 75–6.

Laor N, Woolmer L, Mayes LC, Gershon A, Welzman R, Cohen DJ (1997) Israeli preschool children under Scuds: a 30 month follow-up. J Am Acad Child Adolesc Psychiatry 36: 349–56.

Locke CJ, Southwick K, McCloskey LA, Fernandez-Esquer ME (1996) The psychological and medical sequelae of war in Central American refugee mothers and children. Arch Pediatr Adolesc Med 150: 822–8.

Lykes MB (1994) Terror, silencing and children: international, multidisciplinary collaboration with Guatemalan Maya communities. Soc Sci Med 38: 543–52.

Machel G (2001) The Impact of War on Children. New York: UNICEF.

Macksoud MS, Aber JL (1996) The war experiences and psychosocial development of children in Lebanon. Child Dev 67: 70–88.

Magnus RH, Naby E (1998) Afghanistan: Mullah, Marx and Mujahid. New Delhi: Harper Collins.

Miller LC, Timouri M, Wijnker J, Schaller JG (1994) Afghan refugee children and mothers. Arch Pediatr Adolesc Med 148: 704–8.

Morikawa M (2001) Upper respiratory infection in acute pediatric care in internal conflict, Kosovo, 1999. J Trop Pediatr 47:379–82.

Munczek DS, Tuber S (1998) Political repression and its psychological effects on Honduran children. Soc Sci Med 47: 1699–713.

Qouta S, Punamaki RL, El Sarraj E (1995) The impact of the peace treaty on psychological well being: a follow up study of Palestinian children. Child Abuse Negl 19: 1197–2208.

Rasekh Z, Bauer HM, Manos M, Iacopino V (1998) Women's health and human rights in Afghanistan. JAMA 280: 449–55.

Rashid AA (2000) Vanished gender: women, children and Taliban culture. In Rashid A (ed.) Taliban: Islam, Oil and the New Great Game in Central Asia. London: Tauris, pp. 105–16.

Rashid A (2002) Jihad: The Rise of Militant Islam in Central Asia. Lahore: Vanguard.

Sack WH, Clarke GN, Seelev J (1995) Post-traumatic stress disorder across two generations of Cambodian refugees. J Am Acad Child Adolesc Psychiatry 34: 1160–6.

Selimbasic Z, Pavlovic S, Sinanovic O, Vesnic S, Petrovic M, Ferkovic V, Cipurkovic-Mustacevic A (2001) Posttraumatic stress disorder – effects of psychosocial treatment in children. Med Arh 55(suppl. 1): 25–9.

Sellick P (1998) The Impact of Armed Conflict on Children in Afghanistan. New York: Save the Children Alliance/UNICEF.

Southall D, Abbasi K (1998) Protecting children from armed conflict: the UN convention needs an enforcing arm. Br Med J 316: 1549–50.

Southall D, Carballo M (1996) Can children be protected from the effect of war? BMJ 313: 1493.

Stover F, Keller AS, Coby J, Sopheap S (1994) The medical and social consequences of land mines in Cambodia. JAMA 272: 331–6.

Summerfield D (1998) Children affected by war must not be stigmatized as permanently damaged. Br Med J 317: 1249.

Sundelin Wahlsten V, Ahmad A, Von Knorring AL (2001) Traumatic experiences and posttraumatic stress reactions in children and their parents from Kurdistan and Sweden. Nord J Psychiatry 55: 395–400.

Ugalde A, Selva-Sutter E, Castillo C, Paz C, Canas S (2000) Conflict and health. The health costs of war: can they be measured? Lessons from El Salvador. BMJ 321: 169–72.

UNICEF (1994) Anti-personnel Land-mines: Scourge on Children. New York: UNICEF, p. 6.

UNICEF (1996) State of the World's Children. New York: UNICEF.

Yip R, Sharp TW (1993) Acute malnutrition and high childhood mortality related to diarrhoea: lessons from the 1991 Kurdish refugee crisis. JAMA 270: 587–90.

SECTION 3

GENERAL ISSUES RELATED TO CLINICAL PRACTICE

CHAPTER 10

Children and families: human rights and evidence-based practice

LIZ GOLDTHORPE

Introduction

Many of the rights in the European Convention of Human Rights and Fundamental Freedoms 1950 ('the Convention'), enshrined in the Human Rights Act 1998 ('the Act'), have implications for health and social care policies and service delivery, from end-of-life decisions to the sensitivity of care provided to individuals, and have consequences for the relationship between professionals, their patients or clients, as well as other individuals and agencies

A comprehensive, definitive guide to human rights law is well beyond the scope of this chapter. A more detailed guide can only set out statements of principle, accompanied by case law that may well be out of date soon after publication. In any event, each case must be treated on its own merits and facts and professionals should seek case specific advice in each instance.

This chapter is designed to identify the main areas that clinical practitioners are likely to encounter, without necessarily being able to provide comprehensive answers. It indicates further sources of material and more detailed advice where relevant, and focuses on:

- *confidentiality,* including exceptions to the basic duty, access to records, disclosure of abuse and sharing information with third parties;
- *consent to, and refusal of, treatment;*
- *access to services and resources,* including constraints on professional or patient choices, and rationing; and
- *standards of practice and procedure,* including commonality and consistency in decision-making processes, delays and potential negligence in diagnoses.

Readers should note that the law is that which applies to England and Wales as of July 2002.

Enforcing Convention rights

Taking a case to the European Court of Human Rights (the 'ECtHR') in Strasbourg is a cumbersome, expensive and time-consuming process. The Human Rights Act 1998, which came into force on 2 October 2000, now enables individuals to enforce the Convention in the UK courts, if they think a public authority has breached or is likely to breach a Convention right or freedom affecting them.

The Articles of the Convention set out specific defined, fundamental rights and freedoms, which concern issues of fairness and justice. These can be found in the Schedule to the Act. They have been described by the ECtHR as a living instrument, which must be interpreted in the light of present day conditions. The Act does not take away or restrict any existing human rights already recognized, and the Convention acts as a yardstick by which all legislation must be measured.

The rights of children and young people

The Convention on which the Act is based does not specifically refer to children and young people. But since the rights of everyone within the jurisdiction must be guaranteed (Article 1) and (Article 14) respected without discrimination on any ground, including sex, race, colour, religion, opinion, origin, property and birth 'or other status', this implicitly covers childhood (*Nielsen v Denmark* 1998 11 EHRR 175).

It is important to remember that children and young people have a right to be considered as separate individuals, and to be consulted if of sufficient age and understanding, regardless of whether they are living with their own families or not. Indeed, most of the new guidance referred to in this chapter takes this approach to the position of children and young people.

The Human Rights Act

Threat or opportunity?

Much of what the Act says should come as no surprise, despite the media's predictions of the courts being swamped with wild challenges, sweeping changes in the law and a new era of judicial power. As John Wadham of Liberty said in 2001, 'the doom-merchants have been proved wrong. Cases have been few and judges cautious.'

As a signatory to the Convention since 1951, the UK's expectation is that legislation and best practice already respects the Convention: as the Health Service Circular, HSC 2000/025 put it:

> The Human Rights Act is an opportunity to build on this in a way that respects fairness and dignity of the individual... Health authorities, NHS Trusts and Social Services Departments should actively develop existing good practice in a manner suited to the new human rights culture, linking as appropriate to the equality and race-relations agenda.

Wholesale, sweeping changes to our laws, professional policies and procedures are unlikely in the immediate future. Lawyers have been warned by the judiciary to be responsible when raising human rights arguments. This is not to diminish its importance: the Act affects almost every aspect of the business of public authorities and professionals must absorb its impact throughout their practice.

Any rise in claims (whether successful or not) in an increasingly litigious society may not be welcome to already overstretched professionals and legal budgets. European experience, however, suggests that Convention rights have not resulted in the destruction or undermining of good practice: according to a study by Markesinis 'the potential of civil liability has not made continental police, local authorities or social security agencies less prompt, less efficient or less effective' (Markesinis et al., 1999).

In a climate of growing scrutiny of health, social and education service delivery and decision-making processes, however, the number of test cases seems likely to rise, especially in a climate of resource constraints. Of late, the courts have become more critical of policies concerning priorities: now they must be sure all the relevant evidence has been considered and given proper weight. This sits well with their new powers under the Act, where they must assess not only the *reasonableness* of the authority's decision, but also the Convention rights of the individual.

How does it affect clinical governance?

Department of Health Circulars in 2000 required the NHS and local authorities to ensure that all staff (including contractors and independent or private providers of their public services) were made aware of the duty placed on public authorities by the Act, and all local policies, operational procedures and practices continued to be compatible with the Convention.

All senior managers must demonstrate that organizational policies, procedures and decision-making show regard for, and take account of, the Act. Decision-making, in individual cases and especially in the making of policies, must be transparent and show consideration for Convention rights has been given at all levels.

Implementing the Act

Potential areas requiring action should already have been identified, especially where important policy or operational considerations are at stake. The NHS's guidance suggests that where there are *significant* operational or policy implications, it is probably better to wait for a court case to argue the issues rather than making hasty and unnecessarily elaborate policy changes (my emphasis). The NHS Litigation Authority has also issued guidance.

In any event, proactively building on existing good practice and procedures, and using these to resolve difficulties, is obviously preferable to risking valuable resources on fighting rearguard actions against costly legal challenges. Challenges should be seen not as obstacles to practice but opportunities to learn: monitoring and evaluation are essential in order to identify and urgently address bad practice.

The Act has contributed to an emphasis on conducting early investigation into disputes, early resolution, and, in consequence, significant financial benefits, including savings on legal budgets, as well as advantages for public and staff relations. Litigation should be the last resort: speedier resolution of disputes and the use of alternative dispute resolution are all being actively promoted by the civil courts. There is also a new Pre-Action Protocol for the Resolution of Clinical Disputes, which contains a sequence of steps for patients and healthcare providers to follow when a dispute arises. Many NHS trusts are changing claims management practices to meet these requirements and those that have not yet done so have seen increases in legal costs.

The Act and the courts

The Convention's provisions now apply in proceedings, and the relevant ECtHR case law must be followed. If there is a conflict between the Convention and UK law, the court must have regard to the Convention. Other conventions to which the UK has signed up, such as the UN Convention on Human Rights, can also lend force to legal arguments because the ECtHR has cited some of these with approval. The House of Lords and Court of Appeal have also referred to decisions in other jurisdictions such as Australia and New Zealand, so the legal picture is a complicated one.

Judges can review legislation and, if appropriate, declare it incompatible with Convention rights. But they cannot amend the law. The House of Lords has stressed that it is up to Parliament to change the law, not the judges (see *Re S (Care Order: Implementation of Care Plan); Re W (Minors) (Care Order: Adequacy of Care Plan)* [2002] 1 FLR 815). Parliament is not bound to amend the law, but in most cases it will do so: notably, the Lord Chancellor has said adverse decisions should be seen as opportunities to enhance the protection of rights in the UK.

To whom does the Act apply?

The Act applies to 'public' authorities, i.e. bodies that undertake functions of a public nature, including:

* central government departments, local authorities and the courts;
* National Health Service Trusts and local authorities, including social services – even when they contract private or voluntary bodies to provide the treatment or care;
* primary care trusts, dentists, opticians and pharmacists when undertaking NHS work, general practitioners;
* bodies running nursing and residential homes, and schools;
* a body that has functions of a public nature (for example, a professional regulatory body), even if it also has private functions.

A body with both public and private functions will be a public authority only in relation to its public functions. So, when private health or social care sector bodies contract to provide care for the NHS, they will be public authorities for that purpose. If there is any doubt, advice should be sought as there are some recent cases on the point

Individuals can also exercise public functions: for example, by virtue of their NHS or social care functions. General practitioners are likely to be public authorities, especially as there is an increasingly close relationship created by personal medical services contracts. Other professionals with personal responsibility to act in an official capacity in respect of their judgements about individuals and in their duty to the courts, such as approved social workers appointed under the Mental Health Act, and children's guardians appointed under the Children Act 1989 in care proceedings (even if self-employed) will be in this category.

Who can bring proceedings and when?

Only victims – those 'directly affected by the act in question' – can do so. Alternatively, where a victim dies or lacks capacity to bring a case (for example, a child), relatives can bring proceedings on their behalf. Proceedings must normally be brought within 1 year of the act complained of, but a court has discretion to extend this. Claims can also be made within other legal proceedings, and the periods normally relevant to those will apply.

Children and young people

Children have a right to respect for their private and family life in their own right. The ECtHR has said that consideration of what is in the best interests of the child is in every case of crucial importance and has made it clear that the best interests of the child can be the 'overriding requirement'.

For example, it is a long-established principle in ECtHR case law that where there is conflict between the rights of a parent and a child, which can only be resolved in favour of one of them, then the child's interests and rights must prevail under Article 8(2).

The ECtHR has also attached considerable weight to the UN Convention on the Rights of the Child (the 'UN Convention'). This provides an almost universally accepted code of children's rights from which guidance may be sought where gaps are identified in the European Convention. The following articles are particularly relevant:

- Article 3(1): 'in all actions concerning children, whether undertaken by public or private social welfare institutions, courts of law, administrative authorities or legislative bodies, the best interests of the child shall be a primary consideration'.
- Article 19: requires states to take all appropriate measures 'to protect the child from all forms of physical and mental violence, injury or abuse'.

These principles have been followed in the UK courts, including a recent judgement that the Children Act 1989 applies to children and young people in young offender institutions.

Some key Convention Articles

Article 2: preserves the right to life

This is not about a right to treatment, but is relevant to:

- life saving operations and end-of-life decisions;
- decisions about access to and withdrawal of treatment;

- investigation of suspicious deaths during medical procedures or whilst under care;
- failure to offer proper supervision to a mentally vulnerable patient at risk of committing suicide.

Article 3: prohibits torture or inhuman or degrading treatment or punishment

In health and/or social care, medical or clinical treatment issues and conditions in hospitals or care homes may be relevant, provided there is a minimum level of severity in the alleged breach. The Council of Europe is currently conducting a consultation exercise on the future treatment of mental patients subject to involuntary placement or treatment with this Article in mind.

Restraint techniques used on people who present challenging behaviour may be necessary for their safety and the safety of others, but these have been open to challenge and some new guidance has appeared as a result of the Act. The Mental Health Act is also undergoing revision.

The failure of agencies to take appropriate action to address severe neglect and abuse can also invoke this Article, starkly demonstrated by the case of *Z v UK* [2001] 2 FLR 612, in which the ECtHR also cited Article 19 with approval. Four children suffered for a long period of years, during which the local authority took no effective action. It was held to have failed in its positive obligation to protect the children from inhuman and degrading treatment and damages of £350,000 were awarded.

Article 5: guarantees the right to liberty and security

Detention for the purposes of medical treatment must be carried out in a way that is compatible with this Article and there have been a number of mental health cases, most notably *Stanley Johnson v The United Kingdom* [1997] (1999) 27 EHRR 296. The UK was found to be in breach because the patient's discharge was delayed for a long time due to the inability of the responsible social services authority to find suitable supervised hostel accommodation and the Mental Health Review Tribunal lacked the power to ensure that the discharge conditions were met within a reasonable time.

Detaining a child or young person in secure accommodation will not be a breach, provided the correct legal procedures are followed and the child's right to a fair trial under Article 6 is adhered to. According to *Bouamar v Belgium* (1988) 11 EHRR 1, a failure to provide a detained child with education will not be a breach of this Article.

Article 6: guarantees the right to a fair and public hearing within a reasonable time by an independent and impartial tribunal

This is a 'limited' right, which means breach is only justifiable in certain defined circumstances. Procedural fairness, full disclosure of relevant documents in proceedings, and the hearing of cases within a reasonable time, are all relevant issues:

- in *Darnell v United Kingdom* [1994] 18 EHRR 205, the UK conceded that a delay of 9 years in resolving whether a dismissal from a Regional Health Authority was fair or not was a violation;
- the independence and impartiality of professional conduct bodies responsible for disciplinary issues has been raised in EctHR cases involving the UK;
- the right of mental patients to have the lawfulness of their detention reviewed speedily has been the subject of recent ECtHR litigation.

Article 8: gives everyone the right to respect for his or her private and family life, home and correspondence

This has potentially wide-ranging application to a number of areas of practice, including patient confidentiality and consent to treatment.

'Family life' is widely defined, based on close personal ties. In *R(L) v Secretary of State for Health* [2001] 1 FLR 406, it was said to be an elastic concept, immediately obvious in some cases, but not in others! Depending on the circumstances, it encompasses:

- Unmarried parents even if no longer living together, or never having done so. It is not clear whether the father of a child born as the result of a casual encounter could rely on this.
- A baby and his extended family, even if they do not know of the child's existence.
- An uncle and nephew.
- A grandparent and grandchild.
- Other *de facto* relationships not dependent upon marriage, for example foster parents.

'Private life, home and correspondence' includes medical records and methods of recording patient information. There is now a plethora of law and guidance in this area. For example, under the Regulation of Investigatory Powers Act 2000, covert surveillance in clinical situations must be carried out by the police.

Article 9: preserves the right to freedom of thought, conscience and religion

This is relevant to treatment issues such as blood transfusions for Jehovah's Witnesses, or emergency surgery. For example, it has been held lawful for doctors to carry out an emergency Caesarean despite objections by the mother on religious grounds. However, it is not likely to result in the ability to deny medical care to a child, although, in some circumstances, this can be an area fraught with complications, and legal advice should always be sought.

Article 12: confers the right to marry and have a family

This is unlikely to enable an individual to insist on fertility treatment or artificial insemination, but adoption falls within the scope of this article.

Interpretation of the Convention

Convention rights may be absolute, limited or qualified. Many are not absolute rights – a breach is permissible if it is:

- in accordance with the national laws of the country; or
- necessary in the interests of national security, public safety or the economic wellbeing of the country; or
- for the prevention of crime or disorder; or
- for the protection of health or morals; or
- to protect the freedom and rights of others.

For example, Articles 8 to 10 are 'qualified' rights, which means they must be balanced against the wider public interest. A breach is justified if the interference complained of is *lawful,* in pursuance of a *legitimate aim, necessary in a democratic society* and *proportionate.*

The ECtHR's interpretation is evolving all the time, but it seeks to guarantee practical and effective rights based on the following principles:

Proportionality recognizes that rights may conflict with each other. For example:

- A duty of confidentiality may conflict with the prevention of crime or the protection of the health of others.
- Intervention by the state in family life is a breach of Article 8 but may be proportionate when balanced against the welfare of the child (*L v Finland* 2 FLR 118 ECHR). Action must be a proportionate response to the nature and gravity of the feared harm. Emergency measures should

only be taken where there is an immediate risk of significant harm to that child. Alternative options should be explored with the principle of reunification of child and family firmly in mind (*Re C and B (Care Order: Future Harm)* [2001] 1 FLR 611).

- Prohibiting information about abortion in order to protect morals was disproportionate to the end to be achieved because it was framed in absolute terms (*Open Door Counselling and Well Women v Ireland* [1993] 15 EHRR 244).

The margin of appreciation recognizes that there may be reasonable differences about the identification of priorities, responses and resources. In matters of social and economic policy, a generous margin of discretion is permitted and many cases on health policy and issues of resource allocation have failed because of the ECtHR's view that, as a general rule, it should be slow to interfere in such matters.

As the Open Door Counselling case made clear, however, when a fundamental human right is in issue, the margin may narrow because the courts will subject the lawfulness of the decision to even closer scrutiny. In judging whether the margin has been exceeded, the more substantial the interference with human rights, the more justification will be required by the court before it is satisfied that the decision is reasonable.

Discrimination

Article 14 requires all Convention rights to be respected without discrimination – but this is not a stand-alone right; it must be used in conjunction with other Articles.

ECtHR case law suggests objective and reasonably justified distinctions do not amount to discrimination but, as the ECtHR is not bound by previous judgements, there may be further developments, particularly with regard to treatment decisions and resource considerations.

Discrimination must be a central consideration for those providing health and social care and education: there is now a raft of legislation promoting the rights of the disabled and those with special educational needs to access appropriate services. Professionals should be mindful of the work of bodies such as the Disability Rights Commission, the Equal Opportunities Commission and the Commission for Racial Equality.

Compensation

Damages for breaches of Convention rights can be awarded but in calculating these, account must be taken of the principles of fairness and equity applied by the ECtHR. There have been some high awards in recent child abuse cases, in contrast to the level of previous awards, so professionals should be aware of the financial risk involved in decision-making that is not based firmly on good practice, sound research and clear information.

Other legislation, guidance and policy measures

The government's aim of transforming NHS and social care emphasizes putting patients and clients first as well as effective communication with the public, staff and other organizations. Performance data and an emphasis on greater levels of transparency have increased the availability of information to the public and impacted on clinical governance.

But many of the measures have been a response to rights issues, as well as to concern about the quality and standards of public services. It is arguable that, in addressing rights issues in disputes about quality of services, the onus will be on authorities to demonstrate what steps have been taken in compliance with the Act and these new measures, for example:

- the Health Act 1999, and accompanying guidance, which gives new powers to achieve effective joint working between health and local authorities;
- the Care Standards Act 2000;
- the Quality Protects, Social Care Quality, Integrated Children's Services and other initiatives;
- the consent to treatment guidance, and accompanying patient information, applicable from 1 April 2002;
- the Framework for the Assessment of Children in Need and their Families (DoH 2001), which is being used by a wider group of professionals rather than just social workers;
- the guidance on the approach to be used in interviewing children and vulnerable adults set out in Achieving Best Evidence (DoH, 2002)
- policy and good practice guidance in the provision of mental health services.
- the recommendations adopted from the report of the Laming inquiry into the death of Victoria Climbié (it should be noted that the Social Services Inspectorate intend to issue a document in 2003 summarizing the existing key requirements in child protection).

A wealth of recent legislation and guidance, informed by human rights principles, is likely to affect evidence-based practice and a number of new regulatory and other bodies are now responsible for, or influential in, the setting and monitoring of standards. These include the National Institute for Clinical Excellence (NICE), and its parallel in the social care field, the Social Care Institute for Excellence (SCIE), the Care

Standards Commission and the National Institute for Mental Health in
England (NIMHE). A comprehensive range of information and level of
awareness is now required to meet professional standards of good
practice.

Multi-agency policies and procedures have long applied to child protection and, since March 2000 now apply to the protection of vulnerable
adults from abuse (HSC 2000/007). However, there is an increased
emphasis on this approach in other areas, and for clinical practice, a good
example is the way in which cross-cutting key standards have been set
for Child and Adolescent Mental Health services (CAMH), due to be
introduced in a couple of years. These include a requirement for written
policies on:

- *child protection* guidance, based on Working Together 1999 and related addenda for particular professionals such as doctors, Senior Nurses,
  Health Visitors and Midwives and their Managers (DoH 1997), as well
  as on arrangements between the NHS and other agencies;
- *restriction of liberty,* based on the MHA Code of Practice 1983 and the
  Children Act 1989 guidance on secure accommodation;
- *education of inpatient children* and liaison arrangements for this in
  line with the Education Act 1996;
- *consent of children to treatment* and arrangements to ensure valid
  consent is obtained. This should include the possibility for older children and adolescents to refuse treatment and have their concerns
  heard, and, if refusal is to be overruled, a clear statement that consideration of the issues must be governed by the principle that the welfare
  of the child or young person is paramount.

Better coordination of services is also the aim of the Health Act 1999
Partnership Arrangements, which give permissive powers to secure services across a wide range of NHS and local authority functions.

Finally, professional guidance from the General Medical Council (the
'GMC') and the Royal Colleges is of increasing relevance in judging
whether a public body, or an individual professional, has conducted itself
not only lawfully, but also reasonably. These include specific advice on
good medical and paediatric practice, confidentiality, consent and managing choice.

Key areas to consider

Convention rights affect patient/client, inter-professional and inter-agency
relationships in a number of different and inter-related ways. Two of the
most important topics, confidentiality and consent, are particularly

complex, and often interlinked, areas of law, which have been the subject of much litigation and debate. Changes to the law on access to information by individuals and the public, and comprehensive guidance on consent issues, have all been introduced in the light of the Act.

In a climate of clinical governance, increased regulation and guidance, as well as scarce resources, the Act may also affect service delivery and issues of availability, choice and standards of practice.

Confidentiality

The protection of personal data, not least medical data, is a fundamentally important concept. The confidentiality of health data is a vital principle in all the legal systems of the member states and it is seen as crucial not only to respect the sense of privacy of a patient but also to preserve his or her confidence in the medical profession and in the health services in general.

The impact of the Act depends on the type of information, the context in which it is obtained, and whether there are competing rights to be considered. A failure to keep confidential information gained in the course of the professional relationship with the patient/client in the absence of consent to disclose is, on the face of it, a breach of Article 8. But in certain circumstances, despite the importance of this professional duty, disclosure of personal sensitive information may be permissible, legitimately requested by third parties, or deemed necessary by statutory or professional requirements.

Professionals may encounter a number of situations that raise issues about disclosure of personal information to third parties. Confidentiality also encompasses concepts such as legal professional privilege, litigation privilege and public interest immunity, many of which concern the duties of disclosure in court proceedings. These are complex areas that a single chapter cannot cover and specialist legal advice should be sought.

Guidance from the GMC makes it clear that if a doctor is asked to provide information about patients, s/he should seek the patient's consent and anonymize data where possible, keep disclosures to the minimum, and be prepared to justify their decision in accordance with the guidance. The capacity to give consent should be judged according to the usual principles.

Sharing patient identifiable information with third parties

The duty of confidentiality may be overridden by a public interest in disclosure, for instance where the benefits to an individual, or to society, outweigh the public's, and the client's, interest in keeping the information confidential. Guidance from professional bodies such as the GMC and others makes it clear that disclosure may be made in the patient's medical interests (for example, where s/he is, or may be, a victim of abuse or neglect), or in the interests of others where a failure to disclose information may expose the patient, or others, to risk of death or serious harm.

Therefore, it may not be possible to guarantee confidentiality, particularly in relation to some categories of information. For example:

- Where it is necessary to protect the safety of others, and the danger is sufficiently grave and real to justify it. For example, in *W v Edgell* [1990] 4 BMLR 96 it was held that a psychiatrist had a duty to disclose information that a patient continued to present danger to society.
- The Children Act imposes duties on agencies to share information on children in need (s.27) and in child protection investigations (s.47): further statutory guidance in *Working Together 1999* sets out how such inter-agency work should be conducted. It is clear from research (Falkov, 1995) that a failure of cooperation and information-sharing between adult psychiatrists and child protection professionals has contributed to death or abuse of children. Professionals involved in care proceedings should note that there is a duty of full and frank disclosure of any relevant information held on children and their families, subject to rules on public interest immunity and data protection and legal advice should always be sought in such circumstances.
- The question of whether confidential information about a person thought to be a risk to children can be shared with other agencies outside a local area has been the subject of test cases recently. A local authority is entitled to share information about allegations with others, including parents, where there is a 'pressing need' to do so for the protection of children, and may do so across geographical boundaries. The position of other agencies is less clear. There has to be a particularly careful balancing act between the public interest in the protection of children against the individual's right to a private life, but the first principle should always be the necessary protection of the child: *Working Together 1999* emphasizes proactive sharing of information.
- Breaches of Article 8 are permissible in accordance with the law and if necessary in a democratic society in interests of, for example, public safety, the prevention of disorder or crime, or for the protection of health or morals, or the rights and freedom of others. Disclosure of medical records by one public body to another has been held not to be a breach (see *M & S v Sweden* 1997). Someone who presents a grave risk may fall into the category covered by *W v Edgell* referred to above.
- In view of the highly intimate and sensitive nature of information concerning a person's HIV status, any safeguards designed to effectively

protect information about it or measures compelling communication or disclosure of such information without the consent of the patient will be careful scrutinised by the courts. In the case of *Z v Finland* (1997) 25 EHRR 371, the ECtHR accepted that the interests of a patient and the community as a whole in protecting the confidentiality of medical data may be outweighed by the interest in investigation and prosecution of crime and in the publicity of court proceedings.

• The Health Service (Control of Patient Information) Regulations 2002 also allow information to be shared with certain bodies undertaking health and disease surveillance or for the 'control and prevention of communicable disease and other risks to public health' .

Management of, and access to, patient information

The Human Rights Act has had a considerable impact on the individual's right of access to information. Legislation includes the Access to Health Records Act 1990 (AHRA 1990); the Education (School Records) Regulations 1989; the Data Protection Act 1998 (DPA 1998) and the Freedom of Information Act 2000 (FOIA 2000).

As neither the FOIA 2000 nor the DPA 1998 has yet been fully implemented, the current legal position is in a state of flux. Practitioners do need to be aware of when and how any exemptions apply, and how best they can be used to balance the need to guarantee the right to know against the right to be protected. Weighing up the respective welfare and rights issues is no mean feat and professionals need to apply a combination of principles and good practice in the context of legal requirements and appropriate legal and professional advice.

The Data Protection Act 1998 is the key legislation covering all aspects of information processing, including security and confidentiality of personally identifiable information. It provides safeguards for the processing of personal data, but does not of itself prevent NHS bodies from using personal data for legitimate medical purposes, including the management of healthcare services. The Freedom of Information Act will introduce a comprehensive right of access to information held by a public body and any application for personal information under such provisions will be treated as an application under the Data Protection Act.

Professionals need to refer to HSC 2000/009, *The Protection and Use of Patient Information*, for full guidance. There is also a quantity of useful information on this subject on the departmental Web site, www.doh.gov.uk/ipu/confiden.

Following the 1997 Caldicott review, a framework should now be in place for the management of confidentiality and access to personal information. By 1 April 2002 there should have been a 'Caldicott Guardian' appointed in all health and social services bodies 'to safeguard and govern the uses made of confidential information within NHS organisations' (HSC 2002/003) and 'in order to provide a good foundation for joint working between health and social services, and to help support the fulfilment of the many joint strategies across children's and adult services.'

Professionals should also follow the recent General Medical Council (GMC) guidance on using visual and audio recordings of patients, as well as the guidance from the Department of Health included in the Model Policy for Consent 2001.

Withholding information

Article 8(2) provides for restrictions allowing for the withholding of information where there is a demonstrable clear and immediate need to do so. Therefore, there are exemptions in the various statutes above which entitle a doctor, for example, to withhold disclosure where he or she believes:

* it would cause serious harm to the mental health of the patient or any other person;
* access would disclose information relating to or provided by a third person who had not consented to that disclosure.

The courts have not yet fully explored the precise extent of this 'therapeutic privilege'.

Sharing information with a patient/client

A failure to inform someone of a serious risk involved in treatment may be a breach: as the Court of Appeal said in *Pearce v United Bristol NHS Healthcare Trust* [1999] 48 BMLR 118, 'if there is a significant risk which would affect the judgement of a reasonable patient, then in the normal course it is the responsibility of a doctor to inform the patient . . . if the information is needed so that the patient can determine for him or herself what course he or she should adopt.' Patients are entitled to have any information they ask for, or need to know, about their condition, subject to the provisions on withholding of information referred to above. It is not clear whether this imposes an obligation to notify a patient's relatives or others who may be at risk.

What is not yet clear is whether there is a clear legal right to be told how and why treatment has gone wrong, although the 2001 GMC Good Medical Practice guide advises full explanations and an apology where appropriate. Patients may now have enhanced rights if given incorrect information, so it is advisable to review checks, safeguards and quality governance against best practice.

Patient identifiable information for research purposes

If consent cannot be obtained, and there is no other reasonably practicable way of disclosing the information legally, the procedure under s.60 of the Health and Social Care Act 2001 should be used. This enables the Secretary of State to support and regulate the use of confidential patient information in the interest of patients or the wider public good. The Department of Health Web site, www.doh.gov.uk, gives full details of this process.

The freedom of the press

The right of the press to inform the public and the right of the public to be informed have long been recognised, and the ECtHR has rarely held that interference with media freedom is justified under Article 10.2. But a balancing exercise is required between competing rights under Article 10 and the right of individuals to privacy under Article 8. This has been well illustrated in a variety of cases brought by celebrities, such as *Campbell* v *Mirror Group Newspapers*. However these should be compared with the approach used in cases involving public health issues: for example, in proceedings brought by an HIV positive healthcare worker for an injunction restraining a health authority from taking steps to reveal his identity, a newspaper was prevented from naming him.

Consent

This area has also been heavily influenced by human rights principles. It is obviously one of the most important issues in the relationship with a patient or client, not least because, without it, practitioners may lay themselves open to legal and/or disciplinary action. The factors involved have given rise to a number of difficult decisions for both practitioners and the courts and, like confidentiality, detailed specialist advice and guidance should always be readily available to professionals.

The Department of Health (DH) has now issued a range of guidance documents on consent, and it is extremely important that current policies on ethics and consent are reviewed in the light of these. These helpful documents include:

- a model consent policy;
- guides on seeking consent, which include sample consent forms, and cover particular groups of patients, including specific guidance on people with learning disabilities and on children;
- a reference guide giving a detailed summary of the relevant case law and the guidance issued by regulatory bodies;
- an aide-memoire for clinicians entitled '12 key points on consent'.

All of these documents are available on the Department's Web site at www.doh.gov.uk.

There is also a large quantity of case law, as well as various guidelines available from other professional bodies such as the Law Society, which are of assistance. Choice and the involvement of the patient/client in decision-making can prove very challenging in certain circumstances, even for experienced professionals and they need to be clear about the principles governing assessment of an individual's capacity to consent, and the consequences that flow from capacity or lack of it.

Articles 2, 3, 5, 8 and 9, with consideration of Article 13, may all be relevant. Article 8(2) allows interference with rights 'for the protection of health', but permits adults to refuse life-saving treatment. Legally, competent adults are entitled to decide for themselves what will happen to them, however irrational or unreasonable their decision may be, and therefore they have the right to consent to or refuse treatment. Notably, the general legal principles were restated recently by the President of the Family Division in *Re B (Consent to Treatment: Capacity)* Times Law Reports 26 March 2002, with some additional guidance.

Patients without capacity must have decisions taken in their best interests. The simple fact that someone is suffering from a mental condition does not render him or her incompetent, because he or she may be able to give informed consent to a variety of treatments. For example, an informed decision to cease taking medication for a mental health problem, even though this may increase the risk of a relapse, can be viewed as a rational decision. This is not the easiest of areas, and is best summed up by the principle that an informed decision not to accept psychiatric treatment does not itself indicate a lack of insight, but a lack of insight can mean that such a decision is not properly informed.

The document '12 key points for Health Professionals' (DoH, 2002) recommends the following:

- Obtain consent before examining, treating or caring for competent adult patients.

- Assume an adult is competent unless demonstrated otherwise. In the case of doubt, asking: 'can this patient understand and weigh up the information needed to make this decision?' Unexpected decisions do not prove the patient is incompetent, but may indicate a need for further information or explanation.
- Patients may be competent to make some healthcare decisions, even if they are not competent to make others.
- Giving and obtaining consent is usually a process, not a one-off event. Patients can change their minds and withdraw consent at any time. If there is any doubt, always check that the patient still consents to you caring for or treating him or her.

Children and young people

Particular care needs to be taken in the process of assessment in cases involving children and young people. The principles for adults and children are similar, but separate considerations apply to children.

Section 8 of the Family Law Reform Act 1969 gave minors aged 16 a right to consent to surgical, medical or dental treatment. The wishes and feelings of the child have assumed increasing importance since the case of *Gillick v West Norfolk and Wisbech Area Health Authority* [1986] 1 AC 112 and professionals need to know the principles governing assessment of capacity in this context. In brief, a child with sufficient maturity and understanding can consent to treatment. The child must understand the risk, benefits and consequences of non-treatment and must not make a decision under duress. Variations in developmental rates and levels of comprehension between one child and another, and the type of treatment, are also relevant factors. As long as they are competent with respect to the particular procedure proposed, they are entitled to information and the right to consent. Gillick competence allows the child to say 'this is what I want, ignore my parents/carers' and to have their wishes followed, provided these are in line with the relevant legislation and case law.

But in certain circumstances the courts have overridden the right of a Gillick competent child to refuse treatment, usually in cases where the child's life or long-term health is regarded as being seriously under threat. Although it is the court's duty to listen to the wishes of a child, it is not restricted by them and will disregard them if the child's welfare appears to diverge from those wishes. A good example of this is in relation to eating disorders: in *Re W (a minor): Medical treatment* [1992] 4 All ER 627, the Court of Appeal ordered treatment to take place in the 'best interests' of a 16-year-old.

Parents retain rights to lawfully consent on behalf of their children, even if the child refuses, and treatment may be ordered in the child's 'best interests'. This principle extends to local authorities in respect of looked-after children and young people. In *Re C (HIV test)* [1999] 50 BMLR 283, the decision of a local authority to admit a 12-year-old in its care to hospital for a psychiatric assessment was upheld: the authority was entitled to conclude that she was not 'Gillick competent' and therefore to consent to her admission on her behalf.

In extreme cases, where the child is threatened by a serious and imminent risk of grave and irreversible mental or physical harm, the court has a duty to intervene. Whether the Convention now gives children and young people greater rights in this respect, even when the risk is grave and irreversible, is not clear, although it is likely that the court will need to consider the situation as particularly serious before overriding the child's wishes.

There are of course, other, less dramatic ways in which children and young people can express their views and make choices, which the court may well endorse. A child may exercise a right of veto, to refuse to be involved in a certain course of action proposed. For example, in *Re P (A Minor) (Education)* [1992] 1 FLR 316, the Court of Appeal held that where a 14-year-old boy had formed a strong view that he wished to attend a particular day school (rather than his previous boarding school) and live with his father, his wish should be listened to and proper regard should be paid to it.

Access to services and resource allocation

By Article 1 of the ECHR, states have a duty to provide adequate resources to carry out their obligations. Rationing complaints based on the National Health Service Act 1977 have had poor prospects of success and several cases prior to the Act endorsed the failure of health authorities to provide care on 'resource' grounds. This was because statutes are often imprecisely drafted, the burden of proof on the claimant is heavy, and, because Parliament is supreme, extensive powers could be given to public authorities in contravention of the Convention in any case.

The Act has not changed this position. A person cannot compel the NHS to give him treatment or an operation except through the courts. It is not possible to predict whether challenges to treatment refusals may be successful where they would not have been before but, in cases where resources are an issue, it is unlikely the courts will adopt a very different approach than in past cases involving refusals of treatment.

As already discussed, the margin of appreciation given to contracting states in creating domestic policy, and policies about the level of funding for public services are regarded by the ECtHR as a particularly sensitive area. Unless the circumstances are exceptional, it will be slow to interfere to impose funding obligations that cannot be applied consistently throughout Europe because of different levels of economic prosperity in member states.

Nevertheless, the courts are becoming more critical of health authorities' policies concerning priorities. The Act requires the courts to assess not only the *reasonableness* of the authority's decision, but also the rights of the patient under the Convention. The primary question now is not whether an authority's decision is reasonable, but whether the court can be sure all the relevant evidence has been considered and given proper weight.

The past refusal of the courts to influence the decisions of health authorities on the grounds that they know best how to manage and make use of finite resources may be subject to greater analysis in future.

Discrimination frequently occurs in healthcare in the sense of excluding certain categories of patients from treatment for the purpose of, for example, diverting scarce resources to the least healthy sections of society. Different health authorities are permitted considerable discretion in choosing how to allocate their resources, but discrimination in treatment decisions may give rise to complaints under Article 14. This forbids discrimination that has no legitimate basis and policies that differentiate between people especially where they are based on personal prejudice. However, some forms of discrimination with a legitimate aim and effect are permitted, as long as they are proportionate to the objective sought. There are, as yet, no cases in the healthcare context to give any clues as to how these concepts might be defined. If objective and reasonably justified distinctions do not constitute discrimination for the purposes of Article 14, discrimination on grounds of resources may be lawful, if the reasons are logical and defensible, rather than, for example, arbitrary and irrational.

Again, guidance may prove relevant in assessing whether a decision not to supply a service is reasonable, or even in respect of whether a long delay in treatment to the substantial detriment of an individual patient is justified. Breaches of Article 8 as the result of delays in treatment were claimed in one European Commission case, but the applicant's condition (severe migraine) was not regarded as serious enough to warrant the intervention of the court. However, the Commission did say 'where the State has an obligation to provide medical care, an excessive delay of the public health service in providing a medical service to which the patient is entitled and the fact that such delay has, or is likely to have, a serious impact on the patient's health could raise an issue under Article 8' (*Passanante v Italy* appl. 32647/96).

An example of how clinical governance issues may provide evidence for judging services in future can be seen in the provision of mental health services to people with severe mental health problems and problematic substance misuse. Service models for dual diagnosis are at an early stage of development. However, as stated in the document *Dual Diagnosis: A Good Practice Guide*:

> . . . policy and good practice in the provision of mental health services to people with severe mental health problems and problematic substance misuse. Individuals with these dual problems deserve high quality, patient focused and integrated care. *This should be delivered within mental health services* . . . Patients should not be shunted between different sets of services or put at risk of dropping out of care completely.

This 'mainstreaming' protocol concerned with clinical governance guidelines and good practice in relation to assessment and treatment, advises that 'all mental health provider agencies should designate a lead clinician for dual diagnosis issues and all health and social care economies should designate a lead commissioner'.

Where an individual is refused particular treatment, there is a potential breach of Article 2, but steps can be taken to safeguard a patient's rights by offering an alternative treatment. Refusal to allocate resources to a particular category of patient will require clear, robust and transparent decision-making procedures that make decisions objectively justifiable and have regard to the Convention, that record discussions and conclusions and are supported by detailed financial evidence.

Standards of practice

Much of what has been said already will also be relevant to general questions of practice and procedure but some specific points need to be noted. The Convention itself does not make any specific reference to standards of care, but according to *Tanko v Finland* appl. 23634/94 (unreported) a lack of proper care in a case where someone is suffering from a serious illness could amount to treatment contrary to Article 3. It would probably be necessary to show severe, rather than merely negligent, circumstances and substandard, possibly reckless, treatment over a long period of time.

Clinical governance, the publication of medical performance data and the duty imposed by the Health Act 1999 to monitor and supervise performance are all relevant considerations here. It is conceivable that, for example, a claim for a breach of Article 3 might arise where standards are known to be poor.

A good example of the way in which human rights principles can affect practice is the new guidance from the Department of Health in July 2002 on physical intervention with people with a learning disability and autistic spectrum disorder in health, education and social care settings. This was prepared in the context of the Act and the UN Convention on the Rights of the Child and states that it

> is based on the presumption that every adult and child is entitled to:
> * respect for his/her private life;
> * the right not to be subjected to inhuman or degrading treatment;
> * the right to liberty and security; and
> * the right not to be discriminated against in his/her enjoyment of those rights.

Associated guidance also exists on the care of adults with learning disability and/or autism in the Circular 'No Secrets' and in the report of the Task Force on Violence Against Social Care Staff, 'A Safer Place: Combating Violence Against Social Care Staff'. As previously noted, the Mental Health Act 1983 is currently under review and its associated Code of Practice provides relevant guidance in respect of people who have been detained.

Conclusion

The Act strengthens the application of Convention rights, which may give rise to a new source of legal argument in future cases. Its impact can already be seen in the courts' approach: they are increasingly concerned to be sure, not just that the public authority's final decision is defensible, but that the process of decision-making is logical and sound in the context of a range of rights. Provided the right measures are in place for policies and procedures, which give proper consideration to the Convention, practitioners need not fear the Human Rights Act, but rather welcome it as a long overdue reinforcement of good practice.

Further reading

Goldthorpe L, Monro P (2001) The Human Rights Act 1998. A Practitioners Guide. London: Association of Lawyers for Children

Kilkelly U (1999) The Child and the European Convention on Human Rights. London: Ashgate.

Lilley R, Lambden P, Newdick C (2001), Understanding the Human Rights Act – A Tool Kit for the Health Service. Abingdon: Radcliffe Medical Press.

Starmer K (1999) European Human Rights Law. London: LAG Education and Service Trust.

Swindells H, Neaves A, Kushner M, Skillbeck R (1999) Family Law and the Human Rights Act 1998. Bristol: Jordans Family Law.

Official publications

www.cabinet-office.gov.uk
www.opengov.uk/hmso/stationery office

References

Clinical Disputes Forum (1998) The Pre-Action Protocol for the Resolution of Clinical Disputes. London: Department of Health.

Council of Europe (2000) White Paper on the protection of the human rights and dignity of people suffering from mental disorder CM(2000)23. Strasbourg: Council of Europe

Department of Health (1991) The Children Act Guidance and Regulations. London: The Stationery Office

Department of Health (1993) Code of Practice: Mental Health Act 1983. London: Department of Health, Welsh Office.

Department of Health (1995) Mental Health Act 1983. Memorandum on Parts I to VI, VIII and X. London: Department of Health.

Department of Health (1997) Child Protection. Guidance for Senior Nurses, Health Visitors and Midwives and their Managers. 3 edn. London: The Stationery Office.

Department of Health (1999) Drug Misuse and Dependence: Guidelines on Clinical Management. London: The Stationery Office.

Department of Health (1999) The National Service Framework for Mental Health. London: Department of Health.

Department of Health (1999) Working Together to Safeguard Children. London: Department of Health.

Department of Health (2000) 'No Secrets': Guidance on Developing Multi-Agency Policies and Procedures to Protect Vulnerable Adults from Abuse. Circular HSC 2000/07, LAC (2000)7. London: Department of Health.

Department of Health (2000) After-Care under the Mental Health Act 1983 Circular HSC 2000/003: LAC (2000)3. London: Department of Health.

Department of Health (2000) Data Protection Act 1998: Protection and Use of Patient Information. Circular HSC 2000/009. London: NHS Executive.

Department of Health (2000) Implementation of Health Act Partnership Arrangements. Circular HSC 2000/010 LAC (2000)9. London: Department of Health.

Department of Health (2000) Legislation: Circular HSC 2000/025. London: Department of Health.

Department of Health (2000) The Human Rights Act: LAC (2000)17. London: Department of Health.

Department of Health (2000) Working Together: Safeguarding Children Involved in Prostitution. London: Department of Health.

Department of Health (2001) 'Good Practice in Consent', Circular HSC 2001/023. London: Department of Health.

Department of Health (2001) 12 Key Points on Consent: The Law in England. London: Department of Health.

Department of Health (2001) A Safer Place: Combating Violence against Social Care Staff, Report of the National Task Force and National Action Plan. Brighton: Pavilion.

Department of Health (2001) Building the Information Core: Protecting and Using Confidential Patient Information. London: Department of Health Information Policy Unit.

Department of Health (2001) Consent – What you have a Right to Expect. London: Department of Health.

Department of Health (2001) Reference Guide to Consent for Examination or Treatment. London: Department of Health.

Department of Health (2001) Safeguarding Children in whom Illness is Induced or Fabricated by Carers with Parenting Responsibilities; Supplementary Guidance to Working Together (consultation draft). London: Department of Health.

Department of Health (2001) Seeking Consent – Working with Children. London: Department of Health.

Department of Health (2001) Seeking Consent – Working with Older People. London: Department of Health.

Department of Health (2001) Seeking Consent – Working with People with Learning Disabilities. London: Department of Health

Department of Health (2001) Shifting the Balance of Power within the NHS. London: Department of Health.

Department of Health (2001) The Framework for the Assessment of Children in Need and their Families. London: Department of Health.

Department of Health (2001) The Mental Health Policy Implementation Guide. London: Department of Health.

Department of Health (2002) Guidance for Access to Health Records Requests under the Data Protection Act 1998. Leeds: Department of Health Confidentiality Issues Section.

Department of Health (2002) Guidance on Restrictive Physical Interventions for People with Learning Disability and Autistic Spectrum Disorder in Health, Education and Social Care Settings. London: Department of Health.

Department of Health (2002) Implementing the Caldicott Standard into Social Care. Circular HSC 2002/003; LAC. Department of Health (2002) 2. London: Department of Health.

Department of Health (2002) Model Consent Policy. London: Department of Health.

Falkov A (1995) Study of Working Together. Part 8 Reports: Fatal Child Abuse and Parental Psychiatric Disorder. London: Department of Health.

General Medical Council (1998) Seeking Patients' Consent: The Ethical Considerations, November 1998.

General Medical Council (1998) Maintaining Good Medical Practice.

General Medical Council (1999) Management in Health Care: The Role of Doctors, May 1999.

General Medical Council (2000) Confidentiality: Protecting and Providing Information, September 2000.
General Medical Council (2000) Priorities and Choices, July 2000.
General Medical Council (2001) Good Medical Practice 3 edn, May 2001.
General Medical Council (2002) Making and Using Visual and Audio Recordings of Patients, May 2002.
General Medical Council (2002) Good Practice in Paediatrics and Child Health (consultation draft).
Markesinis BS (1999) The Tortious Liability of Statutory Bodies: A Comparative and Economic Analysis of Five English Cases. Oxford: Hart Publishing.
Wadham J (2001) The Human Rights Act One Year On. Times 2 October 2001.

Legislation

European Convention on Human Rights and Fundamental Freedoms 1950.
Family Law Reform Act 1969.
Local Authority Social Services Act 1970.
Mental Health Act 1983.
Access to Personal Files Act 1987.
Access to Medical Reports Act 1988.
Children Act 1989.
UN Convention on the Rights of the Child 1990.
NHS and Community Care Act 1990.
Access to Social Services Records Act 1990.
Access to Health Records Act 1990.
Education Act 1996.
European Convention on the Exercise of Children's Rights 1996.
Data Protection Act 1998.
Human Rights Act 1998.
Data Protection (Subject Access Modification) (Health) Order 2000.
Care Standards Act 2000.
Regulation of Investigatory Powers Act 2000.
Freedom of Information Act 2000.
Special Educational Needs and Disability Act 2001.
Health and Social Care Act 2001.
The Health Service (Control of Patient Information) Regulations 2002 SI 2002 No. 1438.

Abbreviations

All ER All England Law Reports.
BMLR Butterworths Medico-Legal Report.
EHRR European Human Rights Reports www.echr.coe.int.
FLR Family Law Reports.
HSC Health Services Circular.
LAC Local Authority Circular.

CHAPTER 11

The contextual influences on practice: managing professional performance

ANTHONY L SCHWARTZ

Introduction

In this book, the focus has been on clinical excellence and the way in which healthcare professionals can assimilate and draw upon evidence of good practice to enhance the treatment and the care of their clients, patients or service users.

This chapter is aimed at redressing the balance through focusing the spotlight on the clinician or health professional. In this chapter, I shall examine the influences acting on the clinician, beginning with the external forces, then examining the professional influences, and finally taking note of the internal factors that affect those working in the health and social care professions. We will then look at ways of examining these pressures and their effects, considering ways of re-energizing and rekindling enthusiasm for people working as 'ordinary people in challenging circumstances'.

Pressure to perform in prescribed ways can be a spur to positive working, it may also be stressful for the caring professionals. In *Beating Stress in the NHS* (Chambers et al., 2003) there is an acknowledgement that the way that we work in the health service is directly influenced by the plethora of initiatives and directives from the government, health bodies, professional groups and consumer associations that create national and local imperatives. How the implications of these initiatives and directives are communicated to the workforce is important because there is often difficulty in coping with the resulting change and uncertainty. This chapter focuses on the importance of recognizing what we need as people and professionals in order to harness good practice and maintain personal effectiveness as well as efficiency amidst change and development.

Influences on professional working

There are numerous factors that affect professional working, at the level of societal influences (for example, politics, economics), at the level of the community (for example, service provision, resources), in the working situation (for example, job clarity, work climate), and at the personal level (for example, skills, attitude). In this chapter we are focusing attention on the person, and asking you to consider how you are affected by these influences. What do you do to maintain a healthy mixture of skills and human factors – the 'tools of the trade'? Whereas the rest of the book highlights the technical and research evidence to promote good practice, this chapter encourages consideration of human factors and your personal 'tool-kit', used for self-management and personal wellbeing. This is represented in Figure 11.1.

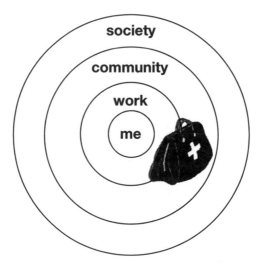

Figure 11.1 Influences on professional working.

As professionals working in the fields of health and social care we need to acknowledge and examine the influences on our working, in order to make decisions about what we can usefully engage in, for our clients and for ourselves.

External environment

The first influence is that of the external environment at large. The societal influences of economics, law and politics have a direct impact on our work in the caring professions. Over the last decades and more particularly the last few years, we have seen the impact of strategic (most often government-led) changes in the health and social services sectors. These changes have had a direct influence on the way in which services are provided (at the operational level) as well as at the professional and personal levels. The government White Paper entitled *The New NHS: Modern, Dependable,* focused on changes that were to affect clinicians directly. For example the importance of clinical excellence and evidence-based treatments can be seen from the guidance published on 'treatment choice in psychological therapies and counselling – evidence based clinical practice guideline'. Consider for a moment the list of words below, what they stand for, and what effect the implementation of these concepts has had in your field of work:

- the NHS plan;
- government legislation;
- modernization of local government;
- clinical governance;
- best value;
- standards and clinical audit;
- National Institute of Clinical Excellence;
- professional bodies' policies and guidelines;
- professional accreditation.

Often this list has the effect of making people sigh, and feel burdened rather than relieved and supported. For many professionals these words are associated with additional pressure, administrative tasks and responsibilities. Although we all recognize the need for codes of professional practice, evidence of good practice, and ongoing development, it is often the manner in which policies are communicated, and their implementation, which provides difficulty at the coalface. A lack of clarity on tasks and goals, uncertainty of how to implement policies, and the seemingly contradictory messages, as well as the number of areas to prioritize, result in uncertainty about direction and how to translate this into action. It is important to remind ourselves to stand back (stepping out of the situation and adopting a hawk's eye view away from the sense of bureaucracy or confusion), in order to plan, act and review. In doing this, we can regain some perspective, control and focus on what it is we can and should do.

Professional influences

The second major influence on working is the NHS plan whose framework focuses on a number of areas for improving patient services and care. The imperative arising from the NHS plan has focused on clinical governance, with the concepts professional accreditation, national service frameworks, clinical excellence, performance assessment frameworks, health improvement and quality having come into everyday use. Standards are included in this drive for efficiency, transparency and best practice, which results in change at a number of levels. Standards require attention to:

- developing, setting and monitoring standards of healthcare;
- partnership working with other agencies (such as local authorities);
- integration of health and social services (such as care trusts);
- cost effective and efficient services;
- quality of care.

Although there is a clear focus on improving services, it is necessary to focus not only the role of the healthcare professional in delivering services *but also on their needs for support, learning and positive affirmation.*

It is recognized that there is low morale amongst staff working in the Health Service and that working in the NHS can be bad for your health (Williams et al., 1998). An insightful anecdote may highlight this issue here. At a recent workshop for staff in primary care, the issue of morale was raised. The question was asked how we might judge whether GPs' morale was as low as suggested by newspaper headlines. One participant observed pointedly that GPs no longer encourage their children to study medicine! This comment was received with a quiet hush in the packed auditorium, with many people nodding their heads in agreement. Whether this is objectively verifiable is less important than the impression that people working in this field are increasingly disillusioned, and that this is shown in a variety of ways (for example, signs of burn-out, symptoms of depression, increased cynicism, a sense of hopelessness).

Job satisfaction is important, and we know that the professional who is motivated is more likely to encourage and enthuse his or her patients, leading to improved rates of concordance or treatment adherence (DiMatteo et al., 1988). Professionals need to be enabled to consider their circumstances and the expectations placed on them, and to make decisions on how best to engage in this new climate in the National Health Service. There will always be change; it is how we see it and respond that allows us to use it as an opportunity to develop and grow. It is up to us to seek out and develop self-management and support structures in order to work more happily. It is also up to the organizations in which we function to promote structures and policies that support staff in a number of ways. Examples of these from both individuals and organizations may be:

- access to confidential support and assistance when necessary (for example, through professional bodies, telephone help lines, employee assistance programmes, therapy networks);

- peer support and supervision;
- ongoing professional development opportunities linked with personal development plans (for example, on managing pressure, people and performance);
- mentoring and coaching opportunities;
- organizations establishing standards on managing pressure and stress at work;
- organizations auditing levels of workplace stress (for example, across different areas of the organization, professional groups) in order to do something about it such as offering preventative or restorative stress-management training programmes;
- setting up peer support groups, coaching and mentoring;
- ensuring that staff have access to confidential and effective support services when they experience difficulties in the workplace.

In considering the influences on us, the concept that behaviour is both a function of the person and the environment is extremely relevant here. Our behaviour (and therefore our professional practice) depends on factors such as knowledge and attitude, as well as on the environment around us; this may include protocols, management structures and the working culture. The equation expressing behaviour as a function of both the person and the environment ($B = f P + E$) permits us to share responsibility for good practice with the organization or team, rather than feel it is all up to us! There is the need for a clear strategic direction that influences the operational, and human resource factors are crucial to this. Workforce planning that focuses on the interdependence of employees and is supportive of staff, is necessary, as Buchan (2002: 751) contends:

> The UK and many other countries need to enhance, reorientate and integrate their workforce planning capacity across occupations and disciplines to identify the skills and roles needed to meet identified service needs. They can also improve the day-to-day matching of nurse (and other NHS workforce) staffing with workload. Flexibility should be about using working patterns that are efficient, but which also support nurses (and others in the NHS workforce) in maintaining a balance between their work and personal life.

Encouraging of the 'human factors' at work means noticing: being aware of the motivational aspects, attending to the small things that make us truly human, recognizing the need to manage and deal with the emotional impact of the work we undertake. We need the organizational structure to recruit appropriately trained staff in sufficient numbers and to provide a suitable workplace in physical terms but we also urgently need to attend to the emotional climate of the workplace. In attending to both the concrete tasks and the emotional processes, we are likely to build interdependent teams. As Druskat and Wolff comment, in the Harvard Business Review

(2001) we need to build trust and a sense of group identity before we can be truly effective. Performance and outcome measures should be assessed using clear behaviours, but results are affected by personal factors as well as environmental ones, as the above equation emphasizes.

Standards

Increasingly our working lives are dominated by charters and standards. These dictate what is expected from individuals, teams, organizations, community and governmental agencies. Yet, so much of what takes place in healthcare is about 'human factors' in addition to the technical skills of the practitioner – the manner in which people work with and for people. Most health professionals fulfil their roles not in order to achieve fame or fortune but because of other people. This important dimension is increasingly being acknowledged in healthcare, because the human factors impact on quality. However, the paradox seems to be that when practitioners see themselves being overwhelmed by administrative data and the requirement to keep proving themselves and their work, they lose the motivation and willingness to do the job.

It can be argued that the culture within the caring professions has changed over recent decades. Previously a culture of 'sociability' existed where there was a sense of sincere friendliness amongst people at work. Increasingly this has been superseded by a 'corporate' culture, which focuses on the ability to pursue shared objectives quickly and effectively, regardless of personal ties. Of course, this is an oversimplification, and all organizations and teams need to have elements of both of these cultures in order to be effective. The challenge is to use the positive concepts of good practice and standards of care in a manner that is flexible and takes into account the critical personal dimensions. It also needs to define standards and targets in ways that more closely approximate what we do as professionals, instead of having a 'one-size-fits-all' measure that appears to favour quantity above quality.

In the NHS quality strategy document *A First Class Service: Quality in the NHS* the focus is on quality and belief that modernizing the NHS requires new, robust systems for quality assurance and quality improvement. This implies significant changes in culture and working practices.

In addition, performance will be assessed using the NHS performance assessment framework. Different and new systems of monitoring and self-regulation are also emphasized, with the Commission for Health Improvement providing independent scrutiny of local efforts to improve quality.

Often neglected, but included in this approach, is the concept of life-long learning for health professionals.

Quality management

Quality is a term used to describe coordinated activities related to staff, patients and management. It involves using methodical processes in a systematic way to build on good practice and to enhance services and ongoing learning. It focuses on both processes and tasks, the practical and the human aspects. Ovretveit (1992: 2) writing about health service quality comments that: 'Successful quality programmes pay as much attention to changing human relations – relations between managers and staff and staff and patients – as to introducing new systems, and to specification and measurement'. In the current NHS context, the term quality is focused on the clinical and cost-effectiveness of treatments and interventions, and the minimization of both clinical and managerial risk (Hall and Firth-Cozens, 2000).

The quality frameworks in health and social care (for example, clinical governance) provide a way to continuously improve the quality of services. Similar principles underpin both:

• active involvement of users and patients;
• clear accountability arrangements for quality; and
• a change in culture to a more active and sustained approach to quality and to staff development.

These situate the user at the centre, with those responsible for service delivery needing to be responsive to those using the service. At the same time, managers are placed in a position where they need to listen to the service users and their employees equally, and in turn need to be listened to by their senior managers. Here too is a complete cycle of communication that affects quality. In essence, each level is a service user of the level above, and a service provider to the level below.

The practical implications of this in the work setting can be seen in the following vignette. Social workers in a residential setting were encouraged by their managers (who had received policies and procedures about greater user involvement) to involve the service users, the children in their home, in order to improve quality and make positive changes. As a result they developed interviews and questionnaires to enquire about what the young people felt about their setting. They received many useful comments and the youngsters were keen to take part. The ideas, views and comments were collated and a briefing document was written. There was, however, no response to this from the more senior staff, and the impact and impetus was lost. The following year, once again, youngsters in the home were asked to share their views. One perceptive voice enquired what had happened to the points they had raised previously, as they had been through this exercise before and it was meaningless and a waste of time because there had been no outcome. The promise had not been kept. Quality at the point of service delivery became a hollow concept. Such experiences (lack of recognition and not being listened to) can result in workers at all levels becoming demoralized and dispirited.

Figure 11.2 shows how each level is accountable to and held accountable by the other levels (for example the client being listened to by their worker, who in turn is listened to by their manager etc.). It is salutary to consider that if professionals are not placed within the quality cycle and do not have their needs recognized, acknowledged and met (for example, their needs for training or support) this has a direct effect on what we produce in terms of quality outcomes.

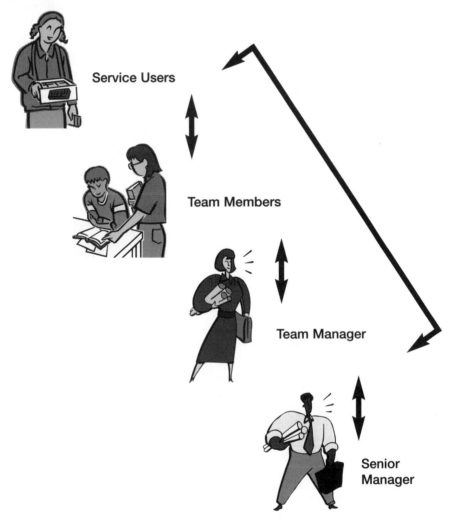

Figure 11.2 Quality feedback and communication links.

When we focus on establishing and monitoring standards, we should be clear about three main aspects of what it is we expect of ourselves and others at work:

* the relevant knowledge and understanding;
* particular skills and competencies; and
* specific behaviours.

This process is represented in Figure 11.3, highlighting the cycle of standards, in which each element is associated with the others, and all are needed. This can be applied in an organization or team, where the emphasis is on our interdependence with other team members – we all have an important role to play, and we all need each other in order to do our job in the most effective way.

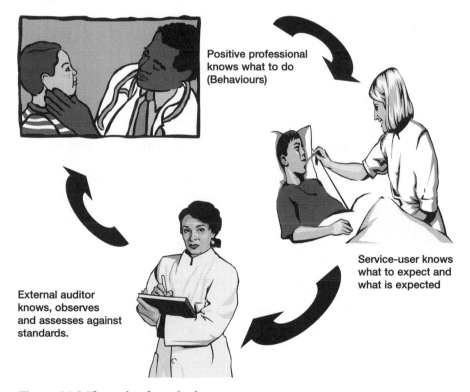

Positive professional knows what to do (Behaviours)

Service-user knows what to expect and what is expected

External auditor knows, observes and assesses against standards.

Figure 11.3 The cycle of standards.

In summary, people and processes together make for quality services, if we intend to improve quality we need to give people the tools and methods, as well as reinforcement and empowerment to do the job. Quality assurance does not happen simply by setting standards, nor does it happen by wishful thinking or 'spin'. *It occurs through having a clarity about building good*

*practices by attending to the human factors as well developing proce-
dures, systems, specifications, and assessing and reviewing them.*
   Ovretveit (1992: 2) points out:

> There needs to be as much emphasis on changing people's attitude towards
> their work as on training them to use specific tools and methods. Tools are
> only used if people want to use them. They are only used properly if peo-
> ple have been trained to use them and have the time to do so.

One of the frequently cited drawbacks to the approach of monitoring
quality is the administrative burden, the ongoing need to account for
what we are doing as professionals, the manner in which data need to be
recorded, and how this links with performance indicators, government
targets and so forth. These are the pressures of professional working that
appear to be increasing and result in 'overload'. Consequently, the issue
of managing pressure and stress in the NHS, is critical.

Managing pressure and stress

When all the external forces are working upon us, what can we do to revi-
talize ourselves? The answer lies not in whether we can escape the demands
or not, as simply moving away from one context does not stop prevent us
responding to other pressures. We take ourselves with us, as Jon Kabat-Zinn
(1995) highlights in *Wherever you go, there you are.* We can often be caught
up in worries, fantasies and anxieties about our working environment, our
colleagues, clients and the service in which we work. Frequently, as we
would comment to our clients, this is not helpful and the mental constructs
simply burden us more. We can be caught up in our internal demands.
What is expected of healthcare professionals? What do we expect from ourselves, and what do others expect? As people, we have a variety of roles and
expectations and within these diverse roles are not only the expectations
that others have of us, but also what we expect and demand of ourselves.
   We are likely to have internal expectations of what we expect of ourselves. These can be linked to our personal vision, the beliefs we hold,
our role models, our need for success and our needs for status. We also
have other, internally driven needs, for instance, to heal, to nurture and
to help. There are also external expectations: the goals or 'mission' of the
organization, the purpose of the team, what users of services at different
levels expect. For example, are we meant to be constantly accessible,
available, infallible, and offer complete cures, and be clinically excellent
at all times! Can we manage this pressure to perform?
   As cited earlier, there are many factors that impact on us, which are
stressful. Some of these are summarized in Table 11.1.

Table 11.1 Factors associated with stress.

Management and Culture	• Unclear vision, goals and objectives • Deficient two-way communication • Poorly trained managers • Inadequate training and development of staff • Lack of humanistic values • Closed and dishonest culture
Relationships at Work	• Unfair and inconsistently implemented personnel and management policies • Unfair systems for dealing with interpersonal conflict and grievance
Job Design	• Inferior training and resources • Role and responsibilities poorly defined • Mismatch between workload and individuals' skills, knowledge and ability
Employee Contributions	• Bad job design • Lack of involvement in change process • Poor consultation • Lack of flexibility
Physical Factors	• Inappropriate environment with excessive noise, heat and cold

Adapted from Howe W (1999) Stress. In Sadhra SS, Rampal KG (eds) Occupational Health: Risk Assessment and Management. Oxford: Blackwell Science.

Management of work-related pressure emphasizes links between the individual and the organization, and the accompanying tensions and opportunities this presents. Pressure at work can be the life-source of an organization when it offers the individual excitement and a chance to achieve and make a difference. This 'buzz-factor' helps to maintain a dynamic and enthusiastic organizational climate. When there is excessive pressure that is negative, the opposite can happen, with decreased performance, stress and burn-out. Managing work pressure is also about placing importance on personal self-management, which includes:

• having a clear vision, role and purpose;
• having an 'uncluttered' mind;
• monitoring quality at organizational and individual levels;
• being actively involved in life-long learning and self-development;
• establishing close 'fit' between the individual and organization;
• using positive interpersonal relating and communication skills;
• having an awareness of our own coping ability;

- being proactive in making choices, rather than being reactive;
- planning, acting on, and reviewing sources of unhealthy stress.

Interventions to manage pressure and stress

Interventions to manage pressure and stress can be targeted at different sources in organizations. Until recently, most interventions focused on stress – the signs, symptoms and effects, as well as on strategies used to manage stress. This approach assumes that all pressure is negative, and ignores the performance implications and the usefulness of positive pressure for achievement. It needs to be acknowledged that not all pressure is productive, and there should be preventative and restorative strategies to deal with stress, but we should consider the need for balance and the recognition of individual difference (what is positive pressure for one person may be negative for another).

Intervention programmes may be targeted at different levels – at the level of the individual, at the organizational level, or at the interface of individual and organization (DeFrank and Cooper, 1987). The most common form of intervention is probably that of stress-reduction activities (for example, stress management training) which are perceived by employers as being less organizationally disruptive (Cartwright and Cooper, 1997). However, it is important for programmes to involve all three dimensions.

It is important to focus on the individual-organizational context and the individual's appraisal of this relationship. This approach examines stress as the reflection of a lack of fit between the person and his or her environment and sees stress as an intervening variable between stimulus and response (Cox, 1978).

In order to manage negative stress at work, interventions are suggested at different levels (Murphy, 1984). Interventions are considered to be primary interventions if they aim to eliminate or at least modify the occurrence of work-based stressors. As such they usually take place at the organizational level (for example, family-friendly policies such as flexible working time, and health at work initiatives such as improved facilities). Secondary interventions (for example, stress management training) help individual staff develop their physical and psychological resources to limit the damaging effects of stress when it does occur, whereas tertiary interventions (for example, counselling, employee assistance programmes) treat or rehabilitate individuals who have succumbed to the negative effects of stress. The majority of stress interventions operate at secondary and tertiary levels of intervention, aiming to reduce the experience of stress rather than tackling the sources of stress (Kompier and Cooper, 1999).

The predominance of secondary and tertiary interventions means that stress management programmes have commonly been run for individuals rather than the workplace or organizations (Geurts and Gründemann, 1999; Kompier and Cooper, 1999). This worker-orientated approach does not prevent the occurrence of stress. It improves the employees' skills so that they are able to manage or resist stress. Such activities, despite being mostly focused on the individuals, also require the involvement of the organization in identifying and modifying workplace stressors (Cartwright et al., 1995; Geurts and Gründemann, 1999) although the degree of organizational change required may vary.

It may be useful to reflect on how stress and pressure are dealt with at the individual level and the organizational level. What does your organization do to manage negative pressure and stress? What do you do? Is stress acknowledged or seen as a sign of personal weakness? Do you see the approach as beneficial? Often organizations prefer to ignore stress ('if we don't pay attention to it, it will go away'). This may be due to the widespread use of stress as an umbrella term, a concept that has lost its meaning, or because there is no clear policy for dealing with it strategically.

The dimensions cited above are summarized in Table 11.2. You could consider which aspects you could fill in for yourself at the various levels and as prevention, restoration or treatment.

Table 11.2 Methods of managing stress log.

	Primary focus: **prevention**	Secondary focus: **restoration**	Tertiary focus: **treatment**
Individual level			
Organizational level			
Individual and organizational level			

So, what have you noticed? How do you or your organization continue to deal with pressure and stress? Can one take a 'stress audit', in order to plan strategically, in order to implement action plans (for example, consultancy input, staff training, workshops to manage pressure)? The first step according to Dr Rob Biner at the Birkbeck College London (Spence, 2002) is to establish organizational standards for managing stress. Without the foundation of established standards, interventions cannot be suitably targeted and training or input that will meet the needs of both the organization and the individuals cannot be identified.

Establishing standards for managing stress

It is important to establish a positive corporate culture within the service sector (be this private or public, such as in the NHS, Social Services or Education) where employers and managers take responsibility for the welfare and wellbeing of the workforce. Practices, trusts or other primary care organizations should look to establishing management standards for communicating with staff, should introduce proactive measures to reduce stress-provoking factors within the organization, should act to boost staff morale, and should maintain rehabilitation programmes for those in whom they have failed to prevent stress. The culture of the NHS as an organization should be such that employees feel that they are able to report feeling stressed or suffering from stress-related illnesses (Chambers et al., 2003).

In the Mental Health National Service Framework for England, Standard 1 requires that 'health and social services promote mental health for all' and that 'action is taken to address the discrimination and exclusion experienced by people with mental health problems' (Department of Health, 1999). Local health-promoting units are reminding employers that people who are satisfied with their jobs are more productive and their organization will therefore be more effective (North Staffordshire Health Authority, 2001). They are encouraging the adoption of mental health policies in workplaces that aim to:

- promote the wellbeing of staff
- support staff returning to work after a mental health problem
- have a positive approach to employing staff who are experiencing, or have experienced, mental distress (Chambers et al., 2003).

In the social care sector, the importance to the modernizing agenda of the workforce is made clear in the statement that 'Social care staff comprise the single greatest asset services possess; to make the most of this asset, staff training and development must be fully overhauled' (Platt, 2000).

The above sits comfortably with the requirement for standards and their implementation. We should expect to set standards for our work and its outcomes for the service users and monitor the quality of our work, but we can only develop our work further by planning investments for staff training and staff management. As an individual, one may need some help in examining the area of stress at work, and undertaking audits in order to set standards, prior to embarking on intervention programmes. It is a huge area, but through linking this to lifelong learning, team and organizational development, and embedding it within the organizational culture, one would hope to find ways of making the NHS a better place to work – which does not damage the health of its workforce.

Its up to you: self-management at work

This chapter has focused on correcting the imbalance. How can you look after yourself in the changing and challenging climate of the modern health service? In personal work as well as input in teams (through workshops or training events)[1] I have come to use this 'mantra': 'stand back, to notice, choose and act'. When we allow ourselves the opportunity to step back from what we are caught up in (crisis management) we become more able to be dispassionate. We can then become more aware and notice what is happening around us and with us.

Once we achieve this awareness, we can then begin to make choices as to where we will put our energy. When we have clarified our options and made a choice, it is imperative to act upon it. Following our action we can then begin the cycle again and observe through standing back:

* Step one: stand back.
* Step two: notice – where are you at now?
* Step three: choose – what are you going to do about it, at what level?
* Step four: act – undertake the action.
* Step five: review through standing back and examining the results.

In order to manage professional performance, you need to focus on yourself first. Notice what gets in the way, what the stresses and positive pressures are. Check the following for ideas:

* recognize the effects of stress and pressure upon you;
* recognize signs of stress and pressure in other people;
* choose from a variety of methods to manage personal stress and pressure (for example, assertiveness skills, visualization, mindfulness training methods, cognitive approaches);
* reinforce what you are doing well;
* encourage members of your team;
* manage your time and include sufficient time for thinking, doing, meeting, developing and learning;
* be assertive, and learn to say 'no' to unnecessary work or other people's jobs and tasks;
* undertake a risk assessment of work related stress in your workplace;

- compose a stress-management policy for your workplace;
- use clinical governance to reduce levels of stress in your workplace;
- work on your personal development plan;
- draw up a logical framework to plan and monitor the achievement of tasks in order to manage yourself and establish yourself at the centre;
- celebrate your successes (as an antidote to the tendency to highlight areas in which we can improve). This is motivating!

See Chambers et al. (2003) for a more in-depth examination of the above issues.

In order to put yourself back in the centre, what do you need to do? There may be workshops you could attend, using a peer group or support network, or personal coaching or supervision just for you. How can you make time for yourself?

A simple exercise may be to get yourself to note all the activities you are currently involved in, say, during a typical week. What does this tell you about where you place yourself, the demands you respond to? Take fifteen minutes to do the following 'Activity Map Exercise' (Schwartz and Dennis, 2002).

The activity map

Take a sheet of A4 paper. Think about how you would divide this, using areas on the page, like a pie-chart, a puzzle, or even graphs, symbols, circles, squares or other shapes or pictures to represent the things with which you are involved that take up your time and energy. If it is a weekday map, does it change at the weekend? Use symbols and images instead of words. You need to produce an impression of what you do on a piece of paper, not a lengthy list of words and sentences.

Can you see anything that is out of line? How big is your TV circle? If you could change anything, what would it be? Assume that it is something within your grasp. Are there things that you can swap around, areas you can ask other people to help you with? How can you achieve this? Take a differently coloured pen to do this. The more detailed this activity map can be, the better able you will be to assess where you are going in your life. Write it down on paper. It is not something that can be made clear in one's head.

Many people who have done this exercise and who have repeated it again after a number of months have made changes to their patterns at work and home. Sometime it is useful to do it with a partner, friend or colleague. In so doing, you can set personal targets to review, and to reinforce your successful achievements.

Recognize that this is the first step in the process. Consider how to maintain what is positive for you in your life – your home circumstances, friendships and relationships, your working situation, your professional endeavours, your hobbies, interests and other pursuits. Think about how you can plan to enhance or increase these – include some of them in your personal development plan for continued professional development.

Summary

As professionals we need to recognize the importance of research, clinical excellence and other important influences on our practice. We should not lose sight of the dream with which we started and the vocation of working as healthcare professionals, but we also need to recognize who we are as people – what we need in order to be fulfilled and in order to be satisfied in our jobs. Personal wellbeing at work is important in order to be motivated and also to reduce the effects of stress. Recognize what it is that will enhance your personal and professional life, and seek ways to be revitalized, restored and reinvigorated. Challenge the organization in which you work to honour the commitments to ongoing development and training as outlined in the NHS plan and be committed to the idea of lifelong learning. Step back and consider which self-management strategies you may use to your advantage, and consider how you may maintain quality in your personal and professional practice.

Note

1. Arcadia Alive Ltd specialises in providing consultancy, training and development within the health and social services sector for personal and management development. Contact: Parkfield Centre, Park Street, Stafford ST17 4AL. www.ArcadiaAlive.com

References

A First Class Service: Quality in the New NHS http://www.doh.gov.uk/newnhs/quality.htm
Buchan J (2002) Global nursing shortages. British Medical Journal 324: 751–2.
Cartwright S, Cooper C (1997) Managing Workplace Stress. London: Sage.
Cartwright S, Cooper CL, Murphy LR (1995) Diagnosing a healthy organisation: a proactive approach to stress in the workplace. In Murphy LR, Hurrell JJ, Sauter SL, Keita GP (eds) Job Stress Interventions. Washington DC: American Psychological Association.
Chambers R, Schwartz AL, Boath E (2003) Beating Stress in the NHS: How to Do It. Oxford: Radcliffe Medical Press.
Cox T (1978) Stress. London: Macmillan.
DeFrank RS, Cooper CL (1987) Worksite stress management interventions: their effectiveness and conceptualisation. Journal of Managerial Psychology 2: 4–10.

Department of Health (1999) National Service Framework for Mental Health. London: Department of Health.

DiMatteo MR, Sherborne CD, Hays RD, Ordway L, Kravitz RL, McGlynn EA, Kaplan S, Rogers WH (1993) Physicians' characteristics influence treatment adherence to medical treatment: results from the medical outcome study. Health Psychology 12(2): 93–102.

Druskat VU, Wolff SB (2001) Building the emotional intelligence of groups. Harvard Business Review 79(3): 80–90.

Geurts S, Gründemann R (1999) Workplace stress and stress prevention in Europe. In Kompier M, Cooper C (eds) Preventing Stress, Improving Productivity – European Case Studies in the Workplace. London: Routledge.

Hall J, Firth-Cozens J (2000) Clinical Governance in the NHS: A briefing. Division of Clinical Psychology Information Leaflet No. 4. Leicester: The British Psychological Society.

Howe W (1999) Stress. In Sadhra SS, Rampal KG (eds) Occupational Health: Risk Assessment and Management. Oxford: Blackwell Science.

Kabat-Zinn J (1995) Wherever You Go, There You Are. Hyperion, New York.

Kompier M, Cooper C (1999) Introduction: improving work, health and productivity through stress prevention. In Kompier M, Cooper C (eds) Preventing Stress, Improving Productivity – European Case Studies in the Workplace. London: Routledge.

Murphy LR (1984) Occupational stress management. Journal of Occupational Psychology 57: 1–15.

North Staffordshire Health Authority (2001) Promoting Wellbeing in North Staffordshire 2002–2005. Stoke-on-Trent: North Staffordshire Health Authority.

Ovretveit J (1992) Health Service Quality. London: Blackwell Scientific.

Platt D (2000) A Quality Strategy for Social Care. London: Department of Health.

Schwartz AL, Dennis EJ (2002) I Won't Let General Practice Get Me Down: Managing Pressure in Primary Care. Stafford: Staffordshire University.

Spence R (2002) The man who could change your life. Interview with Dr Rob Briner. Guardian, 12 January.

The New NHS: Modern, Dependable. http://www.doh.gov.uk/newnhs/popular/index~1.htm

Treatment Choice in Psychological Therapies and Counselling. Evidence Based Clinical Practice Guideline http://www.doh.gov.uk/mentalhealth/treatment-guideline/

Williams S, Michie S, Pattani S (1998) Improving the Health of the NHS Workforce. London: Nuffield Trust.

Index

United Nations Convention on the
  Rights of the Child 230, 247
United States of America 7, 21, 49, 53,
  70
  adoption 86
  Afghan war 210, 212
  brain tumours 12
  divorce and remarriage 180, 191, 197
  intergenerational relationships
    155–6, 161–2, 164, 167, 173
  perinatal brain insults 18
  self-harm 105, 119

vaccination programmes 212
ventricular enlargement (VE) 18–19
videotapes 57, 61, 65, 67

war 207–20
Wender Behaviour Checklist 23
Wilson's disease 20
withdrawal 37, 40, 182
withholding information 240
Working Together (1999) 2326, 238
World Health Organization 49
  war 211, 212, 214

Youth Offending Teams 50

Zaire 211
Zahir Shah 208
Zia ul Haq, General 208, 209